Faith-Based Health Justice

Faith-Based Health Justice

Transforming Agendas of Faith Communities

Editors: Ville Päivänsalo, Ayesha Ahmad,
George Zachariah, Mari Stenlund

Fortress Press
Minneapolis

FAITH-BASED HEALTH JUSTICE
Transforming Agendas of Faith Communities

Cover image: © iStock 2020; Blue Textured Background by STILLFX
Cover design: Alisha Lofgren

Print ISBN: 978-1-5064-6542-5
eBook ISBN: 978-1-5064-6543-2

Brief Description

This volume provides critical insights into the promotion of health justice across Christian and Islamic faith traditions and beyond. Given the chronic and complex humanitarian crises stemming from natural and man-made disasters and armed conflicts, plus weak and fragile health systems during postconflict and peace rehabilitation periods, dialogues between religion and health are crucial for integration and mediation of core humanistic values and prevention of human rights violations, including the right to health. In light of the pluralistic nature of our global world, in each case, the authors of this volume will ask the following:

- What could health justice mean today if developed in accordance with faith traditions with a commandment to care for the poor, ill, and marginalized?

- What kind of transformation of both faith traditions and public policies would be needed in the face of the acute health justice challenges of humanitarian crises present during our turbulent time?

The idea of justice implies that all people have a right to decent health and well-being, or at least to the central capabilities for healthy living. Accordingly, there must also be identifiable agents who are responsible for securing and fulfilling these rights in a fair manner. Of particular interest in the present volume is the way in which different health-care roles and ideas could influence religious organizations, communities, and individual people of faith to do their fair part in the promotion of the proper health rights of some of the poor and the ill of our time. Indeed, among all the global challenges of the twenty-first century, few are as crucial as the transformation of major, growing monotheistic religions to become increasingly supportive of justice and well-being instead of violence and oppression.

The volume at hand

- demonstrates an illuminating selection of ways in which religious beliefs and practices, such as Protestant Christian and Sunni Islamic ones, are highly relevant to health justice promotion in our global age;

- provides insight into a variety of topical challenges that especially the globally poor and the ill are facing in their search for holistic well-being as human beings, citizens, and people of faith; and

- stemming from the analysis of Christian and Islamic faith traditions as national majorities and minorities and of some other contextually relevant health justice agendas of the twenty-first century, seeks to boost dialogue and cooperation in the field across cultures.

Issues of religion and health justice inevitably take their own forms in each context. The approaches developed in this volume may serve as entry points for the further analysis of its topics ranging from basic health to the promotion of well-being and from HIV and AIDS to mental health. And beyond that, the case studies of this volume, addressing contexts with Christianity, Islam, and Hinduism as the majority faith traditions, pave the way for the development of context-specific models for practical collaboration to make an impact. Thereby, this enterprise can assist individuals from a range of disciplines who are concerned about health justice to understand its forms across cultures, especially when it comes to the religion-related challenges in its promotion of holistic health in our turbulent global age.

Contents

CONTENTS

Preface

This volume is the result of twenty-two contributors' efforts. Ten of them (see the list of contributors) have been based in Europe (six in Finland), nine in Asia (mainly South Asia), and three in Africa. Hence we may confidently say that this project has been a cross-continental venture. Moreover, three of the Europe-based contributors—Ayesha Ahmad (also one of the editors), Josephine Sundqvist, and Auli Vähäkangas—have written on their research performed in Africa. Thus African contexts are well presented in this cross-continental, cross-cultural, and indeed cross-contextual volume on faith-based health justice.

It turned out to be too difficult to write a balanced list of acknowledgments here, for so many senior and junior scholars as well as family members have in some way supported this enterprise. The completion and editing of all nineteen chapters have not been easy tasks! Over the years, extra effort has definitely been needed to push the initiative onward. When it comes to funding and other material resources, the work has been made possible by the institutions mentioned in the list of contributors—as each author relates. Those authors with special acknowledgments have added them at the end of their chapters.

Each reference list consists of all the pieces referred to in the chapter in question. The index of names includes all personal names, references to literature, and a selection of the most frequently used organization names with their acronyms as well as other names. The index of subjects includes a selection of the most important topics/concepts of the volume, albeit not some that have been used often (e.g., *health justice* is included, but *health* and *justice* are not).

All the acronyms are expanded when used for the first time in each chapter. Given that the chapters and their reference lists are relatively short, it should be quite easy to check the acronyms chapter-wise; a separate list of acronyms for the entire volume would hardly have made anything easier.

Despite being a cross-contextual venture in a profound sense, we editors have paid particular attention to the very idea of faith-based health justice throughout the process. Each part of the volume opens with a thematic introduction, which helps the reader follow the underlying greater narrative of faith-based insights into health justice and the practical implications they and the corresponding traditions have had. And given that few challenges could be more important for the human race in the twenty-first century than (re)finding religions as resources for health and well-being instead of those of disruption and violence, we can just hope that the readers will find each part and chapter of this book illuminating and inspiring.

Finally, this volume was written before the outbreak of the COVID-19 pandemic. There is no way we could have predicted it and the sudden escalation of global health concerns in 2020. Indeed, the world has suddenly entered into an age of fragile global health in a more comprehensive way than hardly anyone could have foreseen! Given that it was not possible anymore to add profound discussion of this pandemic to the present volume, we decided to leave the text as it was. However, it is very clear the emergence of this disease urges us to develop, in addition to immediate practical responses, as complete an understanding as possible of the underlying historical, ideological, and religious patterns of health and justice across contexts. And this is very much what *Faith-Based Health Justice* is all about!

V. P.

Introduction

TRADITIONS FOR HEALTH AND IMPERATIVES OF JUSTICE

Ville Päivänsalo

The freedom that is health cannot be found in solitude.
—Alastair V. Campbell, *Health as Liberation*

No blessing other than faith is better than health.
—Prophet Muhammad (as narrated by Ibn Majah),
Health Promotion through Islamic Lifestyles

1. Types of Health Impacts

The international community has been explicitly committed to several broad health rights agendas at least since the adoption of the *International Covenant on Economic, Social and Cultural Rights* in 1966 and *the Alma-Ata Declaration* in 1978. Too often, however, little attention has been devoted to the impact of religious perspectives and initiatives on the implementation of these rights. Yet it is true that today, much more than anyone anticipated some decades ago, religious insights both harm and inspire health-related human progress. The present volume approaches the topic through a number of Protestant Christian contexts of health promotion and service across the globe as well as through some Sunni Muslim contexts. In addition, as South Asia and sub-Saharan Africa are the key regions in the Global South to be addressed, there also is one chapter on Hinduism and another on traditional African religion. All this allows for an analysis that does not lean on particular assumptions about Christianity or Islam as national majority views and that provides entry points for dialogue among many faith traditions.

Typically, media become most alert in this field in the cases of evident *harmful health impacts* of religious beliefs and activities, and often rightly so. When individual religious extremists turn violent, perhaps amid conflicts, or when charismatic leaders of closed faith communities ruin the health of some of their weaker brothers or sisters—for example, through sexual abuses—it is quintessential that media houses and individual journalists unveil such practices. It is highly important, however, also to conduct in-depth analyses of the more subtle harmful effects of religions on essential human health. This has happened worldwide, for instance, when it was shown that many HIV-positive people have feared to test their serostatus because of stigmatizing religious teachings (Gill 2007; Stangl et al. 2010). And across the globe, authoritarian religions unfortunately harm the progress of gender justice in the fields of health and well-being.

At the same time, there is a growing literature on the *positive health impacts* of religions. One such line of argumentation focuses on *mental health*, building on the idea of the inherent capability of spirituality to help—whether through ideas, narratives, rituals, prayers, or communality—distressed people cope with their life challenges (Koenig and Larson 2001; Borras et al. 2007). Religious coping mechanisms certainly do not enhance mental health uniformly: people may, for example, suffer from teachings about God's abandonment or punishment (Pargament and Brant 1998, 119–20). Nevertheless, given the holistic nature of human existence, any positive impacts of religion on mental health tend to entail positive impacts on bodily health as well.

The second type of argument for the positive health impact of religions calls attention to *lifestyles*. Traditionally, religious norms have been hugely important in the regulation of human behavior in many health-related issues ranging from sexuality and family relations to dietary codes and gambling addiction. When rigorously adhered to, such norms can certainly be harmful. But James J. Walsh (2011, 110), in *Religion and Health* (first published in 1920), definitely gave a voice to broad currents of religious thought when he wrote, "The repression of the natural tendencies is an extremely valuable practice for the prevention of the many excesses which have so much to do with the undermining of health." Since then it has become common to recommend the rejection of religious aspirations to control one's natural desires, and emancipatory theologies have frequently contrasted themselves here with traditional ones.

Whereas the health risks connected to extreme religious lifestyles have remained clear enough, disregarding the potential for good health in moderate religious lifestyles would be both unfair and a waste of resources on a global scale. In the context of Islam, for instance, praying five times a day is a moderate physical exercise that helps one's blood circulation and breathing and also supports mental awareness. The ablution ritual before the prayer—comprising washing the hands, mouth, nose, face, arms, and feet—definitely adds to the health impact of the prayer practice as a whole. Furthermore, diets and fasting tend to have positive influences on health when people avoid extreme exertion. One can only imagine the global health impact of such activities within the worldwide Islamic community of some 1.7 billion people, a substantial number of them actively practicing Muslims. Similar lifestyles, beneficial to one's health when moderate, are of course integral to most other religions as well.

Third, when it comes to the positive health impacts of religions, the vastly influential *social engagement* of religion-based agencies across centuries and even millennia cannot be ignored (Rahman 1998; Porterfield 2005). Faith organizations are still coordinating large shares of health and welfare services in a great many regions of the world, and people of faith are active in a variety of initiatives for health, human development, and humanitarian aid, in recent years frequently responding to refugee crises (Jackson and Passarelli 2016). Whereas much of the social engagement stemming from Christian roots has been well known at least since the times of Florence Nightingale (1820–1910) and Albert Schweitzer (1875–1965), there is a growing interest to understand more about, for example, Islamic engagements in this field (Haynes 2007, 150–75; Koenig and Al Shohaib 2014). Perhaps the most common religious precept in the background of, or at least within, Abrahamic religions is the Golden Rule—that is, the command to love others as oneself (Küng 1990; Royal Aal al-Bayt Institute for Islamic Thought 2007). In such contexts of neighborly love, the perspective of eternity is not usually a threat but rather a profound source of motivation—in one way or another, depending on the theologies involved. In Islam, as in Surah Al-Baqarah in the Qur'an (2:25), the baseline belief here is that of reward for just social engagement: "And those who believe and do righteous good deeds, they are dwellers of paradise, they will dwell therein forever."

Yet behind any division of the harmful and beneficial health impacts of religion lurks the question of the very possibility of a cross-cultural understanding of "health" and "well-being" as well as of "justice." How have health-related concepts been framed in religious frameworks, such as Protestant Christian and Sunni Islam, in the first place? Neglecting the religious underpinnings in the quest for just human development would ignore hugely influential understandings of what health, justice, and human development are all about. Indeed, among all the global challenges of the twenty-first century, few are as crucial as the move of major, growing monotheistic religions toward increasing support of justice and well-being instead of violence and oppression. This volume, in turn, provides perspectives on several health justice issues across cultures, taking into account a wide range of faith traditions and their practical impacts. The venture touches upon faith-based ethics and public policies alike in the face of the acute health justice challenges of our time.

2. Faith as a Matter of Health Justice

Not all questions of mental health, lifestyle, or social engagement are really matters of justice. And countless religious agencies throughout history have conceptualized their responses to poverty and illness as matters of care, charity, and aid—and that may be all right in a great many cases. Questions of health justice, in turn, are often depicted as those that concern *the violation of proper health rights* (negative rights) and the provision of *adequate health services and products* (positive rights to the external aspects of health). These rights delineate a kind of "basic health justice."

The provision of any decent standard of basic justice for all necessarily involves *duties* of health justice. If people of faith and faith-based agencies worldwide, for some peculiar reason, simply stopped caring for the health of their neighbors, this would be not only a gross failure of neighborly love but also a matter of neglecting duties of care. We have duties to care for our near ones, but we may also have broader duties of health justice. In our age of modern medicine and global economy, we might expect at least high-income countries (HICs) and middle-income countries (MICs) to meet the essential standards of basic health justice. Globally speaking, impressive improvements have indeed occurred: for example, the total number of under-five deaths dropped from 9.9 million to 5.6 million between 2000 and 2016 (UN 2019, SDG 3). But that also means that some 100,000 children between the ages of zero and five years die *every week* worldwide, often from preventable causes.[1] People of faith must assume a fair share of their global duties of care. One may even argue, akin to Thomas Pogge (2002, 12–14), that the duty to promote human health and development is based—due to many harmful impacts of the present global order on the poor—*already* on the negative rights of the poor.[2]

Particularly since around the 1970s, approaches based on dignity, liberation, justice, and cooperative community life (rather than mere love and care) have indeed found religious expressions as well. Former president of the International Association of Bioethics Alastair V. Campbell (1995, 5), for instance, had both liberation and communality in the core of his account rooted in the Christian theological heritage: "The freedom that is health cannot be found in solitude." More recently, widely influential theologian William T. Cavanaugh from DePaul University has depicted the church that he dreams of in very health-related terms in *Field Hospital: The Church's Engagement with a Wounded World* (2016). Some aspects of such involvement could surely be solid duties as well. When it comes, in turn, to Islamic teachings on health, let us mention here *Health Promotion through Islamic Lifestyles: The Amman Declaration* (1989)—a challenging declaration and a call for action in a global age. Although it takes lifestyles as its focus theme, many of its articles illuminate well the overall framing of health promotion within the Islamic tradition and also the justice perspective. This declaration opens up by stating that "health is a blessing from God, which many people do not appreciate" (World Health Organization [WHO] 1996, 14). Furthermore, it refers to the saying of the Prophet as narrated by Ibn Majah, "No blessing other than faith is better than health" (WHO 1996, 16).[3]

Broad health justice debates have also touched upon *holistic well-being with a spiritual aspect* (positive rights to the internal aspects of health). The WHO famously defines health as "a state of complete physical, mental

---

1 The global under-five mortality rate declined from 90.2 to 42.5 deaths per 1,000 live births from 1990 to 2015 (WHO 2015, 53; WHO 2016, 48, 110).

2 As Pogge (2012, 12) presumes that harming others is wrong, his focus is on challenging the factual claim "that we are not harming the poor by causing severe poverty, but merely failing to benefit them."

3 The appendix of the declaration provides the essential references in the Qur'an and the hadiths to each article.

and social well-being and not merely the absence of disease or infirmity" (WHO 1946). This account resembles an array of religiously informed concepts such as shalom, harmony, and wholeness, many of which largely overlap with each other. For example, in India, the traditional Ashram movement has inspired Christian visions of wholeness (Varughese 1999). Toward the end of the twentieth century, initiated by the Christian Medical Commission (CMC) of the World Council of Churches (WCC), the relevant WHO (1997, 2) bodies actually considered redefining health as a "dynamic state of complete physical, mental, spiritual and social well-being." Although the WHO retained its original definition, the spiritual dimension has continued to affect the health of billions in dynamic manners, and the discussion of definitions is far from over (WCC and DIFAEM 2010, 14–18).

Amartya Sen (2009, 284–86), the pioneering theorist of the so-called capabilities approach to human development, has reminded us about the difficulties of measuring the internal aspects of health and thus overemphasizing them as policy guidelines. Yet Sen's account leaves room for the discussion of internal well-being as a matter of health justice as well. And due to the return of religion to the entire human development discourse (Deneuline and Bano 2009; Fountain 2013), the conceptualization of the internal aspects of health in the discourses of justice has become increasingly topical.

Whenever the target has been set on complete or holistic health, or when the aim is an extensive provision of health services beyond basic health rights, it has commonly been a practical necessity to understand the right to health in a progressive manner (Wolff 2012, 9–12). Between the requests of universal basic health justice and puzzlingly high ideals of complete well-being and all-around healthy spirituality, there is plenty of room for intriguing mediating definitions of health and approaches to health justice. And here it is important to see faith or spirituality not only as an aspect of internal well-being but also through its impacts on public health—as, for example, Gary R. Gunderson and James R. Cochrane (2012) have impressively done. Indeed, whenever the internal significance of a religion in a community grows strong, or when faith-based charities are scaled up to become major social institutions, or when faith traditions start to affect the popular understandings of social ideals of entire nations and cultural spheres, then some sort of justice issues are bound to become topical as well.

In this volume, it has been up to each author to define "health" and "well-being" as well as "justice" and the other key terms as they have seen it best. And when it comes to justice, it is of central importance to think of not only the right to health but also the responsibilities for health, for without properly corresponding responsibilities (or duties), any rights may become exposed as an empty manifesto (O'Neill 2000, 126; Sen 2009, 382–89).[4] But again, the approaches of the authors to such problems vary. What is common in this volume is rather the quest itself— that is, the quest of understanding such concepts anew in contexts where faith matters to human progress and indeed to *just* progress.

3. Contexts: Mainly in the Global South

Around the globe, it has been customary to think that the *primary responsible agency* (or the primary duty bearer) of health justice is the non-confessional public health system of each country. But even in such high-income countries as Germany and the United States, church-owned institutions or other faith-related organizations have served in prominent roles as health service providers. Especially the Nordic welfare state model, albeit partly rooted in religious values, has been heavily focused on the public sector.

In most countries of sub-Saharan Africa, some 30–50 percent of health services are provided by faith-based organizations (FBOs), predominantly Christian ones (Olivier et al. 2015). This state of affairs stems from the history of the medical mission that once was in a pioneering role in importing modern medicine to Africa (Grundmann 2005). In the postcolonial age, both missionary and political paradigms have been profoundly transformed, but the need to understand the role of faith organizations in the health-care provision and the promotion of essential human well-being has remained topical. As the public health services have still remained seriously deficient in most low-income countries (LICs) and also in many MICs and HICs, and as the expanded business sector has had little to provide to the poor—for example, in Africa and India (Oxfam 2014; Kurian 2015)—the nonprofit sector with its large share of faith agencies is not to be overlooked.

The current edited volume has been designed to provide quintessential perspectives on Christian and also Islamic engagement in the promotion of health justice across cultural spheres, especially among the globally poor and the ill. Its primary focus is thus on the "two-thirds world" that

---

4 Sen (2009, 382–79) has argued, though, that Onora O'Neill's account about the correspondence between rights and responsibilities or duties is somewhat too straightforward.

has experienced significant progress over the past few decades but must still struggle hard to keep on track. For this major part of the human race, it usually appears not strange at all to see religious agencies as cooperation partners in the implementation of health rights, although particularly in India, the official secularism has not been very flexible in this respect.

The key *country contexts* to be explored are Tanzania, Bangladesh, India, and South Africa. Tanzania and Bangladesh are very poor countries and are still dependent on international support to be able to guarantee proper health rights to their citizens. India and South Africa are comparatively wealthy but also highly unequal countries. As a matter of justice, prima facie, many have expected them to invest quite a bit more in the health and welfare of their citizens—India's less than 1 percent governmental budget of its gross domestic product (GDP) to health has evoked serious concerns (Drèze and Sen 2013; Kurian 2015, 3; WHO 2019, "India").[5]

Certain features in some other countries, including the United Kingdom and Finland, will also be looked at in order to provide intriguing reference points. As the debt crisis has driven several governments in the Global North to adopt public sector austerity programs, the world has become flatter in this sense: most states around the world must struggle to find their own paths of health justice under relative scarcity with support to their ventures from the civil society. For instance, Saudi Arabia has not really suffered from economic scarcity, but it has had persistent difficulties meeting the international gender justice standards.

It is true that the most shocking health justice challenges often occur in the world's conflict zones that do not belong to the focus areas of the current volume. However, plain conflict resolution as a means to secure health rights would shift the discussion largely to another topic. The focus of this volume is deliberately on contexts in which certain basic requirements of social stability for the promotion of health justice prevail. We should also bear in mind that although the media tends to report more from conflict zones, hundreds of millions of people live in

---

5 In India, the current health expenditure shifted from 4.0 percent of the GDP (current health expenditure per capita USD) as of 2000 to 3.7 percent, but this consists predominantly of out-of-pocket spending. The domestic governmental health expenditure rose slightly from 0.8 percent of the GDP (per capita USD) in 2000 to 0.9 percent in 2016 (WHO 2019, "India").

the midst of health crises every day in the more neglected contexts of poverty and misery.

In terms of *religious contexts*, Protestant Christianity is the main heritage to be looked at, but also several Islamic contexts are included. This emphasis reflects the traditional high-level involvement of Christianity in the promotion of health and well-being in three of the focus countries of this volume: Tanzania, South Africa, and India. Indeed, also in India, where Christianity has always been clearly in a minority position, Christianity has been very influential in some fields of health. In the 1940s, for example, no less than 80 percent of the nurses of the country were reported to be "Christian girls who had been trained in church-related institutions" (McGilvray 1981, 4). And today, there still are hundreds of Protestant and even thousands of Roman Catholic hospitals in the country. India indeed provides a pivotal context where Christian faith-based ventures for health have been pursued from the minority position onward. This complements quintessentially the analyses that assume a multidimensional impact of Christianity either through the majority culture (as is usual in the Western countries) or where the state has regarded faith-based service providers as their important health and social sector collaborators (as is often the case in Tanzania).

An endeavor to provide equal attention to all religions of the focus countries in a balanced way would have required another volume—or even separate volumes—for example, on Buddhism as well as on Western and Eastern Catholic thought. And putting together a handbook of the insights and impacts of all religions in all regions would have been an even more grandiloquent effort, and one that could have dismissed the power of tradition through a sort of detached bird's-eye view on all traditions everywhere. Yet Islamic insights and activities—for instance, in the contexts of Bangladesh and the Bangladeshi diaspora in London as well as Saudi Arabia—are addressed here quite intriguingly. They illuminate faith-related health issues among the globally poor and under quite pressing patterns of inequality or asymmetric pluralism. In addition, a look at Hinduism and the traditional South African healing practice illuminates contexts and vocabularies well beyond both secularism and Christianity.

As a matter of *diseases*, particular attention is called to HIV/AIDS and mental disorders. HIV/AIDS has simply been such a devastating pandemic, and the relevance of religious teachings in encountering it has been so obvious that special attention to it here hardly needs further justifications. Mental health deserves particular attention as well. Whenever life challenges seriously upset a human mind or the entirety of the human body/mind, this also frequently brings about questions of a religious nature.

4. Aims: To Understand and to Advance Dialogue

This volume aims at providing *critical insights into the promotion of health justice across Christian and Islamic faith traditions and beyond.* In each case, its authors will ask the following:

- What could health justice mean today if developed in accordance with faith traditions with a commandment to care for the poor, ill, and marginalized?

- What kind of transformation of both faith traditions and public policies would be needed in the face of the acute health justice challenges of humanitarian crises present during our turbulent time?

The idea of justice implies that all people have a right to decent health and well-being, or at least to the central capabilities for healthy living. Accordingly, there must also be identifiable agents who are responsible for securing and fulfilling these rights in a fair manner. One question of particular interest in the present volume is, In which roles and through which ideas could faith-based organizations, faith communities, and individual people of faith do their fair part in the promotion of the proper health rights of some of the poor, ill, and marginalized of our time?

If successful, the volume at hand will

- demonstrate an illuminating selection of ways in which religious beliefs and practices are highly relevant for health justice promotion in our global age;

- provide insight into a variety of topical challenges that especially the globally poor and the ill have to face in their search for holistic well-being as human beings, citizens, and people of faith; and

- stemming primarily from the analysis of Christian and Islamic faith traditions as national majorities and minorities and of some other contextually relevant health justice agendas of the twenty-first century, seek to boost dialogue and cooperation in the field across cultures.

This enterprise, so we hope, can help anyone concerned about health justice understand its forms across cultures and numerous religion-related challenges in its promotion in our turbulent global age—and to make an impact.

5. Some Achievements and Challenges

One of the most encouraging global health development measures is life expectancy at birth. The *Global Strategy for Health for All by the Year 2000*, published in 1981, reports that life expectancy in the developed countries then was 72 years on average. In the least developed countries, it was no more than 45 years, indicating overwhelming basic health challenges (WHO 1981, 24).[6] By 2017, however, the *global average* life expectancy at birth had risen to as high as 71.5 years and even in low human development countries up to 60.8 years (United Nations Development Programme [UNDP] 2019, table 1).[7] In this light, humankind has progressed remarkably in one of its most ambitious ideals—health for all!

Especially in countries where life expectancy is still under 70 years, however, large portions of the population must struggle hard for their very basic health rights. Now we are talking about countries like Tanzania—68.1 years in 2017. In India, life expectancy at birth indeed rose from 55.4 years in 1980 (through 62.1 in 2000) to 70.4 in 2017. Yet in that vast country, there are a great many people whose basic health rights are guaranteed hardly at all. Poverty does not always indicate low life expectancy, though. Bangladesh, which is poorer than both India and even Tanzania in economic terms, had achieved as high a life expectancy

---

6 The global goal by 2000 was sixty years (WHO 1981, 76). Fully consistent global measurements—for example, by the WHO and the United Nations Development Programme (UNDP)—are available from 1990 onward.

7 By 2013, this development indicator had amounted globally up to 70.8 years. In the countries of low development, it was 59.4 in that year; in those of medium development, 67.9; and in the countries of very high development, 80.2 (UNDP 2014, 160–63).

level as 74.6 years by 2017 (World Bank 2017; UNDP 2019, "Health: Life Expectancy at Birth")![8]

Of all the broad regions of the globe, health challenges have remained the greatest in sub-Saharan Africa (or the African region, as defined by the WHO). The neonatal mortality rate (per 1,000 live births) there, as of 2016, was 27.2. This particular figure was on the same level only in the conflict-torn Eastern Mediterranean (27.7), followed by the South East Asia (22.6) region in the same year. It was below 8 in the other regions of the world (WHO 2018, 67).[9] The special challenges of the African region are striking in the overarching ways of comparing the achieved health levels, ways that take into account communicable and noncommunicable diseases as well as injuries.[10] The number of direct deaths from major conflicts was on an entirely different level in the Eastern Mediterranean region (19.5 per 100,000 population in 2011–15) than elsewhere (the African region as the second in this respect with figure 1.4; WHO 2016, 119).

Figures like this confirm that although major progress has occurred, there still remains a whole lot to do in order to reach even the basic health justice threshold in any universal sense. Fortunately, initiatives have been launched to understand religious involvement and to enhance cooperation—health issues are strongly on the agenda of, for example, the International Partnership on Religion and Sustainable Development (PaRD 2018), which brings together governmental and intergovernmental entities with civil society organizations across the globe. Nevertheless, as Christianity and Islam are growing world religions with long traditions of engagement in health-related fields, it surely is worth exploring further what kind of resources these traditions might include in face of the health justice challenges ahead.

---

8 *Human Development Report 2015* announced, "Life expectancy at the age of 60, the world average being 20.7 years" (UNDP 2015, 241). There are minor differences in the UNDP and the World Bank figures themselves. In 1960, according to the World Bank (2017), the life expectancy at birth was 43.7 years in Tanzania, 41.2 in India, and 45.8 years in Bangladesh.

9 One of the explaining factors here is the percentage of births by caesarean section, which was 10 in the Southeast Asia region and well over 20 in all the other regions, although in the African region, from 2007 to 2014, it was only 4 (WHO 2015, 98).

10 One measure here is the number of years of life lost per a population of one hundred thousand through communicable and noncommunicable diseases as well as through injuries. It was on average, globally, 28,311 years in 2012. The regions with somewhat worse figures as of 2012 were Southeast Asia (29,553) and the Eastern Mediterranean region (30,396). In sub-Saharan Africa, in turn, this indicator was as high as 63,153 years (WHO 2015, 72).

6. Synoptic Outline

Part 1, "Toward Basic Health Justice," focuses on the roles of faith organizations in securing every human being some kind of minimum standards of health rights (theme introduction by Ville Päivänsalo and Ayesha Ahmad).

Ville Päivänsalo opens up this chapter with a brief historical review of the development of Protestant health work in India and Tanzania, calling attention to certain key differences in the roles of faith-based health provision in these countries. He indeed anticipates, and argues for, a kind of interdependence model of cooperation for health justice in both of these contexts, across cultures. Josephine Sundqvist and Thomas Ndaluka continue here by presenting an analysis of the grassroots challenges in Tanzanian church-related health services. With examples from health institutions maintained by the Evangelical Lutheran Church in Tanzania, the Roman Catholic Church, and the Free Pentecostal Church of Tanzania, the chapter illuminates how faith organizations can complement the deficient government health-care provision, especially at the grassroots level.

Whereas Tanzania is a very poor country still, South Africa in the twenty-first century has been doing economically better. Elina Hankela's case study nevertheless focuses on the challenges of basic-level health justice. The Methodists' work for justice through health and well-being has included radical ministry among refugees in Johannesburg and impactful social projects involving social housing, home-based care, and HIV/AIDS work—for example, in Pretoria. An analysis of the meanings of "health" and "justice" will form the main bulk of the chapter, while Methodist teaching on justice will offer a theoretical conversation partner to the empirical inquiry. Another context of a relatively advanced economy, albeit accompanied by high inequality, to be looked at in part 1 is India. Alok Chantia and Preeti Misra's chapter approaches this context through an analysis of Hinduism, health, and health justice. Ronald Lalthanmawia and S. N. Among Jamir then provide an updated view on Christian organizations for basic health justice in India.

Part 2, "Faith Traditions for Health and Well-Being," addresses issues of health justice also beyond the most urgent responses to ill health: How might insights and organizations of faith be integrated most appropriately in the health systems of comparatively affluent countries and what further impacts might the faith-sector have also in the conditions of scarcity (theme introduction by Ville Päivänsalo)?

In the first chapter of part 2, Abu Sayem provides an introduction to certain basic Islamic teachings on health and welfare and then discusses their relevance in today's South Asia, particularly in Bangladesh. Thomas Renkert then provides an overview of Christian perspectives on health and elaborates conceptual tools for analyzing it in terms of health justice. Subsequently, the role and impact of Christian Medical College, Vellore, in the promotion of health justice in India is discussed by Arul Dhas T.: How has this prominent institution managed to renew itself so that it has remained among the pioneers of health care in the country for the rich and the poor alike? Henrietta Grönlund, in turn, provides empirical perspectives on justice and well-being in Finland. She shows how attitudes on welfare justice in the Finnish context are changing and debated after decades of strong welfare state ideology and asks, What might be the particular role of religious agents in justice in today's postsecular society?

Part 3, "Transforming Agendas of Faith Communities," highlights, first, transformations in two Muslim-majority contexts and then focuses on encounters of HIV and AIDS in the contexts of faith, mainly Christian (theme introduction by Ayesha Ahmad and George Zachariah).

First, Jibon Nesa and Ville Päivänsalo examine the contribution of two Islamic faith-based hospitals to the promotion of public health in Bangladesh: the Islami Bank hospitals and Ibn Sina hospitals. In which ways might such initiatives contribute to the transforming health sector of the country? Hana Al-Bannay identifies then a number of health justice challenges for women in Saudi Arabia, beginning with social and cultural barriers that intervene with their accessibility to health services and adoption of healthy behaviors.

Sahaya G. Selvam provides next a systematic literature review on the ethical issues underpinning the relationship between HIV/AIDS and religion in Africa. Auli Vähäkangas continues the chapter with her analysis of the Tanzanian context, calling attention to "transforming masculinities" in the era of HIV/AIDS. She distinguishes among hegemonic masculinity, soft patriarchy, and liberation theological masculinity and takes into account the contributions of both southern and northern scholars on the discussion of masculinities in Africa. The concept of health justice in the context of HIV/AIDS in India will be then discussed by George Zachariah. He underlines the importance of a critical inquiry into the theological rationale for Christian engagement in this field, especially insofar as the HIV infection is seen as a result of the irresponsible behavior of the infected persons—who are thereby identified as particularly sinful. He also proposes some alternative ways of discernment and praxis of HIV and AIDS in India.

Part 4, "Mental Health," focuses on the interrelatedness of religion and mental health and explicates what the quest for health rights and health justice could mean in this complex field of research (theme introduction by Mari Stenlund).

Ayesha Ahmad's chapter on traditional South African sangoma consultations introduces an intriguing perspective on religious impacts on mental health, especially through somatization and sharedness. She argues that exploring these concepts against the Western dialectics of cause and symptom, as well as the pathological take on somatization, will highlight an interesting discourse of empathy. The chapter suggests that the narratively embodied sangoma insight into human relations is beneficial to health-care systems that currently and typically attempt to reduce persons to diseases. Furthermore, it brings the value of the human exchange in healing/medicine into the concept of health justice. Khaldoon Ahmed and Simon Dein's account of jinn and misfortune, in turn, is based on ethnographic fieldwork among Bangladeshis in East London. They examine explanatory models of misfortune among members of this community and discuss the implications for health care. The explanations, which centrally involve witchcraft or the evil eye or possession by a jinn spirit, are frequently contested by different members of the family. The chapter points out related problems negotiating between biomedical and folk explanations and closes by exploring the role of imams, prayer, and the Qur'an in the healing process.

Mari Stenlund takes up the issue of possible conflicts between the freedom of religion and the right to mental health. She explicates first different understandings of these human rights and then some central ways as to how these rights may conflict with each other. Finally, Stenlund explores opportunities for reconciliation between the freedom of religion and the right to mental health and suggests that the so-called capabilities approach to human development provides some promising insights forward in this field. Janne Nikkinen, finally, addresses the spiritual dimension in the treatment of addiction. Whereas ideas related to substance abuse have historically originated from religious discourses, today many medical practitioners accept the notion that addiction is a disease, a chronic illness like diabetes or hypertension. However, this view is increasingly being challenged. Beginning with problem gambling as his case example, Nikkinen points out ways in which many recovery programs today are either religious or at least ideological in a quasi-religious manner.

As a whole, all four parts to this volume thereby highlight the importance of religions both as causes of major health challenges, and as sources of inspiration for humanitarian as well as for much more far-reaching efforts to support healthy living in broad regions.

References

Borras, L., S. Mohr, P.-Y. Brandt, C. Gilliéron, A. Eytan, and P. Huguelet. 2007. "Religious Beliefs in Schizophrenia: Their Relevance for Adherence to Treatment." *Schizophrenia Bulletin* 33 (5): 1238–1246.

Campbell, Alastair V. 1995. *Health as Liberation: Medicine, Theology, and the Quest of Justice*. Eugene, OR: Wipf and Stock.

Cavanaugh, William T. 2016. *Field Hospital: The Church's Engagement with a Wounded World*. Grand Rapids, MI: William B. Eerdmans.

Deneuline, Séverine, with Masooda Bano. 2009. *Religion in Development: Rewriting the Secular Script*. London: Zed Books.

Drèze, Jean, and Amartya Sen. 2013. *An Uncertain Glory: India and Its Contradictions*. London: Allen Lane / Penguin Books.

Fountain, Philip. 2013. "The Myth of Religious NGOs: Development Studies and the Return of Religion." In *International Development Policy: Religion and Development*, edited by Gilles Garbonnier Houndmills, 9–30. UK: Palgrave Macmillan.

Gill, Peter. 2007. *The Politics of AIDS: How They Turned a Disease into a Disaster*. New Delhi: Viva.

Grundmann, Christoffer H. 2005. *Sent to Heal: Emergence and Development of Medical Missions*. Lanham, MD: University Press of America.

Gunderson, Gary R., and James R. Cochrane. 2012. *Religion and the Health of the Public: Shifting the Paradigm*. New York: Palgrave Macmillan.

Haynes, Jeffrey. 2007. *Religion and Development: Conflict or Cooperation?* Basingstoke, UK: Palgrave Macmillan.

International Partnership on Religion and Sustainable Development (PaRD). 2018. Accessed August 26, 2018. http://www.partner-religion-development.org.

Jackson, Darrell, and Alessia Passarelli. 2016. *Mapping Migration, Mapping Churches' Responses in Europe: Belonging, Community and Integration: The Witness and*

Service of Churches in Europe. Brussels: Churches' Commission for Migrants in Europe; Geneva, Switzerland: World Council of Churches. Accessed August 23, 2018. https://tinyurl.com/y63cxjam.

Koenig, Harold G., and Saad Al Shohaib. 2014. *Health and Well-Being in Islamic Societies: Background, Research, and Applications*. Cham, Switzerland: Springer.

Koenig, Harold G., and David B. Larson. 2001. "Religion and Mental Health: Evidence for an Association." *Internal Review of Psychiatry* 13 (2): 67–78.

Küng, Hans. 1990. *Projekt Weltethos*. Munich: Piper.

Kurian, Oommen C. 2015. *Financing Healthcare for All in India: Towards a Common Goal*. New Delhi: Oxfam India. Accessed October 27, 2015. https://tinyurl.com/yytmfbvr.

McGilvray, James C. 1981. *In Quest for Health and Wholeness*. Tübingen, Germany: German Institute for Medical Mission (DIFAEM).

Olivier, Jill, Clarence Tsimpo, Regina Gemignani, Mari Shojo, Harold Coulombe, Frank Dimmock, Minh Cong Nguyen, et al. 2015. "Understanding the Roles of Faith-Based Health-Care Providers in Africa: Review of the Evidence with a Focus on Magnitude, Reach, Cost, and Satisfaction." *Lancet* 386 (31): 1765–1775.

O'Neill, Onora. 2000. *Bounds of Justice*. Cambridge: Cambridge University Press.

Oxfam. 2014. *Investing for the Few: The IFC's Health in Africa Initiative*. Oxfam Briefing Note, September 2014. Accessed October 27, 2015. https://tinyurl.com/yyqpw3vz.

Pargament, Kenneth I., and Curtis R. Brant. 1998. "Religion and Coping." In *Handbook of Religion and Mental Health*, edited by Harold G. Koenig, 111–129. San Diego: Academic.

Pogge, Thomas. 2002. *World Poverty and Human Rights: Cosmopolitan Reforms and Responsibilities*. Cambridge: Polity.

Porterfield, Amanda. 2005. *Healing in the History of Christianity*. Oxford: Oxford University Press.

Rahman, Fazlur. 1998. *Health and Medicine in the Islamic Tradition: Change and Identity*. United States: ABC International Group.

Royal Aal al-Bayt Institute for Islamic Thought. 2007. *A Common Word between Us and You: 5-Year Anniversary Edition*. English Monograph Series: Book No. 20. Amman, Jordan: MABDA. Accessed October 26, 2015. http://www.acommonword.com/the-acw-document.

Sen, Amartya. 2009. *The Idea of Justice*. Cambridge, MA: Belknap Press of Harvard University Press.

Stangl, Anna, Dara Carr, Laura Brady, Traci Eckhaus, Mariam Claeson, and Laura Nyblade. 2010. *Tackling HIV-Related Stigma and Discrimination in South Asia.* Washington, DC: World Bank.

United Nations. 2019. "Sustainable Development Goals (SDGs) Knowledge Platform." Accessed January 15, 2019. https://sustainabledevelopment.un .org/sdgs.

United Nations Development Programme (UNDP). 2014. *Human Development Report 2014: Sustaining Human Progress: Reducing Vulnerabilities and Building Resilience.* New York: UNDP. Accessed October 27, 2015. https://tinyurl .com/kman8k3.

———. 2015. *Human Development Report 2015: Work for Human Development.* New York: UNDP. Accessed February 17, 2017. https://tinyurl.com/js4 ole7.

———. 2019. "Human Development Reports." Accessed January 22, 2019. http:// hdr.undp.org/en/data.

Varughese, K. V. 1999. *A Vision for Wholeness: Ashrams and Healing in India.* New Delhi: Christian Medical Association of India.

Walsh, James J. 2011. *Religion and Health.* Radford, VA: Wilder.

Wolff, Jonathan. 2012. *The Human Right to Health.* New York: W. W. Norton.

World Bank. 2017. "Life Expectancy at Birth, Total (Years)." Accessed February 21, 2017. https://tinyurl.com/yyl5xy2.

World Council of Churches (WCC) and the German Institute for Medical Mission (DIFAEM). 2010. *Witnessing to Christ Today: Promoting Health and Wholeness for All.* Geneva, Switzerland: WCC.

World Health Organization (WHO). 1946. *Constitution of the World Health Organization.* 45th ed., Supplement, October 2006. Accessed June 17, 2015. https:// tinyurl.com/2yqzar.

———. 1981. *Global Strategy for Health for All by the Year 2000.* Geneva, Switzerland: WHO. Accessed June 17, 2015. https://tinyurl.com/7jc9l62.

———. 1996. *Health Promotion through Islamic Lifestyles: The Amman Declaration.* Alexandria: WHO Regional Office for the Eastern Mediterranean. Accessed January 21, 2019. https://apps.who.int/iris/handle/10665/ 119558.

———. 1997. *Review of the Constitution and Regional Arrangements of the World Health Organization: Report of the Special Group.* November 14, 1997. Accessed October 27, 2015. https://tinyurl.com/y6tyvevo.

———. 2015. *World Health Statistics 2015.* Geneva, Switzerland: WHO. Accessed October 27, 2015. https://tinyurl.com/llnyxmm.

———. 2016. *World Health Statistics 2016: Monitoring Health for the SDGs.* Geneva, Switzerland: WHO. Accessed January 22, 2019. https://tinyurl.com/y3ag4kqp.

———. 2018. *World Health Statistics 2018: Monitoring Health for the SDGs.* Geneva, Switzerland: WHO. Accessed January 22, 2019. https://tinyurl.com/y8rwczhh.

———. 2019. "Health System Financing Profile by Country." Global Health Expenditure Database. Accessed January 21, 2019. https://tinyurl.com/y286tfzq.

PART 1

Toward Basic Health Justice

THEME INTRODUCTION

Ville Päivänsalo and Ayesha Ahmad

1. Contexts of Inequalities and Conflict

Viewing faith-based traditions for health justice is part of a continuum of the fluctuating relationship between religious discourses and conceptualizations of health (provision). The advent of a formalized global health movement around the world emphasizes inequalities and injustice by virtue of trying to tackle these aspects of our contemporary human condition. Although in most countries of the world, people are wealthier and healthier than ever on average, severe poverty and deficiencies in basic health have remained great challenges that call forth vehement involvement of the civil society in addition to the governmental political efforts, often of very fragile states, to heal their nations and the world.

The majority of the countries in the world are currently either experiencing or involved in conflict, and the nature of conflict is changing by lasting longer and involving civilians as targets. Values of human identity in the ways that they become culturally recognized are manipulated and forced into a paradigm of violence as tactics or strategies of the conflict. Our identities betray us and become our vulnerabilities. In parallel, humanitarian crises related to natural disasters, climate change, and the environment are defining the childhoods and futures of significant populations around the globe. The migration and forced movement of communities push minority groups into uncharted territories where they become victims of discrimination on the basis of fear and political instrumentalization.

The question arises on how to operate health care in such challenging circumstances. Could purporting a faith-based value system in health care symbolize processes of mediation, cultural resolution, and peace? These aspects are important for contemporary societies that are faced with challenges such as harmful traditional practices, radicalization, counterterrorism initiatives impacting the physical and mental health of affected populations, and rising discrimination and marginalization based on ethnic and religious identities. Any deeper understanding of faith-related responses to topical health challenges must, on the one hand, come with understandings of the historical roots of the more recent involvements in this field. On the other hand, such insights need to be rethought in the light of solid data on recent development trends.

In the present book, the focus is less on the immediate responses to disastrous health conditions and more on the development of health systems and the related impacts of religious insights and involvement. For as necessary as the humanitarian responses are, sustainable improvements in terms of basic health can come about only through building up stable institutions, long-term cooperation with the civil society, and viable cultures of care. Such developments, in turn, can crucially stabilize nations and thereby also reduce enmities and conflicts and enhance preparedness for humanitarian crises.

2. Major Challenges across Regions

Basic health can be defined in many ways. One approach is that used in *the Alma-Ata Declaration* (WHO 1978, art. 5), according to which all peoples were to attain, by the year 2000, "a level of health that will permit them to lead a socially and economically productive life." But references to different indicators shed light on different aspects of basic health. Let the following figures from selected regions and countries illuminate some essential basic health challenges even in the 2010s, when the world on average was healthier, wealthier, and technologically more advanced than ever before.

Maternal mortality clearly counts as one indicator of basic health. The global trend has been firmly positive: a decline of 44 percent of maternal deaths from 1990 to 2015. In Southern Asia, however, about sixty-six thousand women lost their lives during the delivery and its aftermath in 2015 (WHO 2015, xi, 16–17). A major challenge involved is unattended home delivery, which is a cultural tradition and also a necessity in many rural parts of, for example, Bangladesh, India, Nepal, and Pakistan. But while the corresponding maternal mortality ratio was 176 (per one hundred thousand live births) in Southern Asia, in sub-Saharan Africa, it was still much higher: no less than 546 in 2015 (WHO 2015, 17). And given that most of the maternal mortality is preventable, there definitely are many related justice and cultural issues to be addressed.

Most health indicators tell about more encouraging developments in Southern Asia than in sub-Saharan Africa. But beyond the wealthiest income groups in Southern Asia, poor maternal health, poor access to health-care services, malnutrition, and widespread malaria are common, and chronic diseases are widespread. In general, rural areas do worse than urban ones in life expectancy, immunization rates, maternal health, malaria incidence, and access to almost all health services. Diarrhea, acute respiratory infections, and diseases preventable by vaccines make childhood mortality a continuing public health challenge. So far most of the trends have nevertheless been positive.

3. Trends in Selected African Countries

In Tanzania from 2000 to 2016, the *under-five mortality rate* (per 1,000 live births) lowered from 132 to 57. The achieved level is not very far from that of medium human development countries on average (43 in 2016), although it is still well below the average levels in high human development countries (13) or the very high ones (6) in the same year. In South Africa, a much wealthier country than Tanzania, the under-five mortality rate was 43 as of 2016 (UNDP 2018a, 50–53).

One of the really troubling challenges in Tanzania is its relative *number of medical doctors*. Whereas, for instance, in South Africa, there were 0.82 physicians per 1,000 persons as of 2016, in Tanzania, there were no more than 0.02 of them in 2014—according to the most recent available WHO (2018, "Data by Country") estimate.[1] The corresponding figure in Switzerland was 4.2 in 2016 (WHO 2018, "Data by Country"). This comparison

---

1 African Health Observatory (2019) does not give a figure for the density of medical doctors in Tanzania at all but indicates that there were 0.43 nurses and midwives per a population of 1,000 as of 2012. The corresponding figures for South Africa according to this source are 0.74 (medical) doctors and 4.84 nurses and midwives per a population of 1,000.

actually indicates that health worries are still largely encountered in Africa without much aid from scientifically trained medical doctors.

Among the mixed trends in Tanzania has been its *health expenditure per capita*. It rose from circa US$13 to $40 between 2000 and 2012 but then declined to $32 in 2015. Similarly, from 2012 to 2015, the health expenditure in the percentage of Tanzania's GDP dropped from 6.7 percent to 6.1 percent. Although this level is still higher than the 5.4 percent for sub-Saharan countries on average, the downward trend is to be noted in analyses of health justice (World Bank 2019).

4. Trends in Selected Asian Countries

In India, the *under-five mortality rate* (per 1,000 live births) decreased from 126 to 43 in the period of 1990–2016. The positive development in this respect has been even more impressive in Bangladesh: from 144 (in 1990) to 34 (in 2016)! This compares strikingly with Pakistan, where 79 of every 1,000 children died by the age of five in 2016 (WHO 2018).

Most sources set their estimates about the *number of physicians* per 1,000 persons in India to circa 0.76 as of 2016—resembling the level of South Africa. In Bangladesh, this number was only 0.47 (in 2015). Both countries still lag far behind China, with its 1.8 physicians per 1,000 persons in 2015 (WHO 2018, "Physicians Density").

Despite rather positive developments in India, Jean Drèze and Amartya Sen (2013) have argued that health care, in the country is in crisis. Although India's economy has boosted in almost all vaccines covered by a particular UNICEF report from the year 2012, India is doing worse than sub-Saharan African countries on average and also worse than Bangladesh. Whereas poor Bangladesh had reached, for instance, the rates of 95 percent for polio, 94 percent for measles, and 95 percent for hepatitis B by 2012, in India, the corresponding percentages were 70, 74, and only 37 (144–45). In general, whereas the relatively well-off Indians can buy treatments in private clinics, Drèze and Sen (149) lament that the public health facilities of the country "are very limited, and quite often badly run." And also in the private sector, the lack of regulation can subject the clients to "fraud, over-medication, exploitative pricing and unnecessary surgery" (151).

Health expenditure per capita has increased in India between 2000 and 2016 dramatically: from $19 to $63. Nonetheless, as of a percentage of GDP, India's health expenditure has declined from 4.2 percent to

3.9 percent during the same period of time, thereby hovering at a level much lower than that of Tanzania (World Bank 2019).[2]

In Bangladesh, the total health expenditure rose remarkably but at a lower level than in India, from $8 to $32 between 2000 and 2016 (World Bank 2019). The levels of expenditure here are intriguing. Recall that, as of 2017 (UNDP 2018b), the life expectancy at birth in Bangladesh is 72.8 years, compared to only 68.8 years in India! Such perceptions invite us to look behind numbers at the political, cultural, and also religious dynamics in the countries in question.

5. Christian Approaches across Regions

When the "health for all" idea emerged in the 1960s, Christian approaches to basic health were strongly involved. Stemming from the foundational insights of faith for caring for the suffering and the oppressed, church-related organizations had been globally active in the field already for decades and even centuries. Indeed, the traditional medical mission approach, which had been in a salient role in the initiation of modern medicine almost all over the globe, was already in decline. While the financial support from many mission organizations was diminishing, maintaining mission hospitals had become increasingly costly. On the other hand, as the public sector health provision had started to catch new international attention, new ideals and forms of the implementation of the basic health rights for all were at hand.

In many parts of the Global South, including India and many countries of sub-Saharan Africa, a really significant progress occurred toward the turn of the millennium and thereafter. But how were Christian faith-based organizations involved in this progress? The following chapters shed some light on such developments and issues. In addition, they provide perspectives on the issues of health justice in the twenty-first century through introducing some organizations active in the field—such as the Christian Social Services Commission (CSSC) in Tanzania and the Christian Medical Association of India (CMAI).

Although Christian diakonia organizations still deal with the issues of basic health even in the Global North, it is clear that the challenges are of a different scale in the Global South. In a country like Tanzania, the

---

2 See also WHO (2019) about health expenditures by country and by the type of expenditure.

scarcity of resources is still so severe that the public sector acutely needs the involvement of the voluntary sector, largely consisting of Christian faith-based agencies. In India and in South Africa, in turn, the economic progress has been rapid enough that in principle, the state could fulfill a lion's share of the responsibilities for basic health. The inequalities of both income and health, however, have been huge in these countries, and poverty and illness have been persistent. So far, it has seemed that any models of implementing basic health rights in countries like Tanzania, South Africa, and India definitely need to include viable forms of coordination and collaboration with the faith-based sector.

6. Contemporary Initiatives in Islamic Contexts

Several faith-based organizations within the broadly Islamic framework have become pioneering civil society agencies in the arenas of international humanitarian and development work, not least in the field of basic health and well-being. One of these agencies is Islamic Relief Worldwide (2019, "History"), which was established in 1984 by Dr. Hany El-Banna and others in Birmingham, United Kingdom, as a response to the famine in Africa. Having explored issues of religion and development broadly, Jeffrey Haynes assigns particular credit to a project by the United Nations Population Fund (UNPFA) in collaboration with Muslim scholars in Uganda. The involvement of the great mufti of Uganda in this program on reproductive health was reported to be progressive and of high value to culture-sensitive health promotion (UNFPA 2004, 40–44; Haynes 2007, 160–63).

Turkish humanitarian aid organization Kimse Yok Mu, established in 2002, used to serve on a truly global scale. Since 2016, though, it has run into problems due to President Recep Tayyip Erdoğan increasing pressure on any organization with connections to widely influential Turkish imam and scholar Fethullah Gülen. Although Kimse Yok Mu was not a religious organization as such, it has been largely inspired by Gülen's teachings and the related Hizmet (service) movement.

Let one more example here be Aga Khan Development Network (AKDN), stemming from the Shia Muslim heritage. Since assuming the office of imamate in 1957, Aga Khan IV, with prestigious Iranian roots and an international life story, became increasingly concerned about the well-being of all Muslims and thus engaged himself in development work (AKDN 2019, "His Highness the Aga Khan"). Further examples, rooted in Islamic as well as in any faith tradition, can be found through the International Partnership on Religion and Sustainable Development (PaRD n.d.), a Germany-based, increasingly influential initiative.

We have to beware, however, of thinking about Islamic or any religious contributions to health too much through individual organizations. To start with, the case is rather that faith traditions influence the values prevalent in each society on a broad front and thereby affect virtually anyone working within the health and social sector in the countries and regions in question. Indeed, Islamic insights and impacts will be discussed further in the beginning of part 3, through the case of Bangladesh, which endeavors to guarantee its citizens basic health rights and beyond. In part 1, we will enter in the basic health discussion first through Christian perspectives in Tanzania and South Africa and then open up our endeavor to South Asia through Hindu and Christian perspectives in India. Thus in part 1, we will get started with Christian faith traditions in quite different contexts of scarcity and inequality and also familiarize ourselves with the South Asian context through its majority faith.

References

African Health Observatory. 2019. "Data and Statistics: Health System." World Health Organization Regional Office for Africa. Accessed January 12, 2019. http://www.aho.afro.who.int/health-workforce.

Aga Khan Development Network (AKDN). 2019. "About Us." Accessed January 15, 2019. https://www.akdn.org.

Drèze, Jean, and Amartya Sen. 2013. *An Uncertain Glory: India and Its Contradictions.* London: Allen Lane / Penguin Books.

Haynes, Jeffrey. 2007. *Religion and Development: Conflict or Cooperation?* Basingstoke, UK: Palgrave Macmillan.

International Partnership on Religion and Sustainable Development (PaRD). n.d. Accessed January 15, 2019. http://www.partner-religion-development.org.

Islamic Relief Worldwide. 2019. "About Us." Accessed January 15, 2019. https://www.islamic-relief.org.

United Nations Development Programme (UNDP). 2018a. *Human Development Indices and Indicators 2018: Statistical Update.* New York: UNDP. Accessed January 12, 2019. https://tinyurl.com/yacktsr3.

——. 2018b. "Human Development Reports: Human Development Data (1990–2017)." Accessed January 12, 2019. http://hdr.undp.org/en/data.

United Nations Population Fund (UNFPA). 2014. *Culture Matters: Working with Communities and Faith-Based Organizations: Case Studies from Country Programmes.* New York: UNFPA. Accessed January 15, 2019. https://tinyurl.com/y2zu3vd7.

World Bank. 2019. "Data." Accessed January 12, 2019. https://tinyurl.com/y77s8f8z.

World Health Organization (WHO). 1978. *The Declaration of Alma-Ata: International Conference on Primary Health Care, Alma-Ata, USSR, 6–12: September 1978.* Geneva, Switzerland: WHO. Accessed June 11, 2015. https://tinyurl.com/3ghddfo.

———. 2015. *Trends in Maternal Mortality: 1990 to 2015 Estimates by WHO, UNICEF, UNFPA, World Bank Group and the United Nations Population Division.* Geneva, Switzerland: WHO. Accessed January 12, 2019. https://tinyurl.com/y5w434k4.

———. 2018. "Health Work Force: Density per 1000." Global Health Observatory Data Repository. Accessed January 12, 2019. http://apps.who.int/gho/data/node.main.A1444.

———. 2019. "Health System Financing Profile by Country." Global Health Expenditure Database. Accessed January 21, 2019. https://tinyurl.com/y2g8qkxw.

2

Transformations of Protestant Faith-Based Health Work in an Age of Fragile Development

Ville Päivänsalo

ABSTRACT

Over the past half century, human development in terms of health has been impressive but far from uniform. Simultaneously, the visions and functions of voluntary sector agencies have been transformed. This chapter focuses on certain changes in the insights and practices of globally responsible Protestant Christian health work, mainly from the 1960s until approximately the end of the millennium. In what sense did basic health deficiencies count, on average, as issues of justice in the improving conditions? And how did the roles of Christian, mainly Lutheran, health agencies change over these decades of fragile development? Special attention is called to the contexts of India and Tanzania: whereas in the former, Protestant health agencies were left to survive largely on their own (the independence approach), in the latter, both the government and international mission organizations were more supportive of the work (the collaborative approach). The preferred approach discussed in this chapter (the pluralist interdependence approach) is presumably relevant, especially when states face persistent difficulties in securing basic health rights on their own. In this approach, the emphasis is on the health results and on the mutual learning stemming from supportive integration of faith organizations in the promotion of basic health rights.

1. Introduction: Toward a Great Ideal

During the 1960s and 1970s, Christian insights into health and justice were deeply occupied with constructing the ideal of "health for all." Since that time, human development in terms of health has been impressive in several respects, yet in large regions, the basic health rights of the poor are still at stake.

The current chapter provides a look at certain transformations of Protestant Christian health work in conditions of fragile development in the Global South, mainly from around the mid-1960s to the year 2000. During this period, the old-style mission hospital approach to Christian health work could no longer be taken for granted. In this chapter, the time span in question will first be discussed at the level of global insights, beginning with the so-called Tübingen I consultation in 1964. Then two contextual approaches will be introduced with an emphasis on the Lutheran branch of Protestantism.

One of the focus contexts of this chapter is India, where Christianity has clearly been in a minority position. After the heyday of mission hospitals, Protestant health work in India largely continued in terms of the so-called *independence approach*: neither international mission organizations nor the government has provided crucial resources for this work. The Tanzanian context, in turn, represents a kind of *collaborative approach*: there the state has basically welcomed faith-based voluntary services to the system, and characteristically, international mission organizations have continued as partners in this collaboration.

In our new millennium, it appears that, on the one hand, state governments such as those of India and Tanzania still need faith traditions and organizations to support their endeavors to achieve the great health-for-all ideal. On the other hand, few faith organizations can maintain health programs focused on the poor without public support. Here, an approach that acknowledges this kind of mutual dependency will be called the *pluralist interdependence approach*. The present chapter will encourage a search for additional ways to integrate faith organizations into public sector collaborations. In addition to the services themselves, both formally and informally enhanced partnerships could also scale up mutual learning about what truly serves basic health needs efficiently.

2. Global Turns in Protestant Health Work

Probably the most important single event in the history of global Prot-estant health work in the 1960s was the Tübingen I consultation, which took place in 1964 under the auspices of the German Institute for Medical Mission (DIFAEM) in Tübingen, Baden-Württemberg. This consultation was initiated by the Commission on World Mission of the LWF and the director of DIFAEM, Dr. Martin Scheel. The key recommendations stem-ming from this international consultation begin as follows: "The Chris-tian Church has a specific task in the field of healing" (WCC 1965, 34). This task is also understood here as a Christian duty "to support all that contributes to the welfare of man." While the consultation report stressed that the Christian ministry of healing is the responsibility of the whole congregation, it also assigned a particular duty to those "who have been trained in the techniques of modern medicine" (WCC 1965, 35).

The emphasis on the entire congregation in the Tübingen I declara-tion, which emerged from the previously mentioned consultation, is striking against the background of earlier Christian medical mission initiatives, which worldwide had been heavily centered on curative services in hospital settings. The process of establishing the Christian Medical Council (CMC) within the World Council of Churches (WCC) in 1968 continued along the same lines. The task of the CMC stemmed partly from the observation that over 90 percent of medical mission activities were hospital based and partly from the need for a broader understanding of the healing ministry (McGilvray 1981, 50). Such percep-tions anticipated the kind of health-for-all approach characteristic of the later *Alma-Ata Declaration* (1978), in which primary health care and communities played key roles.

With its establishment in 1968, the CMC explicated the theological understanding of its own task with references to (1) Christ's compas-sion for the suffering, (2) the commandment of love, and (3) seeing the dignity of neighbors as created in the image of God. In accordance with these foundational insights, Christians were to serve their fellow men and women in imitation of Christ (McGilvray 1981, 49). The CMC also encouraged the congregation to witness "the salvation which Christ offers to man whether in health or in death and [to testify] the unshaken hope in the resurrection of Christ" (qtd. in McGilvray 1981, 50).

The idea of justice in the field of health was already central to the early discussions in the CMC. In 1973, the CMC published its paper on "Health Care and Justice." This statement is strikingly critical of the hospital-centered paradigm of Christian health work, which it portrays as responding to the health needs of the population both ineffectively and unjustly. In the CMC's view, Christian hospitals had become expensive to maintain, owing to the rising costs of medical technology and wages. Instead, there should be more preventive work beyond the hospitals and more attention paid to the 90 percent of illnesses that the auxiliary personnel can care for "as effectively as physicians" (CMC 1973, 3–4). It was believed that a truly collaborative approach would also help people solve their health problems on their own (5). In sum, the statement underlined injustices related to the inequitable distribution of scarce resources, the lack of opportunities for communities and individuals to participate in health-care decisions, and the need for the health-care system to "promote the wholeness of individual, family, and community life" (6).

This approach promoted a people-centered paradigm that was still emerging in the more general discussion that eventually led to the *Alma-Ata Declaration*. It also included a concern for distributive justice and opportunities for participation that resonated smoothly with many later declarations and theories of universal health justice. "Health Care for All: The New Priority" was indeed the motto of the first issue of *Contact* (April 1975), CMC's magazine.

Later, because of economic difficulties related to the eighth assembly of the WCC held in Harare, Zimbabwe (1998), the WCC dramatically diminished its support of health work, ending the story of the CMC as such (Benn and Senturias 2001, 24). The Health and Healing Division of the WCC has continued to coordinate a wide range of initiatives: its HIV/AIDS program has been especially extensive. By the dawn of the new millennium, the still-extensive global Protestant health work was coordinated less and less from Geneva or any other city. Nevertheless, during its heyday, this work was at the heart of the rising global health movement, including grand initiatives to achieve health for all and address health issues from the perspective of justice.

3. Earlier Developments and Insights in India

The beginning of the Protestant medical mission in India is usually dated to 1730, when Caspar Gottlieb Schlegelmilch, who held a licentiate degree in medicine, was engaged by the Danish-Halle Mission and arrived in South India. Subsequently, in the late eighteenth century, Dr. John Thomas (1757–1801) managed to initiate health work in the Kolkata region. His companion, William Carey, a Baptist missionary, was able to maintain this practice by founding a leprosy clinic. Carey also contributed to the defense of health rights—and indeed the right to life—by opposing *sati* (widow burning), which was officially banned in 1829.

During the first half of the twentieth century, among the successful Protestant health initiatives in India were the treatment of tuberculosis and leprosy as well as measures in preventive medicine and community health. Nursing, one of the least appreciated jobs in traditional Indian culture, was of special importance: it has been estimated that around 1940, approximately 80 percent of nurses in the country were trained in Christian institutions (McGilvray 1981, 4). When India gained its independence in 1947, however, the government left Christian health work largely on its own, and gradually the support from Western missionary societies declined. Often this was a deliberate aim of the missionaries. For example, in 1950, as reported by the Norwegian medical missionary Olav Hodne (1976, iv, 105–13), the Ebenezer Evangelical Lutheran Church was founded to replace the older Santal Mission and realized the long-term vision of an independent Lutheran Church with health facilities. These included several hospitals and schools for nursing and midwife training.

In addition to the work in permanent health facilities and training centers, another type of Protestant work for basic health rights in India has had a humanitarian profile. For example, during the Bangladesh Liberation War in 1971, more than seven million refugees (and perhaps as many as ten million) poured through the Indian side of the border. Both the Indian government and international humanitarian agencies were overwhelmed by the needs of the refugees. Olav Hodne was there to do what he could, invited to the area by the Lutheran World Federation (Kruse 1971, 7). In the huge resettlement work over the coming years, Hodne and the Lutheran World Service India (LWSI) collaborated closely with the Indian government.

The fieldwork of the LWSI was basically nonconfessional in character from the beginning. However, in the LWSI annual report in 1978, titled *Recovering a Lost Dignity*, Hodne (1979, 4) explained the motto of the work "PREM CELL": it comes from Bengali and means roughly the idea that "we love because God loved us first." In 1979, LWSI (1980) was five years old and had been very active in community health work in such things as immunization, nutritional supplements, health education, and home visits.

Speaking more generally, Christian medical work came to the country largely as a response to the "terrible inadequacy of medical facilities in

India" (Jeyakumar 2009, 37). This approach has often been accompanied by demands for the government to assume greater responsibility for health development. Such requests were expressed, for instance, in 1973 in the Gurukul Lutheran Theological College and Research Institute in Madras (Chennai), South India. There, in a seminar on social justice, democracy, and religion, the director of the institute, Dr. P. David (1973, 10–11), pointed out that both political and religious ideas needed to be tested in social life. True democracy as well as true religion must serve the people and advance social justice. The goals of the government and faith organizations thus appeared very similar in this field. In a development workshop held in the institution five years later, Eugene Ries (1978, 13), the director of the Lutheran World Service (LWS), emphasized the importance of listening to and learning from the priorities of the LWF member churches. The agenda for health work should not come essentially from Geneva but rather from the actual health needs of Indians as understood at the grassroots level.

In the 1960s, rising trends in Protestant health work in the country significantly included preventive medicine, community health, training in pharmacy, and family planning (Padmanabha 1997, 15–17). The Christian Ashram movement, which endeavored to transform the traditional Indian idea of Ashram communities to fit Christian theology, was viable as well (Varughese 1999). In the early 1970s, however, several grants stopped, which profoundly transformed the work by the Christian Medical Association of India (CMAI) as well as by the Protestant health agencies in India generally.

4. Later Developments and Insights in India

The paradigm change in Protestant health work was authoritatively addressed in 1990 by Jacob Chandy, a pioneering Indian neurosurgeon and the deputy director of the Christian Medical College and Hospital in Vellore (CMC). Chandy (2001, 7–12, 16–17) reiterated then that at the heart of the old paradigm until the 1940s were medical doctors who were trained to cure diseases and were supported by mission organizations. Then the support diminished, and the Indian government often refused to renew the missionaries' visas. However, no one seemed to remember that new health work models needed funding. Chandy stressed that Christian doctors, nurses, and paramedical workers alike would need to be paid a salary equivalent to those at other institutions. In addition, viable health work needed high-tech hospitals. In retrospect, we may say that Chandy defended the importance of both fairness and economic sustainability, even when close collaboration with either the state or the missionary agencies was not possible or at least not easy.

How then to conceptualize the roles of Christian health work anew? In 1992, the eminent Indian ecumenical theologian M. M. Thomas (2001, 22–23) reminded that the Constitution of India assigns the primary responsibility for medical and health services in the country to the state. Thomas saw clearly the potential of modern science and technology but lamented that the accompanying ideology lacked the vigor to serve the people with justice and dignity. In such a context, Thomas (22, 35) suggested that the Christian healing ministry could promote "medical technology with a human face" as well as community health as aspects of a new wholeness approach.

Indeed, in the early 1990s, the key projects of the CMAI included community-based family planning and community-based primary health care. In addition, its many other projects, such as those promoting child survival and women's health and combating substance abuse, had strong community aspects (Padmanabha 1997, 22–28). In *Health: Everyone's Birthright*, Rev. A. C. Oommen (1997, 18–19) made it clear that, without support, Christian primary health-care centers would have to be closed down. In any case, he added, more could be done to address health challenges—such as those related to broken families, suicide mania, alcoholism, and drug addiction—beyond health institutions. Yet we can say with some degree of certainty that the dependency of Protestant health work on foreign support remained a fact. Meanwhile, the Indian government was still far from being capable of providing basic health rights to all the country's citizens.

A commercialization process characterized the Indian health sector in the 1990s. Dr. Raj S. Arole (1997, 20–28) of the Society for the Comprehensive Rural Health Project of CMAI reminded health workers and decision-makers about the Alma-Ata (1978) vision of primary health care under such conditions. He elaborated on the community health approach by requesting the provision of food and water along with basic curative services, particularly in poor communities, and advocated enabling community members to attend decision-making processes. The leading ideas—in contrast to the commercialization process—would include responding to the real needs of the people and providing the poor with information to defend their causes. As the goal of such work in theological terms, Arole (1997, 33) highlighted *shalom* with its aspects of peace, health, wholeness, and harmonious relations. Such an approach definitely promoted justice, at least insofar as we understand it as a provision of basic services to the poor and oppressed and the enhancement of their opportunities to participate in related decision-making on all relevant levels.

One highly elaborated model of congregation-based health care was subsequently developed in a collaborative process between the CMAI and the Presbyterian Church in the United States. In the year 2000, these partners organized a joint meeting in New Delhi on the theme of "Congregations in Health: Making Community-Based Health and Development a Reality." In the resulting publication, the leading image had changed. Whereas formerly it had been that of the mission hospital on the hill, now the idea was to come down to the grassroots level in order to respond holistically to the population, especially to the needs of the poor, who cannot afford the costly treatments of commercialized care. The approach provided a matrix for prioritizing health problems (Booth et al. 2002, 99–101) by means of three questions: How serious and how common are the health problems in question? How easy are the apparent solutions? How strong is the community's interest in solving these problems?

With different partners, however, the CMAI adopted different approaches. This was reemphasized by Dr. Vijay Aruldas (2005, 22–23), the general secretary of the CMAI in 2005. Aruldas (2005, 23) called further attention to the idea of creating the ability to respond, which he wanted to encourage, especially at the local level. This would accord with the idea of diversity as a strength rather than a weakness of the CMAI. And we could reemphasize that this approach definitely addressed many issues of basic health rights.

5. Earlier Developments and Insights in Tanzania

Among the most admired Christian missionaries of all time was David Livingstone (1813–73), who famously met Henry Stanley on the shores of Lake Tanganyika in 1871. For Livingstone, a medical mission was an integral part of missionary work. Yet essential progress in medical missions in the region largely took place after the year 1891, when mainland Tanganyika was made a German colony. In 1914, the country became a British colony, but the number of Lutheran Christians in Tanganyika continued to rise—to about 81,000–85,000 in 1939 (Lindquist 1982, 20–24; Bernander 1968, 157). Such a rise in numbers indicates that this type of newly introduced faith indeed attracted many, although it is difficult to differentiate between genuinely religious attraction and that stemming from service provision in health and education by the missionaries. And of course, the complex controversies about outright colonial policies should be taken into account in any broader analysis.

At the outbreak of World War II, in "the Lutheran mission fields in Tanganyika," there were reportedly 132 missionaries, 6 medical doctors, and 48 nurses as well as 1,780 teachers and teacher-evangelists (Bernander 1968, 157). These numbers plummeted during the war but began to rise afterward, eventually restoring and stabilizing salient roles in Lutheran health services alongside their counterparts from different denominational backgrounds, most of whom were Roman Catholics.

It has been natural in Tanzania to see faith in God and Christ as connected with liberation from all kinds of problems, including illness. To be a healer or "medicine man" (*mganga* in many Bantu languages) is traditionally very much appreciated among Tanzanians. Often Christ is seen to fit smoothly into the role of "supreme healer" (Svensäter 2002, 118, 135). Such a belief appears to be on a continuum with the belief in the love of God that "does not want anything higher than to deliver people from all kinds of burdens, whether in sickness, spiritual oppression or material shortage" (Svensäter 2002, 125). Christian health workers could not, however, take for granted that the newly independent United Republic of Tanzania (1964), a socialist regime, would welcome the faith-based sector as an integral part of its social service system.

In 1967, the Evangelical Lutheran Church in Tanzania (ELCT) served as the key organizer of the conference called Consultation on Health and Healing, chaired by Dr. John Wilkinson from the East African Presbyterian Church in Makumira.[1] Bishop Stefano R. Moshi, *Mkuu* (head) of the ELCT, emphasized in that context that the church does *not* do medical work in order to win more converts. This would "not show God's love and compassion for man in his suffering" (Moshi 1967, 2). Rev. Cuthbert K. Omari from the University of Dar es Salaam, in turn, underlined the need for a holistic understanding of each person. Originally created as body, mind, and spirit in equal parts, any person who is sick needs healing in all these respects, but not only for oneself. Here on earth, said Omari (1967, 87), Christians are to seek health "in order to live for the service of God" and thereby for the service of their neighbors as God's coworkers. Dr. Aart van Soest (1967, 87–90) from Tübingen focused in this consultation on the practical planning of church-related medical work.

---

1 This consultation was one of the follow-ups to Tübingen I, 1964.

He urged recognition of unmet needs as the guides to action. Hospitals should not be maintained as monuments to prestigious service.

The international Lutheran community had its chance to come up with prophetic perspectives in the country, especially in the fifth LWF assembly in Dar es Salaam in 1977. The main theme of the conference was "In Christ: A New Community." The concept of communion (*koinonia*) used there had a prophetic edge that also allowed the quoting of the president of the country, Julius Nyerere, in a very appreciative spirit in the conference study guide. Nyerere, the champion of Ujamaa socialism in Tanzania, had underlined that a political and economic system must neither lead to "millions being hungry, thirsty, and naked" nor condemn "millions to preventable sickness." Similarly, in the LWF (1977, 43, 63) view, the new community should strive for a better life and a more just social order and declare mankind's liberation through Christ from determinism and oppression. With reference to Paul's letter to the Romans (8:39, 12:9–21), this guide (LWF 1977, 92) explained that the righteousness of God "not only transforms hearts, but by transforming hearts it transforms the world." Such insights paved the way for a collaborative approach to health in Tanzania, exemplifying a very different spirit than that in India in the corresponding relations between the Protestant health providers and the governmental authorities.

Similar to India, however, the central role of hospitals in Christian health work has been challenged time and again, both in Tanzania as well as throughout sub-Saharan Africa. But it has also been often pointed out, as in a WCC study by Rexford Asante (1998, 78–79), that through transparency and active stewardship, many church-related health institutions can remain highly valued in their field.[2] And numerous hospitals owned by local churches have indeed remained viable in Tanzania, although they are supported by the state and international donors. This can be seen as one way of promoting basic health justice in circumstances where health development has remained fragile and does not yet approximate the ideal of universal coverage.

2 Asante (1998, 78) requested improvements in transparency through "periodic, formal, and carefully conducted studies" of church-owned health-care institutions and through thoroughness in the appointments of key persons.

6. Later Developments and Insights in Tanzania

The leading authors on the role of the church in Tanzania in the late twentieth century included the aforementioned Cuthbert K. Omari, a Tanzanian Lutheran pastor and theologian who passed away in 2001. In a book completed in 2000 (and published in 2006), Omari (2006, 20–26) distinguished among four conceptualizations of the church: a building, a denomination, the body of Christ, and a community of believers. In discussing the church as the body of Christ, he emphasized—in terms of Pauline theology—the importance of the functioning of every part of the body. Otherwise, the whole body suffers. Under the leadership of Christ (the head), different parts of the body should function in interdependent harmony. One type of rift in this functioning is denominational arrogance. Another can consist of exaggerated geographical distinctiveness. The church is to be essentially a universal, worldwide body. In Omari's (2006, 26) view, the believers should vindicate their faith through discipleship, witness, and service.

Instead of conceptualizing the church and society as if they were *separate entities*, Omari (2006, 27–30) regarded the church as being *within society*. Within a larger community, the members of the church live up to their calling to witness for Christ and serve society, spreading goodness all around like salt and light. Thereby, the church also "becomes the agent of change through awareness creation" in a process that "aims at promoting equity and social development" (30). An important aspect of this approach is the church's social ministry. Although Omari (104) understood this as a "horizontal ministry," social ministry is rooted in the vertical dimension of faith, which essentially consists of God's work of reconciliation through the work of Christ.

The visions of individual churches shed light on what such dimensions could mean in practice. For example, the vision statement of the health charter of the ELCT focuses on society at large: "A society with healthy individuals and communities whereby physical, emotional, mental and spiritual needs are met and balanced resulting in peaceful and joyful life" (2010, 4). The mission statement of the health section of the ELCT (2010, 4), in turn, opens from the perspective of witnessing through the provision of holistic, affordable, and accessible quality care to all people, supported by the community and other stakeholders.

In 1992, the roles of faith-based organizations (FBOs) in the health sector became clarified, and the entire system transformed in a less state-centered direction when the Christian Social Services Commission (CSSC) was founded in the country. In this process, the government of Tanzania, the Christian Council of Tanzania (CCT), and the Tanzania Episcopal Conference (TEC), a Catholic organization, negotiated a memorandum of understanding (MoU) to provide a formal framework for CSSC-related health service collaboration. Since 2007, so-called service agreement (SA) documents have been used to specify the forms of collaboration between the government and individual hospitals. In many respects, however, the collaboration between public authorities and Christian health organizations has continued to rely on trust-based relationships (Boulanger and Criel 2012, 85–87, 91–93).

Although the challenges of maintaining church-related health institutions have remained pressing in Tanzania, the supportive approach for this sector by the government and by numerous international donors has provided some prospects for the legacy to continue to be viable. At least the history of this cooperation, although sometimes mutually suspicious, provides ingredients for further conceptualizations of the interdependence approach and its implementation.

7. Toward a Conscious Interdependence Approach?

In the late twentieth century, as Jeffrey Haynes (2007) puts it, faith-based organizations "were often explicitly excluded from national development programs by modernization processes often led by secular states in many parts of the developed world" (4). It has been shown earlier, however, that Christian churches and agencies have often been willing to question at least their hospital-centered health work. Yet Protestant Christian traditions, among others, continue to include a great deal of potential as effective partners for basic health rights in pluralist settings. This potential is rarely so vigorous that it could make impressive responses to the health needs of the poor without any external support. It is rooted, however, in such a long and intriguing history and theology that simply to disregard it would be odd in the face of the transforming basic health challenges of the twenty-first century, challenges that still are both profound and broad. Much of this potential has also been recently mapped both broadly and systematically (Päivänsalo 2020).

Indeed, the aforementioned DIFAEM institution, the same one that in 1964 hosted the meeting that led to the Tübingen I declaration, organized another conference in 2014 on the present and future of Christian responsibilities for global health. In the resulting document, "A Call to

Health and Healing: Declaration"—or the Tübingen III declaration—the conference participants affirmed that "the Christian Church continues to have a unique, relevant and specific role to play in Health, Health Care, Healing and Wholeness, in changing contexts and in all regions of the world" (DIFAEM 2014, 93).[3] While the conference presentations confirmed that a great deal of important health work is still carried out by particular Christianity-rooted organizations, even without major external support as happens in India, it also urged churches at large and state governments to reflect on their responsibilities for global health.

The conditions of mutual interdependence can easily be overlooked. Individual voluntary agencies could be expected to produce major results simply on their own, even under very challenging conditions, or secular states could be imagined as being capable of providing universal health coverage unassisted. This chapter reminds us of a variety of impressive faith-based initiatives of the past for the right to health and encourages the further elaboration of pluralist, collaborative schemes for basic health justice in the spirit of mutual learning.

Acknowledgments

I am grateful to the University of Helsinki, my employer for most of the time of this entire project, for providing the basic facilities for this research and to the Business Ethics Research Group (Aalto University) for travel funding. I am also thankful to the Finnish Evangelical Lutheran Mission, the Evangelical Lutheran Church of Tanzania, the Gurukul Lutheran Theological College and Research Institute, the Lutheran World Federation (Geneva), the German Institute of Medical Mission, the Nordic Africa Institute, the University of Heidelberg, and the United Theological College (Bangalore) for providing me material for this research chapter (and the related broader research project).

---

3 Right after this affirmation, Tübingen Declaration III (DIFAEM 2014, 93) begins an explication of the foundational insights involved as follows: "Every human being is made in the image of God, created with dignity in diversity irrespective of any personal circumstances, and this is equally true in suffering, disability or when living with chronic disease."

References

Arole, Raj S. 1997. "Beyond Maternal and Child Health." In *Health: Everyone's Birthright*, edited by Santosh Gnanakan, 20–33. New Delhi: Christian Medical Association of India.

Aruldas, Vijay. 2005. "CMAI in a Nutshell: General Secretary's Report." *Christian Medical Journal of India* 20 (3): 20–23.

Asante, Rexford Kofi Oduro. 1998. *Sustainability of Church Hospitals in Developing Countries: A Search for Criteria for Success*. Geneva, Switzerland: World Council of Churches (WCC).

Benn, Christoph, and Erlinda Senturias. 2001. "Health, Healing and Wholeness: Concepts and Programmes in the Ecumenical Discussion." In *Neglected Dimensions in Health and Healing: Concepts and Explorations in an Ecumenical Perspective*, edited by Beate Jakob, Christoph Benn, and Erlinda Senturias, 8–27. Tübingen, Germany: German Institute for Medical Mission (DIFAEM).

Bernander, Gustav. 1968. *Lutheran Wartime Assistance to Tanzania Churches, 1940-1945*. Uppsala, Sweden: Gleerup.

Booth, Beverly, Carl Taylor, Cherian Thomas, and Dorothy Brewster-Lee. 2002. *Congregation-Based Health Care: Making Community-Based Health and Development Reality: A Resource Book for Congregations Working with Communities*. New Delhi: Christian Medical Association of India.

Chandy, Jacob. 2001. "The Concepts of the Ministry of Healing (1990): The Responsibility of the Congregation in the Healing Ministry of the Church." In *The Healing Ministry of the Church of India: A Compilation of the Jacob Chandy Orations*, edited by Vijay Aruldas, 5–18. New Delhi: Christian Medical Association of India.

Christian Medical Council (CMC). 1973. "Health Care and Justice." *Contact* 16 (August): 2–6.

——. 1975. "Health Care for All." *Contact* 26 (April): 1.

David. P. 1973. "Welcome Speech." In *Seminar on Social Justice, Democracy and Religion*, 9–12. Madras: Gurukul Lutheran Theological College and Research Institute.

Evangelical Lutheran Church in Tanzania (ELCT). 2010. *Health Service Charter*. Arusha, Tanzania: ELCT.

German Institute for Medical Mission (DIFAEM). 2014. "A Call to Health and Healing: Declaration." In *Christian Responses to Health and Development: German Institute for Medical Mission (DIFAEM): Symposium at Tübingen, June 2014, Documentation*, 91–95. Tübingen, Germany: DIFAEM.

Haynes, Jeffrey. 2007. *Religion and Development: Conflict or Cooperation?* Basingstoke, UK: Palgrave Macmillan.

Hodne, Olav. 1967. *The Seed Bore Fruit: A Short History of the Santal Mission of the Northern Churches 1867-1967.* Dumka, Santal Parganas, India: Santal Mission of the Northern Churches.

———. 1979. "To Our Friends." In *Recovering a Lost Dignity: Annual Report 1978*, 4. Kolkata, India: Lutheran World Service India (LWSI).

Jeyakumar, D. Arthur. 2002. *History of Christianity in India: Selected Themes.* Delhi: Indian Society for Promoting Christian Knowledge.

Kruse, Rainer. 1971. "Bei den Flüchtlingen aus Ostpakistan." *Nachrichten aus der Ärztlichen Mission*, December, 6–9, 1971.

Lutheran World Federation (LWF). 1977. *In Christ: A New Community: A Study Guide in Preparation for the Sixth Assembly of the Lutheran World Federation in June 1977 in Tanzania.* Edited by Risto Lehtonen and Gerhard Thomas. Geneva, Switzerland: General Secretariat of the LWF.

Lutheran World Service (India) (LWSI). 1980. *Preparing the Ground . . . : Annual Report 1979.* Kolkata, India: LWSI.

McGilvray, James C. 1981. *In Quest for Health and Wholeness.* Tübingen, Germany: German Institute for Medical Mission (DIFAEM).

Moshi, Stefano R. 1967. Foreword to *Health and Healing: The Makumira Consultation, February 1967*, 1–2. Arusha: Medical Board of the Evangelical Lutheran Church of Tanzania.

Omari, Cuthbert K. 1967. "Health and Healing in the Creation." In *Health and Healing: The Makumira Consultation, February 1967*, 28–33. Arusha: Medical Board of the Evangelical Lutheran Church of Tanzania.

———. 2006. *The Church in Contemporary Africa: Issues, Problems and Challenges in the Eighties and Nineties.* Neuendettelsau, Germany: Erlanger Verlag für Mission und Ökumene.

Oommen, A. C. 1997. "Rebuilding the Healing Ministry." In *Health: Everyone's Birthright*, edited by Santosh Gnanakan, 15–19. New Delhi: Christian Medical Association of India.

Padmanabha, A., P. Ramachandran, and Sukant Singh. 1997. *Christian Medical Council of India: Comprehensive Evaluation: Summary of Findings and Recommendations.* New Delhi: Christian Medical Association of India.

Päivänsalo, Ville. 2020. *Justice with Health: Faith in Support of Progress across Contexts.* Uppsala, Sweden: Acta Universitatis Upsaliensis.

Ries, Eugene. 1978. "Dr. Ries' (November 20, 1978) Address to UELCI Development Workshop, Gurukul, Madras, India." In *Development Workshop*, by the United Evangelical Lutheran Churches in India (UELCI), 9–15. Madras: UELCI.

Svensäter, Frederic. 2002. "Concepts and Practices of Healing within the Lutheran Church in Tanzania: With a Special Focus on Iringa Diocese." In *Church Life and Christian Initiatives in Tanzania: A Report from a Field Study 2001*, edited by Klas Lundström, 117–140. Uppsala: Swedish Institute of Missionary Research.

Thomas, M. M. 2001. "The Church's Healing Ministry in India (1992)." In *The Healing Ministry of the Church of India: A Compilation of the Jacob Chandy Orations*, edited by Vijay Aruldas, 19–35. New Delhi: Christian Medical Association of India.

Van Soest, Aart. 1967. "The Strategy of the Healing Ministry of the Church." In *Health and Healing: The Makumira Consultation, February 1967*, 85–91. Arusha: Medical Board of the Evangelical Lutheran Church of Tanzania.

Varughese, K. V. 1999. *A Vision for Wholeness: Ashrams and Healing in India*. New Delhi: Christian Medical Association of India.

World Council of Churches (WCC). 1965. *The Healing Church: The Tübingen Consultation, 1964*. Geneva, Switzerland: WCC.

3

Toward Basic Health Justice

GRASSROOTS CHALLENGES IN CHURCH-RELATED HEALTH SERVICES IN TANZANIA

Josephine Sundqvist and Thomas Ndaluka

ABSTRACT

This chapter aims at providing insight into the development and emerging role of church organizations in health sector developments and, consequently, mutual partnership with regard to the realization of basic health rights and health justice. Health as a right of every human being is a key indicator of development. In this context, church organizations have, since their establishment, been providing health services to people living in poverty. This chapter has a focus on three church organizations engaged in health sector development: the Roman Catholic Church in Tanzania (Tanzania Episcopal Conference), the Evangelical Lutheran Church in Tanzania, and the Free Pentecostal Church of Tanzania. The argument of this chapter is that in entering into public-private partnerships (PPPs) with the Tanzanian public authorities, church organizations have increased their potential to contribute to the realization of health rights following the latest political and economic reforms. Their attraction as service providers follows from their existing infrastructure and previous experience and capacity in the health sector. The chapter further shows that church organizations are also becoming more vulnerable financially, as they are not compensated according to the PPP contracts at the local level. The agenda is also to a large extent set by external donor agencies and brings distinct grassroots challenges on both the Tanzanian model of secularism, with its emphasis on Muslim and Christians being treated equally, and the local governments' efforts toward national ownership with their favoring of public health care over private alternatives.

1. Trends and Pattern of Christian Church Organization in Tanzania

This chapter examines and reflects upon three case studies on the role of Christian church organizations and local public authorities with regard to the realization of basic health justice in Tanzania. The chapter draws from data generated through interviews with different key informants, participant observation, and policy reviews in Tanzania. Empirically, the chapter examines health-care delivery by three church organizations within the framework of public-private partnerships (PPP) in Tanzania. These partnerships are defined and understood as an arrangement between the public and the private sector (Itika 2009). The focus is on the pooling of resources (financial, human, technical, and information) from the public and private sector in order to achieve a commonly agreed-upon social goal, such as health-care delivery and the realization of health rights at large (Bandio 2012).

Since the early years of Christianity in Tanzania, the contribution of the provision of health by the Christian churches to people living in poverty is significant. This contribution has remained significant throughout the country's modern history through today, despite the changing political environment (Leurs, Tumaini-Mungu, and Mvungi 2011). Religion in Tanzanian society is generally also characterized by high visibility. Religion is deeply embedded in the lives of people (Jones and Petersen 2011; Ndaluka 2012, 2). Religion forms the basis of living, helps determine attitudes and decision-making, and is the foundation in life and the root of the Tanzanians' search for well-being (Mushi and Mukandala 2006, 533–39). Religion, power, and governance are also interconnected and have been since kings and chiefs traditionally ruled by divine right, combining the functions of providing spiritual and political leadership (Mhina 2007; Mukandala and Heilman 2015, 4). Affiliation-wise, Tanzania is characterized by a multireligious context, and ever since independence, religious pluralism and the harmonious coexistence among indigenous believers, Muslims, Christians, and other faiths have been promoted by the Tanzanian state (Ndaluka 2012, 2). The majority of Tanzanians are either Muslims or Christians who practice their faith with integrated forms of African traditional religions (Bakari 2012; Richebächer 2007). African traditional religions are particularly influential, as they affect how most Tanzanians relate to one another in extended families and in the larger community (Mhina 2007; Lawi and Masanja 2006, 112; Magesa 2010, 45).

The concept of health justice is central to both economic development and the realization of human rights in Tanzania today (Päivänsalo 2013). Health justice has emerged as a concept within sociological and developmental discourses as a critique of top-down approaches in policy making as well as governments' and private actors' limited capacity to ensure health rights and implementation of health policy in remote and poor areas. Under the framework of global health governance, shared health governance (public and private) is defined in universal human rights terms. Full knowledge and mutual understanding of global health objectives are considered preconditions for the realization of health justice (Ruger 2012). The global right to health has been further promoted through its inclusion in the UN 2030 Agenda for Sustainable Development. Health is seen as both a contributor to development and a key indicator of what people-centered, rights-based, inclusive, and equitable development seeks to achieve. Sustainable Development Goal 3 of the aforementioned agenda has also brought a stronger focus on universal health coverage (UHC) as an overarching theme, with a greater emphasis on the social, economic, and environmental dimensions of sustainable development as central features of health. The 2030 agenda is also framed in such a way that the attainment requires shared solutions across multiple public sectors (WHO 2018).

Basic health justice in this chapter is defined as the common key health goals that involve a broader spectrum of health and development indicators, including child/maternal health, alleviating hunger, and supplying safe drinking water. Health as a concept is understood as being essential to an individual's well-being, quality of life, and ability to participate in society (Venkatapuram 2011). Health is central to the existence of any individual, while collective action to decrease health injustice is perhaps the greatest project for social cohesion (Ruger 2012). The PPP reform in health in Tanzania carries the potential to facilitate the development of effective health institutions to achieve health justice through mutual partnerships between public authorities and church organizations. However, the current alignment process of public and private health institutions in Tanzania is characterized by multiple grassroots challenges, and it is necessary to overcome these in order for basic health justice to be achieved (Sundqvist 2017, 17).

2. Christian Churches in the Provision of Health-Care Services

The health sector in Tanzania has gone through large top-down structural changes and has adopted numerous divergent policies over the last decades. Existing literature on the development and the role of church organizations in the health sector in Tanzania dates back to the colonial period, the early years of Christian missions in the country (mid-nineteenth century; Sundqvist 2017, 76).

Since the early years of Christianity in Tanzania, the contribution of Christian churches to the provision of health care to the poor and marginalized has been significant. This contribution has remained important throughout the country's modern history and is still today despite the changing political environment (Leurs, Tumaini-Mungu, and Mvungi 2011). When European missionary societies arrived, they began to establish health institutions in collaboration with the colonial rulers of East Africa, where colonialism created the preconditions for the kind of political and economic context in which European missionaries could work with health sector development unchallenged (Green, Mercer, and Mesaki 2010). Christianity in general became increasingly associated with social service provision and received public recognition. This was particularly evident in the case of Catholic missions where health-care delivery was prioritized, together with the expansion of the church and the gospel. Wherever there was a mission station, there was also a dispensary or hospital providing missionary societies with an opportunity to have direct contact with the population (Sundkler and Steed 2000). Gradually, the Christian missions moved into the center and advanced in their capacity as development collaborators in the delivery of social services (Leurs, Tumaini-Mungu, and Mvungi 2011).

Tanganyika gained its independence in 1961. Most foreign missions handed over the ownership and part of the administration of hospitals to the independent Tanzanian church organizations during the years following independence (Yates 1994). In this process, foreign missions were integrated with native church organizations (Jennings 2008), even though church-based health institutions and schools were still financially dependent on foreign missions and the international donor community. In the years following independence, the Tanzanian church organizations developed into self-governing organizations (Pallant 2012). In general, during this period, church organizations continued to play a dominant role in the health sector. Following independence, the Tanganyika African National Union (TANU) came to control the economic and political spheres (Fouere 2015). In 1964, Tanganyika united politically with Zanzibar and was renamed Tanzania, with Julius Kambarage Nyerere as its first president. Shortly after, the Tanzanian government introduced a development model based on so-called African socialism, or *Ujamaa*, as it was termed in Kiswahili (Havnevik and Isinika 2010; Ndaluka 2012, 31). During this time, the Christian churches started showing a growing concern with regard to the development process. The response of church organizations to the policy of Ujamaa was somewhere in between full acceptance and resistance (Ndaluka 2012, 33). The Protestants and the Catholics agreed to commit their resources to support the government's development objectives, where the nature of an appropriate church-state relationship formed the core of their strategies (Kijanga 1978). Several of the church leaders were not particularly committed to Ujamaa and feared a Marxist and atheist drift (Westerlund 1980). Critics within the churches also questioned the nationalization of the major means of production and the state taking over the ownership of several Christian health facilities (Leurs, Tumaini-Mungu, and Mvungi 2011; Ngowi 2009). The resistance to Ujamaa was particularly strong among the Pentecostals and the Seventh-day Adventists, even though regional differences probably played a more important role than differences between various Christian denominations (Westerlund 1980). Despite the mistrust of Ujamaa exhibited by mainstream church organizations, a majority of Catholic and Protestant bishops eventually agreed to support the policy and decided to reorient their institutions in line with the public development policy (Mhina 2007; Ludwig 1999). The most common view is that the church-state partnership during Ujamaa remained relatively stable while to some extent being weakened as part of the nationalization process (Bakari 2012; Mallya 2006, 397–98).

Nyerere stepped down as president in 1985, a time of serious economic crisis. The government was under pressure from the donors and the international community, forcing him to change from the Ujamaa policy and instead implement structural adjustment programs (SAPs) of the World Bank and IMF (Leurs, Tumaini-Mungu, and Mvungi 2011). Most government health facilities ran into difficult conditions with an insufficient supply of drugs and a lack of important facilities and health personnel (Green 2005). As a consequence, the government appointed some faith-based hospitals to become district and regional referral hospitals. This health-care reform enabled them to sign District Designated Hospital (DDH) agreements. DDH was implemented to make up for the shortage of public facilities and to prevent the risk of duplication at places where the church already had established hospitals. These types of contracts or in some cases just agreements were established between the owner of the hospital and the government (Boulanger and Criel 2012).

In 1992, the Roman Catholic Church (TEC) and the Protestant Christian Council of Tanzania (CCT) established the Christian Social Services Commission (CSSC). The TEC and the CCT had two executive organs—namely, the Christian Education Board of Tanzania (CEBT) and the Christian Medical Board of Tanzania (CMBT)—that emerged into one ecumenical body. The same year, a memorandum of understanding between the government and CSSC was agreed upon. Church organizations gradually changed their social mission to integrate further with the public development policies (Boulanger and Criel 2012). The government agreed to share with the churches grants from foreign governments and assured them they would not nationalize institutions owned by Christian churches. This collaboration developed further and later took the shape of the PPP reform (Sundqvist 2017, 17).

3. PPPs Introduced in the Health Sector

The current institutional framework for PPP in health is a complex reform that includes a PPP policy, a PPP act, and PPP regulations. The PPP policy was introduced by the Tanzanian government in 2009 and includes a comprehensive overview and description of the PPP mechanism (Phares, Mujinja, and Kida 2014). In 2010, the PPP act was approved by the parliament and specified the purpose, role, terms, and conditions for these types of partnerships in health. The first Strategic Public-Private Partnership Health Plan (2010–15) was launched in 2010. Through the 2011 PPP regulations, church organizations were offered the possibility of entering into subcontracting and receiving funding for operating costs in a more structured way, such as basic salaries for employees, medicine, and infrastructure by the local government. In return, church organizations were responsible for operating the health facilities, including the maintenance of buildings and new investments in health infrastructure (Ministry of Health 2011). The current PPP framework allows for different forms of collaboration between the government and church organizations. This is based on the nature of the contract, on the parties involved, and on the types of service delivery (World Bank 2013). The PPPs are classified into three main categories: (1) delegation of responsibility, (2) purchasing of services, and (3) cooperation. The first category, contractual relations based on delegation of responsibility, refers to when the state delegates the task of operating health-care facilities to another agent. The second category, contractual relations based on an act of purchase, is when a health actor entrusts a partner with providing services in exchange for payment. Finally, a contractual relation based on cooperation refers to sharing the resources needed to work together with a partner toward a common goal while respecting each other's identity (Sundqvist 2017, 91). In relation to the different forms of collaboration, there were three main types of collaborative contracts introduced: (1) council-designated hospital contracts, (2) service agreements, and (3) grants-in-aid (National PPP Steering Committee 2009). Some of these contractual models may be combined, while others may only be entered into separately. It is important to note that not every hospital can be granted the status of CDH. Nevertheless, every dispensary, health center, hospital, and any other facility can technically enter into a service agreement with a district council. With regard to the staff grants, these are paid out directly to the church-based hospitals by the national treasury. However, both the council-designated hospital contracts and the service agreements are examples of collaborative forms of PPPs that increased in numbers (Sundqvist 2017, 96).

4. Three Case Studies

This chapter contains three thematic case studies in Tanzania examining three local health units as part of national church organizations, the Roman Catholic Church in Tanzania (Tanzania Episcopal Conference), the Evangelical Lutheran Church in Tanzania (ELCT), and the Free Pentecostal Church of Tanzania (FPCT). The church organizations were strategically selected for the case studies based on their status with regard to membership, levels of institutional public partnership, health-care provision, number of members, and theological doctrines (Sundqvist 2017, 52). This was done in order to cover the broadest spectrum of church organizations—namely, Catholic, Lutheran, and Pentecostal (Afrobarometer 2008).

However, it is important to note that the selected church organizations do not serve as a statistically representative sample and also that there are other prominent church organizations in the health sector, such as the Anglican Church, not included in the study. I selected the church organizations with support from the Ministry of Health and the CSSC's database for church health facilities. Together these church organizations account for about 35 percent of health-care services in Tanzania (Ministry of Health 2016). For each church organization, a corresponding church-based hospital was included as part of the respective case study at the local level. I also engaged in a dialogue with additional stakeholders, including the National Public-Private Partnership Unit and the prime minister's Office of Regional Administration and Local Government, several nongovernmental organizations (NGOs), international faith-based organizations (FBOs), and the World Bank (Health Unit). These formal and informal consultations resulted in the first selection of the three church-based hospitals and corresponding local governments (Sundqvist 2017, 52).

The study includes national and local public authorities and their relationships to, and views on, the related church organizations, thereby capturing a mutual perspective and a more comprehensive understanding of the contractual partnerships (PPPs) in the health sector. Furthermore, in order to ensure that the study captured Tanzania's unique institutional contexts, the Local Government Reform Programme was taken into consideration. Since contractual partnerships are concluded at the local level, I was open to the possibility of variances in local collaborative forms, subcontracting, and informal stakeholder relationships. The financial policies and subcontracts concluded between the church organizations and the local government authorities were also analyzed. The empirical results from the local case studies served as a foundation for gaining deeper insights into the PPPs in health and local grassroots challenges. Relevant national policy documents and strategies on PPPs and positions adopted in health policy formulation were also analyzed.

Triangulation was applied through the use of multiple data sources and a qualitative method mix, comprising qualitative text analysis, semi-structured interviews, and participant observations. The identification of interviewees was carried out through strategic selection (Bennett and George 2005). Interviewees were selected from four categories: (1) public authorities at the national level and related stakeholders, (2) church organizations and related NGOs/FBOs at the national level, (3) public authorities at the local level, and (4) church-based hospitals at the local level. The focus was on key informants with specific information on PPPs in the health sector with regard to the role of church organizations. The pilot study clarified the management structures at the church hospitals and within the local government while allowing for the identification of key individuals in the respective management groups.

The selection of interviewees began after formulating the research questions, constructing the interview guides, and selecting cases to study. Interviewees on policy and legal issues from the Ministry of Health were included. At the council level, Council Health Management Teams (CHMTs) were included, as were district medical officers. The official representatives from the church organizations or the public health authorities participating in the case studies were not considered the voice of the entire membership of these church organizations or the Tanzanian government but rather as key individuals within these institutions (Sundqvist 2017, 51).

5. Dependency on External Donor Agencies

There are several identified grassroots challenges in the local governments' and church organizations' struggle to realize health rights and basic health justice in Tanzania. The first challenge is of aid dependency in health policy making. More often health policy making is still conducted in an aid-dependent context whereby actors at the local level have little influence over health planning, budget priorities, and the development of health units (Sundqvist 2017, interview 13). CHMTs and church health facilities at the district level become in these arrangements almost entirely dependent on the agenda set by the national government and external donor agencies. Earlier studies have also pointed to the fact that the growing focus on collaborative partnerships between church organizations and public authorities with regard to health care has come as an externally driven global reform agenda (Itika et al. 2011).

It's evident that the foreign missionary societies still impact the development of church-related health services at the grassroots level in Tanzania. Following a sharp reduction in the financial aid to the health sector from the outside since the 1990s, external actors are still involving themselves in strategic planning for the long-term development and sustainability of the church-related health services. Faith-based hospitals are situated in remote areas but are far more globally connected than what has been formerly recognized in related field studies.

Moreover, missionary societies still play an important role in developing and maintaining the church-related health facilities in Tanzania. Even though missionary societies handed over their health institutions, assets, and ongoing health programs to national church organizations more than thirty years ago, they still involve themselves to a high extent. Church health facilities strive to promote local ownership and bottom-up development. At the same time, due to a shortage of human resources, financial resources, drugs, and specialist competence, the external support is still perceived as a necessity. However, at the Selian Lutheran Hospital in Arusha, district external support has declined partly due to disagreements between hospital management and external partners (Sundqvist 2017, 116, interview 42). In the other two cases, the involvement of external actors is rather on the way up. In all three cases, I argue that a grassroots challenge occurs when the involvement of external missionary societies is not officially recognized and fully integrated into the local health planning done by the local CHMTs. The key informants express a situation where church-related health facilities are influenced strategically from two sides. Church health organizations are sometimes torn between the external demands of missionary societies at the global level and the directives from CHMTs at the local level. These strategies might be complementary but can also contradict each other.

Despite agreements concluded between the government and church hospitals, external donors still play an important role in developing and maintaining church-related health facilities. This needs to be analyzed further and taken into consideration in future developments of the PPP reform.

6. Government Financial Support to Church Health Facilities

The discussions and negotiations around the future development and sustainability of the church-related health services involve stakeholders ranging from the village to the international stakeholders. Church-related health facilities are claiming that the local governments are not delivering financial support to their health facilities in accordance with the agreed contracts. Funds from the government were delayed and sometimes not delivered at all. This frustrated functions of church health facilities and affected the quality of service delivery.

At the same time, local governments have questioned why external partners have provided church organizations with additional external financial support that has remained largely outside the planning and priority structures at the local level. The local government further questioned the lack of transparency on the utilization of foreign financial supports. These funds were often not reported or disclosed to local government authorities because church facilities are not responsible to the local government. Such a lack of mandate frustrates the local government authorities and leads to a difficult and complex contractual relationship.

CHMTs argue that vertical health programs need to be more integrated into the planning and programming systems for the purpose of improving transparency and subcontracting at the local level and in order to enable local government to realize health rights. At the same time, some representatives of church-related health facilities argue that if all funding goes through the local government, less will trickle down to the population on-site (Sundqvist 2017, 181).

What is seen, though, is that under the current PPP reform, church organizations are in fact collaborating more closely with the local governments. In this process, they have moved from partly reducing their financial dependency on international partners to increasing their financial dependency on the state. The partnerships aim for further integration of the church health facilities into the public health system. Nevertheless, the argument here is that all three church organizations were still only to a small extent involved in comprehensive health planning in the local districts.

Most church representatives stressed the fact that local public authorities do not involve private actors, such as church-based facilities, the way they are supposed to according to the contractual agreements with regard to the full process of local health policy making. According to several local key informants, the partnership dynamics are top-down, where church health facility representatives are not perceived as local key stakeholders but rather as executors on someone else's behalf. CHMTs, on the other hand, argue that church health facilities lack the capacity or interest to engage in health planning at the local level. They accuse church-related health facilities of being more loyal to foreign partners than to the CHMTs.

In relation to these claims, the analysis indicates that church leaders and hospital directors mainly address the public-private partnership in financial terms. A core principle in these partnerships is delivering services for free to vulnerable groups (children under five, pregnant women, and elderly people). This is referred to by the CHMTs as a regulation of patient fees. When this principle is implemented by the three church-based hospitals, it leads to a loss of income in terms of patient fees, for which they do not receive the compensation they are entitled to. All three hospital management teams express that they are not receiving compensation in accordance with the PPP contracts and the formula stipulated for block grants and basket funding.

Lack of financial compensation (for these patient groups) has been closely related to a lack of comprehensive health insurance for the population, in addition to the fact that church-related hospitals mainly serve the rural poor population. There also seems to be a lack of trust and financial transparency in church-state-donor relationships. Local governments have not disbursed agreed-upon funds, resulting in church hospitals subsequently not receiving any patient fees or service compensation.

Moreover, many CHMT members seemingly exhibit a lack of trust in church-based hospitals, and this is partially due to an absence of comprehensive financial reports and related comprehensive audits of church-based hospitals. CHMT members request that they are given an overview of the inflow of all funding to the church-based hospitals, which the hospitals are generally unable or unwilling to provide. This lack of trust has prompted the government to embark on a megaproject of building public hospitals in all districts in the country. The success of the government project will mean that automatically church-designated district hospitals will be phased out in the long run.

CHMT members furthermore argue that in order to build trust, vertical health programs need to be more integrated into planning and programming systems to improve transparency and subcontracting at the local level. However, this might work itself out in the long run, as the current government wants to introduce comprehensive health insurance for the whole population.

Still several representatives of the church hospitals consider the partnership with the local governments important for the long-term security and stability in running the hospitals (Sundqvist 2017, 152–248, interview 27). Through the partnership, the church-related hospitals are expected to receive important funding and contributions. Some of the respondents in my study even expressed a wish for the local government

(CHMTs) to fully support the hospitals in financial terms beyond the existing levels of basket funding (10–35 percent), service agreements, and DDH/CDH contracts (Sundqvist 2017, 171, interview 44). This not only points to stability but could also be seen as an absence of inspiration and future vision to run and develop the hospital organizations and mission.

The PPP reforms have aimed for health sector development in general but have also meant a strengthening of church organizations' responsibility in the realization of basic health justice. Representatives of the Catholic Church tend to relate to this model, whereas representatives from ELCT and in particular the FPCT argue that they play a complementary role in relation to the Tanzanian public authorities when it comes to enabling health rights. In some instances, all three church organizations describe themselves as a parallel resource to the state within the framework of PPP regulations by offering increased choices for health care on the road to health justice.

For decades there has been a rather acute awareness of the difficulty of maintaining church health facilities without support from the outside. This has been a concern raised in all conducted interviews by both the church organizations' headquarters and the local governments (CHMTs). Several key informants have suggested that church organizations should strive to identify a business model where the services could be completely free to poor and marginalized groups and more economically sustainable. A key concern in the PPP policy is that it is not clear how the government should act in order to support church-related health activities in relation to simply investing more in the public sector. Several respondents believe that some politicians think of them as competitors (Sundqvist 2017, interview 25).

Several church-based hospital managers in the study bring forward criticisms of local politicians who, instead of strengthening the already existing church health infrastructure, advocate for the establishment of new public health facilities (Sundqvist 2017, 204, interview 3). These managers maintained the assertion that local politicians advocate for the establishment of new public health facilities. The critique of the local governments might stem from the fact that the idea of PPP was never initiated by them but was brought to them from the national level and international actors. Moreover, the local government has limited influence over the health facilities. Local government representatives on the other hand argue that they are implementing the national health policy containing the vision of establishing one health unit per village and district.

Representatives of church organizations refer to themselves as doing the duty of the government. Few respondents argue that the government should be responsible for the whole hospital, staff salaries, and expenses for drugs. In all local cases, the doctor in charge is a member of the district medical board and the district medical officer (DMO) is a member of the hospital board.

Through this close and ongoing relationship, the representatives from church organizations are perceived to have influence in some sort of way or at least can express what they think, and the DMO has a possibility to gain insights into how church-related hospitals are functioning. Through CSSC, the influence on a national and regional level is strong—for example, membership in various committees and groups on the national level. There is an indication in the study that the relationship is highly based on resource dependency. Church-related health facilities are mainly seeking to collaborate strongly with the local governments because they are lacking finances. The relationship between the hospitals and local governmental authorities in this sense is a resource exchange partnership. The respondents claim that hospitals could survive without the contribution from the government, though it would be hard. Moreover, the respondents claim the government is absolutely dependent on them in fulfilling the services.

Here we argue that church leaders challenge state legitimacy, in particular at the local level, and several church-based hospital managers in the study are critical of local politicians who instead of strengthening the preexisting church health infrastructure advocate for the establishment of new public health facilities. It is demonstrated that CHMTs wish to strengthen their legitimacy by expanding public health care instead of funding existing private services. Here, an existing tension between the public and the private within the PPP reform itself was identified. It seems as if some CHMT officials perceive the strong influence of church leaders on people's thinking, decisions, and behaviors as a potential threat or as competition.

The case studies demonstrated that the relationships between church organizations and the state are closer at the national level, through the Christian Social Services Commission. Most interviewees find the collaborations with national public authorities (Ministry of Health) to work better than those with local governments (CHMTs). The ownership debate was brought up in several interviews and conversations concerning PPPs, and several church leaders consider the partnership with local governments important for the long-term security and stability of operating their hospitals. However, the analysis also shows that local governments do not deliver financial support to church-based hospitals in accordance with agreed contracts. It is hard to determine the amount of funding originally planned to reach the FBOs that does not arrive due to this local resistance.

There even seems to be ideological resistance from local governments in relation to partnerships with FBOs that most likely affects the level of funding redistributed at the local level. Local governments question why the external financial support through "global health initiatives" has largely remained outside the planning and priority structures at the local level. This shows an inconsistency between the national and the local governments and the agendas that are pushed on the one hand and those implemented on the other. But personal relations and the quality of these relations remain a key to success for collaboration. Hospital managers emphasize the importance of the personal factor, such as the religious background of the respective partners in the contractual partnership, something that might indicate an unhealthy dependency on interpersonal relations. The DMO is often favored by the church-related hospitals. Still, the executive powers of the DMO seem limited compared to the district executive director (DED).

Church-based hospitals look upon external funding from global health funds and other vertical health funds as crucial, as the public funding within PPPs is less than expected and agreed upon and does not arrive on time. Interviewees from all three church-based hospitals perceive these direct links between local church-based hospitals and global actors as crucial for their operations, even though they operate outside state structures and the PPPs.

What was again evident at church health facilities are staff departures and the national shortage of doctors, nurses, assistant medical officers, and so on, which leads to increased competition for human resources in the health sector. Churches are rarely able to offer competitive wages, and staff at church-based hospitals increasingly look for better terms in the public sector. The obvious differences in social benefits for church-based staff compared to civil servants are a major source of frustration at church-based hospitals. Social benefits for civil servants include retirement allowances, health insurance, and a social protection fund. However, my analysis shows that visiting nurses, midwives, and medical students from abroad in several cases offset the human resource gap.

Another crucial grassroots challenge that the study identified was the fact that church organizations were better equipped when it comes to entering into contractual partnerships in the health sector in comparison to Muslim organizations—which has led to increasing tensions and frustrations. This might also partly explain why some CHMT members are critical of the PPP policy in itself.

In some informal discussions, the state has been accused of actively favoring church organizations. "State favoritism of Christianity" (Mfumo wa Christo) is a common slogan that refers to the national debate on religious pluralism. A few critics argue that colonial patterns are reproduced through the partnerships, since they often require existing infrastructure. The result is that PPP reforms are becoming more provocative and complex in religiously diverse countries, such as Tanzania, compared to countries with a Christian majority, such as Zambia.

Another way of looking at this is that the PPPs have enabled the state to gain more control and also affiliate itself more strongly with moderate religious groups, such as mainstream churches willing to deliver services to everyone, regardless of religion. However, it is important to note at this juncture that the PPP reform is not sufficiently understood nor sanctioned by the broader population (Sundqvist 2017, 250, interview 13).

7. Conclusions and Theoretical Implications

The principle of health justice demands that we strive to reach all individuals with health services necessary to maintain and promote community health. In this chapter, we have argued that the right to health is still unrealized even after the introduction of PPP reforms in Tanzania.

We come to the conclusion that church organizations are bridging the gap as complementary agents to the Tanzanian government under the PPP initiative, especially in remote areas where public health facilities were underdeveloped. There are severe grassroots challenges, though, facing church-related health facilities and the current local governments with regard to collaborative models, global-local partnerships, trust, and the implementation of health policy in general.

The agenda is still to a large extent set by external donor agencies and not understood properly or sanctioned by the broader population. Church hospitals are torn between the external demands of missionary societies at the global level and the directives from CHMTs at the local level.

For the realization of health justice and sustainability in the case of Tanzania, it is important to design a policy addressing this reality. The church leadership sometimes regard the church-related hospital services as a potential resource for the organization. At the same time, church-related hospital management at the local level claims that health facilities run services with a deficit. It is therefore crucial that all stakeholders involved in the running of the church health facilities engage in an enhanced dialogue where they develop a comprehensive response to the challenges presented in this chapter.

The PPP reform in health in Tanzania carries the potential to facilitate the development of effective health institutions to achieve justice through mutual partnerships between public authorities and church organizations. However, as the data reveal, the current alignment process of public and private health institutions in Tanzania is characterized by multiple grassroots challenges, and it is necessary to overcome these in order for basic health justice to be achieved.

References

Bakari, M. 2012. "Religion, Secularism, and Political Discourse in Tanzania: Competing Perspectives by Religious Organisations." *Interdisciplinary Journal of Research on Religion* 8 (1): 1–34.

Bandio, E. 2012. *CHAs Partnering with Governments through MoUs—the DDH (CDH) Model of Partnership*. Dar es Salaam, Tanzania: Christian Social Services Commission.

Bennett, A., and A. George. 2005. *Case Studies and Theory Development in the Social Sciences*. Cambridge, MA: Belfer Center for Science and International Affairs.

Boulanger, D., and B. Criel. 2012. "The Difficult Relationship between Faith-Based Health Care Organisations and the Public Sector in Sub-Saharan Africa: The Case of Contracting Experiences in Cameroon, Tanzania, Chad and Uganda." *Studies in Health Services Organisation & Policy* 29:1–227.

Fouere, M. ed. 2015. *Remembering Julius Nyerere in Tanzania: History, Memory, Legacy*. Dar es Salaam, Tanzania: Mkuki na Nyota.

Green, M. 2005. "Priests, Witches and Power: Popular Christianity after Mission in Southern Tanzania." *Canadian Journal of African Studies / Revue Canadienne des Études Africaines* 39 (1): 167–165.

Green, M., C. Mercer, and S. Mesaki. 2010. *The Development Activities, Values and Performance of Non-governmental and Faith-Based Organisations in Magu and Newala Districts, Tanzania*. Birmingham: University of Birmingham, Religions and Development Research Programme.

Havnevik, K., and A. Isinika. 2010. *Tanzania in Transition—from Nyerere to Mkapa*. Dar es Salaam, Tanzania: Mkuki na Nyota.

Itika, J. 2009. *Public Private Partnership in Health Services Management: Some Experiences from Decentralized Health Care Systems in Tanzania*. Cologne, Germany: Lambert Academic.

Jennings, M. 2008. *Surrogates of the State: NGOs, Development and Ujamaa in Tanzania*. New York: Kumarian.

Jones, B., and M. Petersen. 2011. "Instrumental, Narrow, Normative? Reviewing Recent Work on Religion and Development." *Third World Quarterly* 32 (7): 1291–1306.

Kijanga, P. 1978. *Ujamaa and the Role of Church in Tanzania*. Arusha, Tanzania: Makumira.

Lawi, Y., and P. Masanja. 2006. "African Traditional Religions in Tanzania: Essence, Practice, and the Encounter with Modernization." In *Justice, Rights and Worship: Religion and Politics in Tanzania*, edited by Rwekaza R. Mukandala, Saida-Yahya Othman, Samwel S. Mushi, and Laurian Ndumbaro, 97–113. Dar es Salaam, Tanzania: E & D.

Leurs, R., P. Tumaini-Mungu, and A. Mvungi. 2011. "Mapping the Development Activities of Faith-Based Organisations in Tanzania." Working Paper 58, University of Birmingham, Religions and Development Research Programme, Birmingham.

Ludwig, F., ed. 1999. *Church and State in Tanzania: Aspects of Changing in Relationships, 1961–1994*. Studies of Religion in Africa, Book 21. Leiden: Brill.

Magesa, L. 2010. *African Religion in the Dialogue Debate: From Intolerance to Coexistence*. Berlin: Lit Verlag.

Mallya, E. 2006. "Religion and Elections in Tanzania Mainland." In *Justice, Rights and Worship: Religion and Politics in Tanzania*, edited by Rwekaza R. Mukandala, Saida-Yahya Othman, Samwel S. Mushi, and Laurian Ndumbaro, 395–416. Dar es Salaam, Tanzania: E & D.

Mhina, A. 2007. *Religions and Development in Tanzania: A Preliminary Literature Review*. Birmingham: University of Birmingham, Religions and Development Research Programme.

Ministry of Health. 2011. *Public Private Partnership in the Delivery of Health Services in Tanzania*. Dar es Salaam, Tanzania: Ministry of Health.

———. 2016. *Service Provision Assessment Survey 2014-2015*. Dar es Salaam, Tanzania: Ministry of Health.

Mukandala, R., and B. Heilman. 2015. Introduction to *The Political Economy of Change in Tanzania: Contestations over Identity, the Constitution and Resources*, edited by Rwekaza R. Mukandala, Saida-Yahya Othman, Samwel S. Mushi, and Laurian Ndumbaro, 1–12. Dar es Salaam, Tanzania: Dar es Salaam University Press.

Mushi, S., and R. Mukandala. 2006. "Religion and Plural Politics in Tanzania: Conclusions and Recommendations." In *Justice, Rights and Worship: Religion and Politics in Tanzania*, edited by Rwekaza R. Mukandala, Saida-Yahya Othman, Samwel S. Mushi, and Laurian Ndumbaro, 534–141. Dar es Salaam, Tanzania: E & D.

National Public-Private Partnership Steering Committee. 2009. *Public Private Partnership for Improved Health Services in Tanzania: Joint Annual Health Sector Review*. Dar es Salaam, Tanzania: National PPP Steering Committee.

Ndaluka, T. 2012. *Religious Discourse, Social Cohesion and Conflict: Muslim-Christian Relations in Tanzania*. Berlin: Lit Verlag.

Ngowi, H. 2009. "Economic Development and Change in Tanzania Since Independence: The Political Leadership Factor." *African Journal of Political Science and International Relations* 3 (4): 259–267.

Päivänsalo, V. 2013. "Fragile Health Justice: Cooperation with Faith Organisations." In *Religion and Development: Nordic Perspectives on Involvement in Africa*, edited by T. Sundnes, 109–125. New York: Peter Lang.

Pallant, D. 2012. *Keeping Faith in Faith-Based Organisations*. Eugene, OR: Wipf and Stock.

Phares G., M. Mujinja, and T. M. Kida. 2014. *Implications of Health Sector Reforms in Tanzania: Policies, Indicators and Accessibility to Health Services*. Discussion Paper 62. Dar es Salaam, Tanzania: Economic and Social Research Foundation (ESRF).

Richebächer, W. 2007. *Religious Change and Christology*. Arusha, Tanzania: Makumira.

Ruger, P. 2012. *Health and Social Justice*. Oxford: Oxford University Press.

Sundkler, B., and C. Steed. 2000. *A History of the Church in Africa*. Cambridge: Cambridge University Press.

Sundqvist, J. 2017. *Beyond an Instrumental Approach to Religion and Development: Challenges for Church-Based Healthcare in Tanzania*. Uppsala, Sweden: Uppsala universitet, Humanistisk-samhällsvetenskapliga vetenskapsområdet, Teologiska fakulteten, Centrum för forskning om religion och samhälle.

Venkatapuram, S. 2011. *Health Justice: An Argument from the Capabilities Approach*. 1st ed. Cambridge: Polity.

Westerlund, D. 1980. "Christianity and Socialism in Tanzania, 1967–1977." *Journal of Religion in Africa* 11 (1): 55–30.

World Bank. 2013. *Private Health Sector Assessment in Tanzania*. Dar es Salaam, Tanzania: World Bank.

World Health Organization (WHO). 2018. *Health and the Sustainable Development Goals*. https://tinyurl.com/y5mvndbv.

Yates, T. 1994. *Christian Mission in the Twentieth Century*. Cambridge: Cambridge University Press.

4

———

Negotiating the Healing Mission

SOCIAL JUSTICE AND BASIC HEALTH AT TWO
METHODIST INNER-CITY MISSIONS IN SOUTH AFRICA

Elina Hankela

ABSTRACT

This chapter approaches the relationship between social justice and basic health through a case study of two Methodist city missions in two South African cities. The discussion centers on the notion of mission, which at these two locations was understood as being open and responsive to the needs of the surrounding city and was implemented in the form of social projects. In line with the broader Methodist vision in South Africa, mission is discussed as the church's healing task in society. At the two city missions, the process of missionization—that is, being consciously reorganized as a mission—highlights the potential that local faith communities have to address issues concerned with both basic health and social justice. Within that framework, social justice (understood as the actualization of respect for human dignity) and basic health emerge as organic, nonhierarchical aspects of a single mission. It is argued that while there could be basic health services without a social justice emphasis, a social justice approach cannot exist in the given inner-city contexts without attention also being paid to basic health needs. The chapter also urges such contemporary healing missions to learn from the mistakes of the healing missions of the colonial era. This would mean, at the least, taking a self-reflective approach to questions of power both within and beyond the faith community itself.

1. A Vignette

In July 2009, a small group of people gathered at a Methodist church in Braamfontein, Johannesburg, to participate in the Wednesday-evening outreach of the Paballo ya Batho (Sesotho: "Caring for People") initiative that operated under the umbrella of the Central Methodist Mission (called Central from now on), a Methodist circuit located in inner-city Johannesburg. The group of volunteers visited a few spots in the inner city weekly to meet with homeless people, serve soup, and provide basic health care. The latter was possible courtesy of volunteers from a local medical school.

At the given street corners, in a city marked by socioeconomic inequality, people lined up to receive a cup of soup and a few slices of bread. Some of these people slept on the street or in homeless shelters. Others stayed in abandoned buildings, a feature of this part of the city since the 1970s and increasingly the 1990s, when apartheid's racial segregation lines began to break down in the inner city and capital escaped into the northern suburbs (Murray 2011, 87).[1]

Before the group headed out to the streets, Unathi,[2] the then leader of Paballo ya Batho, reminded those who came regularly and instructed the first-timers, "Some people call this a feeding scheme, but it is not one. A soup kitchen is a feeding scheme; that is where you serve soup and people come to you. But here, we go out to them. Thus, this is an outreach. This is about affirming human dignity."[3] Unathi surely knew he was fighting against common, deep-seated perceptions about the poor when he reiterated that we go out to the streets to meet "our friends."

The vignette illustrates a dynamic that is at the heart of the discussion in this chapter—namely, that between, on the one hand, concrete service, such as basic health care, and, on the other, the broader social justice goal of tangibly affirming human dignity. The chapter is based on ethnographic engagement with two South African Methodist inner-city missions: Central in Johannesburg between 2009 and 2014 and the Pretoria City Mission (called Wesley from now on)[4] in Tshwane in 2014. The

---

1 Based on field notes by the author, July 22, 2009, and an interview with Unathi, July 23, 2009.

2 The names of research participants, except the superintendent ministers of the city missions, are pseudonyms.

3 Reconstructed based on field notes by the author, July 8, 2009.

4 A nickname by which some know the Pretoria City Mission. Used here for readability. Tshwane was formerly called Pretoria, and the center of Tshwane still is.

vignette thus introduces the reader not only to the theme of the chapter but also to the kind of engagement upon which the analysis is based.[5]

2. Introduction

The objective of the chapter is to provide an understanding of the nature of the healing mission in the contemporary South African city context. The task is approached through interrogating the relation between social justice and basic health in Wesley and Central in which the two elements emerge as organic and nonhierarchical, even if not uncontested, components of the "healing mission" in a socioeconomically unequal world.

For the sake of conceptual clarity, it should be noted that social justice is here understood to refer to the actualization of respect for human dignity among and between social groups and persons in society, informed by the demands of both redistribution and identity politics (see Fraser 1999). A social justice approach aims to "avoid the pitfalls of an individualistic charity," meaning that a person is seen not only as an individual but also "in the fabric of social relationships" (Gutiérrez 1988, 116). Gustavo Gutiérrez, instead of renouncing charity, reinterprets its meaning in the context of justice (Hankela 2017, 53–54). At the heart of such an approach to mission is the affirmation of humanity, which cannot be achieved in isolation from political and socioeconomic realities.

The term *mission* is used to refer to a mission as an institution as well as to mission as holistic *missio Dei* in which that institution and its membership participate. It is not an innocent term in postcolonial Africa due to the role of Christian missions in the westernization and colonization of the continent (e.g., Pawliková-Vilhanová 2007; Comaroff and Comaroff 1986). The "healing mission" of the nineteenth and twentieth centuries claimed to bring not only the gospel—and Western medical care—to the African continent but also "civilization" shaped in a Western image (see, e.g., Flikke 2003). Shokahle Dlamini (2018) shows how medical missions helped legitimize colonial authority in Eswatini, while Rune Flikke

---

5 I here use the term ethnography in a broad sense, as theologians often do (see Ward 2012). As much as the work I have done on Central would also qualify as ethnography in a more specific usage of the term, my engagement with Wesley was short term. I conducted extensive fieldwork at Central for most of 2009 (see Hankela 2014) and some further research in 2013 and 2014. With Wesley, I was involved as a researcher for a limited period of time in 2014; I conducted qualitative interviews with four staff members, visited a couple of worship services, and spent some time observing at the Mahube testing and counseling center.

(2003, 7) points out that, although some early missionaries were open to local African ways of healing, in the years of the Scramble for Africa and after developments in bacteriology, the zeitgeist instead deemed the African the source of disease—thus compromising the dignity of the African person. Moreover, many Black churches in Africa, with roots in Western missionary activity, were historically called "missions," not "churches": "The adjective 'African' would only gradually and with care be placed alongside terms such as 'church', 'Christian', or 'theology'" (Maluleke 1997, 7). This human factor necessitates attention to power as an aspect of mission, particularly here, in the context of postapartheid South Africa, where apartheid, colonialism, and the memory of oppression under a Christian banner continue to impact on the present.

The trajectories of the two city missions have much in common in terms of the relation between social justice and concrete service in their work and are discussed as similar cases that build on the same argument. Nonetheless, although Central and Wesley, both comprising more than one society or local congregation, belong to the Methodist Church of Southern Africa (MCSA)—a large mainline denomination in South Africa (see Forster 2008 on the 2001 Census)—and are thus a window into the Methodist presence in South Africa, the intention is not to make claims of the MCSA at large.

After a brief look into selected research on health, justice, and religion in South Africa and an outline of the two city missions, the chapter engages with the connection between social justice and concrete service, such as basic health care, at these missions. The social projects[6] run at the missions are examined as a dimension of healing society. The founding of the projects is portrayed as illustrating the (re)surfacing of societal and justice-driven interpretations of faith. After linking the projects to a conscious shift of focus on the needs of the surrounding city, the perspective is narrowed down to the basic health aspect of the praxis of these city missions. The resonance between Central and Wesley and the broader denominational landscape is established by looking briefly at the concept of healing in the vision and mission statements of the MCSA. Finally, questions are raised about the lack of involvement on the part

---

6 The projects running at Central, when I conducted research there in 2009, 2013, and 2014, included a crèche called For the Love of Children, the Paballo ya Batho street ministry, the Urban Institute, the Ray of Hope Refugee Ministry, and the Albert Street School. Similar projects were run at Wesley in 2014, organized under the umbrella of Wesley Community Centre (WCC), including initiatives such as the Mahube testing centre, the Salem Children's Centre, and the Salem Aftercare Centre.

of the church membership in the projects and, related to this, the power dynamics in the defining of a church's vision/mission.

3. Health, Social Justice, and Religion in Academic Discourse

Religion is historically closely connected to human understanding of health (Green 2013), and in the recent past, religion has attracted keen interest among scholars who work on development and public health. A few years ago, Jill Olivier (2014, 252) spoke of "a massive surge of publication" in the niche area of religion and development and/or public health. Theologians too have addressed issues related to health, exemplified by the work of the Circle of Concerned African Women Theologians on HIV and AIDS (e.g., Hinga et al. 2008). Out of this broader body of writing, for the purposes of this chapter, the work of two South African scholars, Steve de Gruchy and James Cochrane, who both participated in the African Religious Health Assets Programme (ARHAP 2002–11[7]), is revisited, as their focus on justice and health provides conceptual pointers for the discussion on the relationship between social justice and basic health at Central and Wesley.

De Gruchy (2007) argues that there is a weak link between health and justice in African Christian communities based on the results of research undertaken by the ARHAP in Zambia. The study suggests that health and healing play an important role in ordinary Christians' expressions of faith, but on the other hand, social justice is not seen as having significant theological importance. Thus the role of religion in matters of health could be described as addressing the needs and lifestyle of individuals, not healing and change at the collective and policy levels. In line with this separation, religious people and bodies have, for instance, been "deeply involved in responding to the [AIDS] pandemic, but the response is characterized by a focus on coping with the crisis rather than on defeating it" (53). De Gruchy further argues that attending to the public health discourse could help theologians in Africa connect questions related to healing with those related to social justice, as the public health discourse, for instance, emphasizes the health of collectives and the prevention of diseases; learning from these priorities could help the

---

7 In 2012, the ARHAP collaboration was relaunched as International Religious Health Assets Programme (IRHAP).

Christian community relearn the central importance of social justice to their own discourse—their "mother tongue" (49)—in relation to health.

While de Gruchy approaches the relationship between health and justice from the perspective of a lack to be addressed, in Cochrane's argumentation, one may read a call for a deeper understanding of the inner logic of faithworlds themselves in order to identify points of connection and, perhaps, to strengthen them. One could indeed argue that a social justice focus has been part of the South African theological scene—even if not specifically in relation to health—in academia but also in certain churches (for instance, through the different liberation theologies born in the struggle years). More specifically, Cochrane (2006, 2010) has drawn attention to the intangible religious health assets embedded in faith communities or faith-based organizations. These include aspects of worldview and self-understanding that explain attitudes and actions: the "volitional, motivational and mobilizing capacities" embedded in religious beliefs and practice (2006, 117). Thus the value of tangible religious health assets (such as some of the projects at Central and Wesley), Cochrane (2006, 117) argues, "depends upon understanding the less visible, intangible elements." He does not ignore the problematic roles played by religion in society but also suggests that religious frameworks, from which faith communities draw, could have a remarkable positive effect on given public health issues (2006), while harnessing the existing religious health assets to serve society could encourage and emphasize the participation and agency of ordinary citizens, a politics from below (2010).

The journeys of Central and Wesley speak to the difficulty of organically linking social justice—and, in particular, a social justice approach to health—to the religious life of a local church but also to the practical potential to address societal healing that lies in faith communities.

4. Two Missions in Changing Cities

Central and Wesley, both now predominantly Black missions, were once White, middle-class churches (Venter 1994; Taylor 2008), just as the inner cities of Johannesburg and Tshwane, where they are located, used to be largely White, middle-class areas. In the late apartheid years and increasingly in the first decade of the new dispensation, these neighborhoods experienced racial and class desegregation faster than White suburbs away from city centers and became predominantly Black localities. Both inner cities are now working-class areas in a socioeconomically highly unequal country (see Hamann and Horn 2015; Murray 2011).

According to Gavin Taylor, the conversion of inner-city churches in South Africa, which used to be "white prestigious conventional family type congregations," into "missions" took place due to radical urban changes rather than voluntary theological reflection—even if the MCSA did take a resolution at the 1987 conference that provided an avenue for developing city missions (Taylor 2008, loc. 1017, 1053). Taylor, who has also worked as the superintendent minister of Wesley, defines city missions as "those congregations that have been forced into *journeys of transition* that will lead to them discovering *new and alternative* forms of mission and ministry" (loc. 1103; italics in original). He argues that in changing inner-city settings, churches have faced a choice between closing, relocating, or changing and being shaped by the social context (loc. 1128).

The leadership of Central and Wesley opted for the third alternative, which was defined by an attempt to keep the church doors open to the streets. As much as this choice could be based on intangible theological assets that resonate with the Methodist doctrine of social holiness and the way in which it has been historically shaped in South Africa, the transformation of these churches draws attention to the role of social context in defining how intangible assets materialize in the social world.

5. Missionization and the Emergence of Social Projects

De Gruchy's findings on the separation between personal and social dimensions of health among people of Christian faith in Zambia resonate with a broader trend in Christian communities of dividing ethics between public and private matters, with the consequence that the emphasis is often on the latter (see, e.g., De la Torre 2014; Gutiérrez 1988). To an extent, the missionization (the term here used to refer to a process of a local church being consciously reorganized as a mission) of Wesley and Central can be read as an attempt to address this division and bring the social (back) into the center of the faithworld of a local church.

Purity Malinga, the superintendent minister of Wesley (2009–15) at the time the fieldwork for this chapter was conducted, offered an account of the meaning of a mission (station) based on her personal history and experience in rural areas. Her recollection illustrates the meaning of a mission that is also reflected in the transformation of

Wesley and Central: "What used to happen always in the rural black areas was that there would be a manse, a house where the minister lives and then there would be a church and . . . a school. [Elina: And a clinic?] And then a clinic and so on. . . . But in terms of . . . the black understanding of the word, mission was where everything was happening, surrounding the church. You'd go to the mission for the service, you'd go to the mission for school, you'd go to the mission for . . ."[8]

With no intention to romanticize the missions of the past, in line with Malinga's recollection, the process of missionization, or organizational transformation, at Central and Wesley can be thought of as aiming to produce a holistic center of life, a nexus where different human needs are taken seriously, at the level of both individual and public discourse.

The missionization of Wesley is reflected in the emergence of various social projects in the early 1990s in Gavin Taylor's time as superintendent. Malinga describes Taylor's then aim as having been to "open this church to the community" and to deal with "the needs of the city." The projects that were established addressed "a separation that had happened in the thinking of people to say that when you go to church, you're going only to worship."[9] Opening the church meant, in other words, working against a separation depicted between the sacred space and the economic, social, and political realities of the street. The attempt to bridge this gap through a world-affirming theological vision—and by extension, a vision that affirmed the dignity of a person inside and outside the church—links to a long and varied history of negotiating the relationship between the church and the world by Christian churches, one shifting between domination, separation, and synergy. In this process, seemingly characterized by synergy (see Hankela 2014, 168), the name of the church was changed to Pretoria City Mission.

While the missionization of Wesley thus clearly coincided with the desegregation of the surrounding city, at Central the process had started prior to the more radical phase of social change in the inner city (Venter 1994, 123–29). The push for a missionization of Central appears to have been dependent more on the leadership and its theology and politics—starting in Peter Storey's time as the superintendent (1976–92)—than pressure from the immediate context. Yet 1976 was also the year of the Soweto uprisings, and in the 1980s, Soweto, half an hour's drive away

---

8 Interview by the author with Malinga, May 8, 2014.
9 Interview by the author with Malinga, May 8, 2014.

from Central, was a key location of the intensifying struggle against apartheid.

The name of the Central Methodist Church was changed to Central Methodist Mission in 1985 (Venter 1995, 326). Much like at Wesley some years later, Storey describes the name change as "a deliberate signal" to return to "the days of Pat Meara and others—a church with its face turned toward the city and its needs."[10] Storey thus implies not that the shift was new to this particular church or to Southern African Methodism but rather that a world-affirming vision had been lost over the years. According to Storey, "mission" in the name indicated "a strong caring social ministry, strong witness on public questions, and strong evangelical outreach."[11] The focus on the needs of the city and societal justice continued at Central through the eras of superintendents Mvume Dandala (1992–97) and Paul Verryn (1997–2014), the latter having been the superintendent during my engagement with Central (Hankela 2014; Kuljian 2013; Venter 1994).[12] The connection between social justice and health that de Gruchy writes about could be argued to be organic within this framework.

6. Basic Health as an Organic Aspect of Mission

In a vision centered on the needs of the city, basic health has been a natural aspect of mission at both Central and Wesley. While one can imagine basic health services being run by faith communities with different theological underpinnings—or, in other words, being motivated by differing intangible assets—a social justice–orientated approach would also and necessarily include inclusive attention to questions of health. Two projects, Mahube (Wesley) and Paballo ya Batho (Central), highlight this.

Mahube, an HIV testing and counseling center, was established at Wesley in 2004 to "bring comfort and hope to those infected and affected by HIV/AIDS."[13] Mahube's aim is threefold: to educate, support, and offer free testing. In 2014, two counselors, John and Tomas, tested and counseled people from Monday to Friday at the clinic, apparently attending to 350 to 400 people per month. Most clients were in their twenties or thirties, and John estimated that 80 percent of them came regularly. Mahube

10 Personal email, July 9, 2012.
11 Personal email, July 9, 2012.
12 I have not followed Central after 2014 and thus do not comment on the current situation.
13 Wesley homepage, accessed October 11, 2014, http://www.weschurch.co.za.

also organized weekly confidential support group sessions directed at those infected or affected.[14]

Religion can be described as absent at Mahube, apart from the clinic being physically located on church property. A theological vision was a source of motivation for offering health services to those who need them, as indicated earlier in relation to the missionization of Wesley, but it did not feature in the concrete work. The support group is not about "what religion is good and which is bad," Tomas explained; instead, "we take out all religions." John concurred that religious customers are accommodated in a "tactful" manner, but the work is done "as scientific[ally] as possible." Moreover, while John and Tomas were both members of Christian churches, neither was Methodist. Rather than explicitly referring to religion as a source of intangible assets, the counselors spoke of the challenge they face with religious people who do not believe that HIV exists or with those who believe that if they test positive, they can go to church and be cured.[15] The work at Mahube as a tangible asset appears to be tailored to affirm human dignity in this particular city; the respectful approach to lived religion seems to have enabled Mahube to attend to the physical health of a multifaith community.

The health care provided by Paballo ya Batho, which was referred to in the opening vignette, followed a similar logic. Religion was not an explicit aspect of the Wednesday-evening outreach, and health care was part of the initiative because it was needed by people on the streets. Yet the case of Paballo ya Batho, even if implicitly, also suggested faith was a source of motivation, the main goal of the initiative being to affirm human dignity, a theme that was, likewise, a constant thread in the preaching at Central. The actual basic health care was rather a subtopic in the dignity framework that addressed a holistic notion of being healthy or being human.

Mahube and Paballo ya Batho responded to concrete needs in the city. Since they were largely geared toward encountering the individual, one may query the distinction between this missionization and a charity response. Based on the reasoning behind the process previously outlined, however, the projects could be thought of as addressing social justice due to their consciously aiming to affirm the dignity of the encountered people (and in the case of some projects, through shifting microstructures; e.g., providing free schooling for refugee children). The thinking

---

14 Interviews by the author with John and Tomas, April 23, 2014.
15 Interviews by the author with John and Tomas, April 23, 2014.

and preaching of the leading ministers—particularly Paul Verryn's, with which I am the most familiar[16]—also suggest that the immediate help offered to the individual was just one facet of the overall vision. Elsewhere (Hankela 2014, 148) I have argued that a given project at Central, for instance, besides encountering those in need, constituted a political statement. Yet if the broader societal implications of affirming human dignity were to be ignored, these missions too could easily, perhaps unnoticed, shift to the liberal or reactionary ends of the social ministry spectrum. Resonating with Cochrane's writing about the value of tangible assets being dependent on intangible assets, these cases emphasize the role of the broader theological framework in the concrete orientation of service projects.

7. Healing as the Mission of Southern African Methodists

At the broader level, the local leaderships' imaginary of a church open to the city is in line with the denominational self-understanding. The two-decade-old vision of the MCSA, to which Wesley and Central belong, sets healing as central to Methodist witness and articulates it as both spiritual and societal. In doing this, it shapes a denominational intangible health asset. The vision statement of the MCSA reads, "A Christ-healed Africa for the healing of nations," and the mission statement, "God calls the Methodist people to proclaim the gospel of Jesus Christ for healing and transformation" (Yearbook 1999/2000, 2). These statements are part of the journey of defining the post-1994 role of MCSA, which, for instance, also involves the Journey to the New Land program of the 1990s and the adoption of a mission charter in 2005 (Bentley 2014; Kumalo 2006). Overall, Wessel Bentley (2014, 5) argues, this centering of social change "is an intentional return to early Wesleyan theology."

The missionization at Central and Wesley could be examined as one operational aspect of this journey. The people under whose leadership such projects emerged and were managed were grappling with the same social context and the theological tradition that was verbalized in the mission and vision statements at the 1998 MCSA conference. Verryn, for instance, referred to the vision as an indication that the Methodist church is a community that focuses on empowerment, engages with the

---

16 I have heard Verryn's preaching extensively (see Hankela 2014) and have also followed his public engagement.

debate on poverty, and creates projects that reflect these priorities;[17] all these emphases have been at the heart of his own ministry and preaching.

Context is key to reading the statements. Dion Forster (2008) writes that a social understanding of holiness, central to John Wesley's theology, needed to be expressed in new ways in post-1994 South Africa. Malinga, for her part, pointed out that the adoption of the vision took place at a time when "as a nation we were still bleeding from the effects of apartheid" and the church was searching for its role in the healing of the country.[18] This is to be understood in a context in which, it is widely agreed, embodying a new active public role after the 1994 transition to democracy was difficult across the board of mainline churches; theologians have spoken of silence or confusion in the ranks of both theologians and churches (Kuperus 2011; Motlhabi 2009; Storey 2004; Maluleke 2000). In the MCSA of pre-1994, social holiness was expressed in statements made from within the church against apartheid, such as the One and Undivided resolution of 1958. Echoing the broader mainline response under the new dispensation, the MCSA sought to shift from the pre-1994 prophetic witness into an era of reconstruction (Forster 2008).

The shift of focus on reconstruction and reconciliation in mainline churches was accompanied by confusion about the place of, and lack of attention to, justice in the discourse, not unlike the reconciliation discourse in the country at large (see Vellem 2012). The vision statement of the MCSA, too, could be read as either reformist or radical.

Moreover, in the 1999/2000 MCSA yearbook, in which the vision and mission statements appear for the first time, it is emphasized that as "the second mission awakening in Africa is beginning to happen, to Africa for Africa by Africa," it is an imperative "for every Methodist Society to be an agency for authentic evangelism, spiritual and moral formation, empowerment of the poor, social action and promotion of inclusive justice" (4). Besides the emphasis on inclusive justice, noteworthy is the will to embrace African agency in mission—in a denomination that was introduced to the land by Europeans. Challenges in the actualization of the social vision over time within the MCSA at large are beyond the scope of this chapter (see, e.g., Mtshiselwa 2015; Forster 2008).

---

17 Interview by the author with Verryn, June 18, 2009.
18 Interview by the author with Malinga, May 8, 2014.

8. Whose Mission?

Missionization has here been translated to mean, among other things, that responding to basic needs is an aspect of social justice (see also Hankela 2017), which in turn is at the heart of Methodist self-understanding. But who defines these parameters for mission? What does the "to Africa, for Africa and by Africa" mean?

At both Wesley and Central, many of the social projects were organized as nonprofit organizations with separate bank accounts. Moreover, some of the people working with the projects were not members of these particular missions, as previously mentioned about John and Tomas. This kind of missionization is thus characterized by what Marian Burchardt (2013, 42) has called FBOization. As nongovernmental organizations have become prominent actors in civil society globally, and international development funders have become increasingly interested in religious actors, FBOs have become a common feature in the religious field, often connected to churches.

An organizational separation between church activities and projects might be a practical choice, but the separation is also reflected at other levels. While the projects, as Malinga suggested, could be seen as an attempt to challenge a separation between the sacred and the social in people's thinking, the material form they took had by and large not managed to challenge this separation in the immediate context of the relationship between the congregations and the projects. Rather, while the projects opened a door onto the street, the backdoor into the church appeared to have been largely closed. I was told that many Wesley congregants viewed the projects as separate from the church and, moreover, did not know much about them. An employee highlighted this when speaking about the past: "The projects were seen to be entirely an entity on its own and there was a lot of suspicion around the projects, that there was money coming from overseas." The separation and suspicion might also be related to the racial shift in the membership and leadership. The now predominantly Black church was still rather White at the time the missionization began, and the projects were linked to the White minister in charge. They were "very misunderstood" in the sense that they were seen as "Gavin's projects," Gavin Taylor having been the then superintendent minister, the interviewee explained, adding that later on, up-to-date, ethnic power politics had impacted on the attitude of the membership toward the projects.[19]

19 Interview by the author with an employee at Wesley, April 23, 2014.

I have written elsewhere about similar dynamics at Central, particularly in relation to the Ray of Hope Refugee Ministry that in 2009 in many ways characterized Central (Hankela 2014). Among the Wednesday volunteers with Paballo ya Batho, according to Unathi, were students, professional people such as doctors, people from other churches and overseas, refugees, and unemployed and homeless people. But members of Central, he said, have "always been a difficult group to attract. . . . There'll be one or two, but they never come in numbers as other groups do." Maybe people "don't see it as part of their church," or, Unathi added laughing, "maybe the gospel, they haven't preached it well to them."[20]

In other words, the materialization of the healing vision in the projects at the two missions depended on the leadership (see also Hankela 2014; Venter 1994). The mission that the projects represented either was not built into the faithworld of the members to the extent that they regarded the projects as theirs or came in a foreign form.[21] The separation between the membership and these projects at Central and Wesley is a reminder that human dignity should be considered in the light of power relations in the church and power in the relationship between the church and other parties in the city that it aims to serve. The separation may, however, also speak to the need for theological conscientization if social justice–orientated mission is to become a stronger Southern African Methodist asset. Overall, if self-critical reflection on power is neglected, contemporary mission of this traditionally hierarchical denomination risks reproducing some of the colonizing aspects of past healing missions.

9. Concluding Thoughts

The missionization of Central and Wesley was a response to what was happening in the surrounding social and political context as well as inside the church in regard to a disconnection between church and society, or the sacred and the sociopolitical. Mission at these two locations

20 Interview by the author with Unathi, July 23, 2009. Also see Venter (1995, 327) on speculation on the impact of class differences on members' perceptions of the programmes at Central in the 1990s, as well as the mention of "the Black congregation's non-involvement in the congregation's programmes" at the time.

21 One needs to add that even if church members were not involved in the projects, this does not necessarily mean that, for instance, the different well-attended church organizations (e.g., Wesley Guild or Women's Manyano) did not have social goals similar to those of the projects. It is a limitation of this chapter that it has concentrated on the projects, not other aspects of church life.

was understood first and foremost as being open and responsive to the needs of the surrounding city, or, in other words, as the church's holistic healing task in society. The homeless person or the poor migrant had been quite literally thrown in the face of these missions, and they responded with various projects that aimed to take the situation of the particular human being or group seriously.

Within this mission framework, social justice and basic health emerge as organic, nonhierarchical aspects of a single mission. While there could be basic health services without a social justice emphasis, a social justice approach could not exist in these inner-city contexts without attention also being paid to basic health needs, when social issues have a human face. Conversely, every personal health problem plays out as part of a broader social structure. Hence questions related to health are at the heart of a healing praxis based on the needs of the city; coping with social suffering and aiming to defeat it are not separate strategies in the context of the mission projects. Thus the chapter also supports the broader argument that true charity forms an important aspect of social justice praxis in an unequal context (Hankela 2017). Yet the relationship between coping and defeating calls for further study, which would carefully analyze what, if any, the broader tangible societal impact of missions like these has been in the cities and societies that they inhabit.

Acknowledgments

I am grateful for the funding received from the Academy of Finland through the Youth at the Margins project led by Professor Auli Vähäkangas in the Department of Practical Theology at the University of Helsinki.

References

Bentley, Wessel. 2014. "Methodism and Transformation in South Africa: 20 Years of Constitutional Democracy." *HTS Teologiese Studies / Theological Studies* 70 (1): art. #2673. http://dx.doi.org/10.4102/hts.v70i1.2673.

Burchardt, Marian. 2013. "Faith-Based Humanitarianism: Organizational Change and Everyday Meanings in South Africa." *Sociology of Religion* 74 (1): 30–55.

Cochrane, James. 2006. "Conceptualising Religious Health Assets Redemptively." *Religion & Theology* 13 (1): 107–120.

———. 2010. "Health and the Uses of Religion: Recovering the Political Proper?" In *Development and Politics from Below: Exploring Religious Spaces in the African*

State, edited by Barbara Bompani and Maria Frahm-Arp, 175–196. London: Palgrave Macmillan.

Comaroff, Jean, and John Comaroff. 1986. "Christianity and Colonialism in South Africa." *American Ethnologist* 13 (1): 1–22.

De Gruchy, Steve. 2007. "Re-learning Our Mother Tongue? Theology in Dialogue with Public Health." *Religion & Theology* 14:47–67.

De la Torre, Miguel. 2014. *Doing Christian Ethics from the Margins*. 2nd ed. Maryknoll, NY: Orbis.

Dlamini, Shokahle. 2018. "The Colonial State and the Church of the Nazarene in Medical Evangelisation and the Consolidation of Colonial Presence in Swaziland, 1903–1968." *South African Historical Journal* 70 (2): 370–382.

Flikke, Rune. 2003. "Public Health and the Development of Racial Segregation in South Africa." *Bulletin of the Royal Institute for Inter-faith Studies* 5 (1): 5–23.

Forster, Dion, 2008. "Prophetic Witness and Social Action as Holiness in the Methodist Church of Southern Africa's Mission." *Studia Historiae Ecclesiasticae* 34 (1): 411–434.

Fraser, Nancy. 1999. "Social Justice in the Age of Identity Politics: Redistribution, Recognition and Participation." In *Culture and Economy after the Cultural Turn*, edited by Larry Ray and Andrew Sayer, 25–52. Thousand Oaks, CA: Sage.

Green, Ronald. 2013. "Health and Disease in Religions." In *The International Encyclopedia of Ethics*, edited by Hugh LaFollette, 2342–2353. Oxford: Blackwell.

Gutiérrez, Gustavo, 1988. *A Theology of Liberation*. 15th anniversary ed. Maryknoll, NY: Orbis.

Hamann, C., and A. Horn. 2015. "Continuity or Discontinuity? Evaluating the Changing Socio-spatial Structure of the City of Tshwane, South Africa." *Urban Forum* 26:39–57.

Hankela, Elina. 2014. *Ubuntu, Migration and Ministry: Being Human in a Johannesburg Church*. Leiden: Brill.

———. 2017. "'There Is a Reason': A Call to Reconsider the Relationship between Charity and Justice." *Exchange* 46:46–71.

Hinga, Teresia M., Anne N. Kubai, Philomena Mwaura, and Hazel Ayanga, eds. 2008. *Women, Religion and HIV/AIDS in Africa: Responding to Ethical and Theological Challenges*. Pietermaritzburg, South Africa: Cluster.

IRHAP. n.d. Accessed September 25, 2019. http://www.irhap.uct.ac.za.

Kuljian, Christa. 2013. *Sanctuary: How an Inner-City Church Spilled onto a Sidewalk*. Auckland Park: Jacana.

Kumalo, Simanga. 2006. "Transforming South African Methodism: The 'Journey to the New Land' Programme 1992–1997." *Missionalia* 34 (2/3): 249–266.

Kuperus, Tracy. 2011. "The Political Role and Democratic Contribution of Churches in Post-apartheid South Africa." *Journal of Church and State* 53 (2): 278–306.

Maluleke, Tinyiko. 1997. "Half a Century of African Christian Theologies: Elements of the Emerging Agenda for the Twenty-First Century." *Journal of Theology for Southern Africa* 99:4–23.

———. 2000. "Black and African Theology after Apartheid and after the Cold War: An Emerging Paradigm." *Exchange* 29 (3): 193–212.

Methodist Publishing House. 1999/2000. *1999/2000 Yearbook of the Methodist Church of Southern Africa.* Cape Town: Methodist Publishing House.

Motlhabi, Mokgethi. 2009. "Phases of Black Theology in South Africa: A Historical Review." *Religion & Theology* 16:162–180.

Mtshiselwa, Ndikho. 2015. "The Emergence of the Black Methodist Consultation and Its Possible Prophetic Voice in Post-apartheid South Africa." *HTS Teologiese Studies / Theological Studies* 71 (3): art. #2897. http://dx.doi.org/10.4102/hts.v71i3.2897.

Murray, Martin. 2011. *City of Extremes: The Spatial Politics of Johannesburg.* Durham: Duke University Press.

Olivier, Jill. 2014. "Mapping Interdisciplinary Communication between the Disciplines of Religion and Public Health in the Context of HIV/AIDS in Africa." *Religion & Theology* 21:251–289.

Pawliková-Vilhanová, Viera. 2007. "Christian Missions in Africa and their Role in the Transformation of African Societies." *Asian and African Studies* 16 (2): 249–260.

Storey, Peter. 2004. *And Are We Yet Alive? Revisioning Our Wesleyan Heritage in the New Southern Africa.* Cape Town: Methodist Publishing House.

Taylor, Gavin. 2008. "City Mission: A Frontier for Mission in the Post-Modern World." In *Methodism in Southern Africa: A Celebration of Wesleyan Mission*, edited by Wessel Bentley and Dion Forster. Kempton Park: AcadSA. Kindle.

Vellem, Vuyani. 2012. "Interlocution and Black Theology of Liberation in the 21st Century: A Reflection." *Studia Historiae Ecclesiasticae* 38:345–360.

Venter, Dawid. 1994. *The Formation and Functioning of Racially-Mixed Congregations.* PhD diss., University of Stellenbosch.

Venter, Dawid. 1995. "Mending the Multi-Coloured Coat of a Rainbow Nation: Cultural Accommodation in Ethnically-Mixed Urban Congregations." *Missionalia* 23(2): 312-338.

Ward, Pete, ed. 2012. *Perspectives on Ecclesiology and Ethnography.* Cambridge: William B. Eerdmans.

5

Hinduism and Health Justice

AN INDIAN PERSPECTIVE

Alok Chantia and Preeti Misra

ABSTRACT

India is the seventh-largest country in the world, consisting of more than 80 percent Hindus. Its roots are more than five thousand years old. In the cultural evolutionary process, *homo sapiens*, besides attaining different socioreligious codes, also developed its health mechanism. Hinduism talks about health not only through medicine but also through yoga and Ayurveda. Hinduism encompasses natural products as medicine and advocates physical exercise for a healthy life. Many forms of spiritual healing also exist in the Hindu tradition. Vedas, as the oldest written texts, exhibit that health justice is nothing but an assurance of Hinduism to make life healthy and wealthy. The present chapter explores health justice in Hinduism from the time of its inception to today. The significance of yoga as a key to a healthy life has been recognized by the United Nations Organization (UNO), as it has declared June 21 as International Yoga Day. This chapter also deals with spirituality as an aspect of good health, which is yet to be included in the definition of health by the World Health Organization.

Sarve bhavntu sukhinh, sarve santu niiramaya.
(May all be prosperous and happy, may all be free from illness.)

Sarve bhadrani pasyantu, maa kaschit dukhbhagbhavet.
(May all see what is spiritually uplifting, may no one suffer.)
Brihadāraṇyaka Upanishad, verse 1.4.14

1. Introduction

The Hinduism[1] of India is the oldest way of living life on this blue planet. It starts from the Indus valley civilization,[2] which is considered a blueprint of human settled life. In the struggle of existence, a human being had to think about himself and his well-being. In this connection, keeping good health was the only way to cope with nature and natural calamities. Hinduism encompasses not only major theistic and atheistic traditions of Indian origin but also numerous folk traditions, tribal practices, and religious customs dating back to prehistoric times. Most of these traditions have been finely integrated into the fabric of Hinduism, so much so that it is difficult to identify and distinguish them without studious effort.

One way of keeping good health was by doing good deeds and having pious thoughts. Hindus believe that every thought, word, and action accumulates karma (deeds), which can affect current and future lives. Hindus believe in fasting, which is seen as a method of purifying the body and soul, gaining emotional strength, and encouraging self-discipline. Though it is not obligatory for a Hindu patient to fast during a hospital stay, one may choose to for various reasons. All illnesses have three components: biological, psychological, and spiritual. Treatments that do not

---

1 Hinduism is an Indian religion and dharma or a way of life widely practiced in the Indian subcontinent. Hinduism has been called the oldest religion in the world, an ancient religion with Indian origin whose characteristics include the worship of many gods and goddesses and the belief that when a person or creature dies, their spirit returns to life in another body. Hinduism is a very complex belief system. It is more than a religion—it is a way of life. Much confusion in the West lies in the fact that core Hindu beliefs are often undermined by social pressures and outside influences. After moving in a direction away from the core beliefs because of foreign influences, there is a worldwide movement among Hindus to return to the basics of their way of life. Hinduism has no one founder, no known origin, and no one holy text. It has been established by a living culture over thousands of years. Hinduism's steadfastness in its core principles and its ability to adapt to modern changes have allowed it to last for many thousands of years. For that reason, there are many personal interpretations of specifics, but the core beliefs remain unchanged.

2 Indus civilization, also called Indus valley civilization or Harappan civilization, is the earliest known urban culture of the Indian subcontinent. The nuclear dates of the civilization appear to be about 2500–1700 BCE, though the southern sites may have lasted later into the second millennium BCE.

address all three of these components may not be considered effective by a Hindu patient. In the Hindu community, physical illness as well as mental illness and cognitive dysfunction have a stigma attached: they have emerged due to bad karma.

Well-being is the prime concern of Hinduism. In the east, and more specifically in the Hindu tradition, spiritual abnormalities and anomalies are often treated using various religious practices and spiritual healing techniques that date back to the time of the Vedas.[3] Vedas, the oldest texts of the entire tradition, elaborate the philosophy of Hinduism. Veda means "science or knowledge" (Crawford 1989, 3). In Vedas, many types of diseases are described. In Western culture, different forms of possession, mental illness, and spiritual disorders are often categorized as pathological and abnormal; these pathologies are usually treated with psychoanalysis, psychiatry, and mass amounts of medication with less frequent attention paid to spiritual treatment (Frawley 1997). Yoga[4] and

3 The Vedas are a large body of knowledge texts originating in the ancient Indian sub-continent. The Vedas are a collection of hymns and other ancient religious texts written in India between about 1500 and 1000 BCE. Composed in Vedic Sanskrit, the texts constitute the oldest layer of Sanskrit literature and the oldest scriptures of Hinduism. Hindus consider the Vedas to be apauruṣeya, which means "not of a man, superhuman" and "impersonal, authorless." There are four Vedas: The *Rigveda* text is a collection of 1,028 hymns and 10,600 verses, organized into ten books (*Mandalas*). A good deal of the language is still obscure, and many hymns as a consequence are unintelligible. The *Yajurveda* is the Veda of prose mantras. An ancient Vedic Sanskrit text, it is a compilation of ritual offering formulas that were said by a priest while an individual performed ritual actions such as those before the yajna fire. *Yajurveda* is one of the four Vedas, and one of the scriptures of Hinduism. The exact century of *Yajurveda*'s composition is unknown and estimated by scholars to be around 1200 to 1000 BCE, contemporaneous with *Samaveda* and *Atharvaveda*. *Samaveda* is the Veda of melodies and chants. It is an ancient Vedic Sanskrit text and part of the scriptures of Hinduism. One of the four Vedas, it is a liturgical text whose 1,875 verses are primarily derived from the *Rigveda*. Three recensions of the *Samaveda* have survived, and variant manuscripts of the Veda have been found in various parts of India. The *Atharva Veda* is the "knowledge storehouse of *atharvāṇas*, the procedures for everyday life." The text is the fourth Veda but has been a late addition to the Vedic scriptures of Hinduism.

4 Yoga is one of the most ancient forms of mystic and human development practice that has originated in India. This practice had been found to be of great reverence in form of a holistic pattern of moral, mental, and physical development. The ancient Hindu text of yoga called the *HathaYoga Pradipka* asserts that Lord Shiva was the first teacher of yoga, while the *Bhagavad Gita*, another sacred text of Hindus, asserts that Lord Krishna was a teacher of yoga. Yoga has been handed down from ancient times in India since the time of Vedas. The great sage Maharishi Patanjali systemized all yoga practices with the advent of their yoga sutras. Many sages have contributed greatly to the development of this field into practices and treatises. Study of this ancient technique for health is divided into three main categories: pre-Patanjali period (before 500 BCE), Patanjali period (500 BCE to 800 CE), and post-Patanjali period (after 800 CE).

Ayurveda[5] are those areas of Hinduism that encompass natural products as medicine and advocate physical exercise for a healthy life. From the time of the Vedas to contemporary Hinduism, many forms of spiritual healing also exist in this long tradition.

2. Vedas and Health Justice

The very first evidence of health justice in Hinduism is in the Vedas, well-written documents encompassing the whole life of humankind to make people different from animals: "Thou, Agni; You are the Protector of the body, protect my body. Thou, Agni, Art the Bestower of long life, bestow on me long life. Thou, Agni, Art the Bestower of intellectual brilliance; Bestow on me intellectual brilliance. Whatever, Agni, Is deficient in my body, make that complete for me" (*Yajurveda* v. 3.17).

Among the diseases, leprosy, hair diseases, and so on were mentioned repeatedly in the *Rgveda*.[6] Ghoṣā (saint girl) was healed from her leprosy and could get married by the grace of the divine physicians *Aśvins* (God physicians). A similar incidence has been mentioned in the hymn I.117.8, where *Aśvins* cured Śyāva of leprosy.

Hymn 50 of book 7 gives a picture of a condition that is very much indicative of the guinea worm disease affecting the skin and other body parts: "Eruption that appears upon the twofold joints, and that which overspreads the ankles and the knees, May the refulgent Agni banish far away: let not the winding worm touch me and wound my foot"[7] (*Rgveda*.VII.50.2).

The word *rapas* (demon) used in these verses was imagined to be an activity of the demon, probably a worm-like creature (guinea worm?) that used to affect the feet and joints, causing a wound.

---

5 Ayurveda texts, considered the fifth Veda in India, begin with accounts of the transmission of medical knowledge from the gods to sages and then to human physicians. In *Sushruta Samhita* (*Sushruta's Compendium*), Sushruta wrote that Dhanvantari, Hindu god of Ayurveda, incarnated himself as a king of Varanasi and taught medicine to a group of physicians, including Sushruta. Ayurveda therapies have varied and evolved over more than two millennia. Therapies are typically based on complex herbal compounds, minerals, and metal substances (perhaps under the influence of early Indian alchemy, or *rasa Shastra*). Ancient Ayurveda texts also taught surgical techniques, including rhinoplasty, kidney stone extractions, sutures, and the extraction of foreign objects. The Sushruta Samhita is an ancient Sanskrit text on medicine and surgery and one of the most important such treatises on this subject to survive from the ancient world.

6 "Ghoṣāyai cit pitṛṣade duroṇe patiṃ jūryantyā aśvinau adattam" (*Rgveda*.I.117.7, 19).

7 "Yadvijāmanparuṣi bandanaṃ bhubadastībantou pari kulphou ca dehaṃ agnistaccho-cannapa bādhatāmito mā māṃ padyena rapasya bidattasaruh."

Some of the hymns like that in 50.11-13 of book 1 are suggestive of the knowledge of heliotherapy, particularly in the treatment of the yellowness of the body, or jaundice, which was mentioned in book 1: "Rising this day, O rich in friends, ascending to the loftier heaven, Surya, remove my heart disease, take from me this my yellow hue"[8] (*Ṛgveda*.I.50.12).

Hair disorders have also found a place in this Veda: in 126.7 of book 1, perhaps it is an example of hypertrichosis—a condition considered an annoying feature in females. Scanty hair was also considered a setback for a lady. Apālā, the *Ṛṣikā* of the hymns, had some hair disease and in the verse could be seen praying for the growth of hair on her body as well as on her father's scalp:

> O Indra, cause to sprout again three places, these which I declare,—
> My father's head, his cultured field, and this the part below my waist.[9]
> (*Ṛgveda*.VIII.80.5)
> Make all of these grow crops of hair, you cultivated field of ours, my body, and my father's head.[10] (*Ṛgveda*.VIII.80.6)

Whether it refers to any genetic hair disease is not conceivable from this text.

The *yakṣmā*, or consumption, had been mentioned in almost all Vedic literature. Therefore, it may be assumed that it was a common disease during the ancient days. A hymn in book 10 mentioned it, describing the affection of the hair and nails:

> From what is voided from within, and from thy hair, and from thy nails, From all thyself from top to toe, I drive thy malady away.[11] (*Ṛgveda*.X.163.5)
> From every member, every hair disease that comes in every joint, From all thyself, from top to toe, I drive thy malady away.[12] (*Ṛgveda*.X.163.6)

In Vedic medicine, the management strategy of diseases was composed of a complicated method of chanting mantras, offering oblations,

---

8 "Śukeṣu me harimāṇaṃ ropaṇākāsu dadhmasi atho hāridraveṣu me harimaṇaṃ ni dadhmasi."
9 "Imāni trīṇi viṣṭapā tānīndra bi rohaya śirastatasyorbarāmādidaṃ mā upodare."
10 "Asau ca yā na urbarādimāṃ tanwaṃ mama atho tatasya yacchirah sarva tā romasā kṛdhi."
11 "Mehanādbaṇāmkaranallaombhyaste nakhebhyah yakṣaṃ sarbasmādātamanastamidaṃ bi brhāmi te."
12 "Angadangallomno lomno jataṃ parvaṇi parvaṇi yaksaṃ sarbasmādātamanastamidaṃ bi brhāmi te."

and performing some intricate rituals. Along with these, there were the use of medicines in the forms of herbs and organic and inorganic materials and some procedures like anointment, hydrotherapy, cauterization, and so on. The physicians were required to have knowledge about the medicinal properties of plants: "He who hath store of Herbs at hand like Kings amid a crowd of men—, Physician is that sage's name, fiend-slayer, chaser of disease"[13] (*Rgveda*.X.97.6).

An ointment was a common method of therapeutic measure practiced by the Vedic physician. It is evident from hymn X.161 that the physician used to recite the mantra and touch the various parts of the body of the diseased with his hands anointed with ritually prepared clarified butter (*ghee*).

In verse VII.50.2, mentioned earlier, the description is very much suggestive of the use of fire for cauterization.

The Vedic seers also used water for the management of various diseases (hydrotherapy):

> Amrita is in the Waters; in the Waters. There is healing balm: Be swift ye Gods, to give them praise.[14] (*Rgveda*.I.23.19)
> Within the Water—Soma thus hath told me—dwell all balms that heal, And Agni, he who blessth all. The water holds all medicines.[15] (*Rgveda*.I.23.20)

A physician used to use his tender touch for remedial purposes. It was of course not very clear if it was a type of massage therapy or part of the hypnotherapy or simply touch therapy (as is used these days in the alternative system of medicine): "Felicitous is this mine hand, yet more felicitous is this. This hand contains all healing balms, and this makes whole with gentle touch"[16] (*Rgveda*.X.60.12).

3. Yoga and Health Justice

Other than *Rigveda*, the fourth and last Veda in Hinduism is *Atharvaveda*. It encompasses health issues through the discipline of the body. Yoga and its medicinal significance have been accepted worldwide, hence the UNO

---

13 "Yatrousadhih samanmataha rājānah samitāmiba bipraha sa ucyate bhishakbaksohamība cātanah."
14 "Apsu antar amṛtam apsu bheṣajam apām uta praśastaye devā bhabata vājinah."
15 "Apsu me somo abravīd antar viśvāni bheṣajā agniś ca viśvaśambhuvam āpaś ca viśvabheṣajī."
16 "Ayam ye hasto bhagavānayaṃ me bhagabattarah ayaṃ me viśwabhesajohayaṃ śivābhimarśanah."

declared June 21 as International Yoga Day for the sake of humanity. Yoga is nothing but the recycling of body energy in an appropriate manner to accelerate its kinetic energy irrespective of the age of an individual.

The etymology of the word *yoga* means "to join or yoke together." It brings the body and mind together in a harmonious experience. Under the pace of health is wealth, yoga is a method of learning that aims at balancing "mind, body, and spirit." Yoga is a practice with historical origins in ancient Indian philosophy. Yoga is an example of how individuals can bring about "balance" between the mind, body, and spirit. In yoga, individuals are taught how to tune out the world and tune in to the "pure" self-consciousness within. What happens is a release of the transcendent spirit that is "free from all the pain, misery, and death characterized by physical existence" (Crawford 1989, 15).

Yoga, as a nonmedicinal technique to make the body healthy, provides a practical method of purification by helping individuals become morally strong, which is a prerequisite for spiritual discipline. There are eight steps of purification: (1) *Yama*, or the sensitivity to the quality of life in the body; (2) *Niyama*, or the sensitivity to the quality of life in the mind; (3) *Asana*, or postures that restore high levels of energy; (4) *Pranayama*, or the control of breathing (enhanced concentration); (5) *Pratyahara*, or complete relaxation; (6) *Dharana*, or attaining the consciousness of the body; (7) *Dhyana*, or controlling the mind without using the body; and (8) *Samadhi*, or psychic powers that maintain the body's vitality.

Yoga relies heavily on discipline, particularly physical discipline. Yogis believe that it is only a fit body that can achieve spiritual well-being. Thus the ability to concentrate is necessary to preserve good health, because disease is a physical, mental, and spiritual liability. The mind as a chief and master organ of the body should be in order and peace. Hinduism talks about meditation, which brings concentration to the mind. It is an elevated state of being where, by completely focusing on a thought, idea, saying, or nothing at all, a person's soul forgets for a time about the physical body, worries, and otherworldly concerns. Meditation involves slowing the breathing and heartbeat and relaxation without falling asleep. Most of all, it requires practice and patience. Meditation is refreshing and brings energy and calmness to a person's daily life. It is also a way to unite with the Absolute Being for a time. It is a system of letting go. Anyone of any faith can meditate.

Sustainability and longevity depend on the health status of an individual. This was understood by a religious person (Rishi) in India, and they understood their natural practice and their uses and codified yoga in different epics in India.

With the practice of yoga, an individual channels their energy according to their choice and requirement in the following different manners:

- Health yoga is the path of physical fitness or the yoga of postures.

- Bhakti yoga is the path of the heart or the yoga of devotion.

- Dhyana yoga is the path of meditation and contemplation.

- Jnana yoga is the path of learning and knowledge.

- Karma yoga is the path of action or selfless service.

- Nada yoga is the yoga of inner sound, the sound of the universe.

- Yoga nidra is the yoga to achieve perfect sleep.

Yoga views the human body as a composite of mind, body, and spirit. In 1946, the World Health Organization (WHO) defined health as "a state of complete physical, mental and social well-being and not merely the absence of disease or infirmity" (WHO 2019, para. 1). Although spirituality is not yet included in the definition of health given by the WHO, it has been, as a fourth dimension of health, proposed by many countries where spirituality is a basic pillar of healthy life, including India (Kiichiro and Asako 2000).

The physical, psychological, and spiritual states of well-being are governed by yoga in the following ways:

Physical

- *Flexibility.* Yoga helps the body become more flexible, bringing a greater range of motion to muscles and joints and a flexibility in the hamstrings, back, shoulders, and hips.

- *Strength.* Many yoga poses support the weight of the body in new ways, including balancing on one leg (such as in the Tree Pose) or increasing the strength in the arms.

- *Breathing.* Most of us don't give much thought to how we breathe and inhale very shallowly. Yoga breathing exercises, called pranayama,[17] focus the attention on the breath, improve lung capacity and posture, and harmonize body and mind, which benefits the entire body. Certain types of breath can also help clear the nasal passages and even calm the central nervous system, which has both physical and mental benefits.

- *Disease eliminator.* Yoga has the power to prevent and eliminate various chronic health conditions in men and women.

- *Heart disease.* With less stress and lower blood pressure, chances of cardiovascular diseases are prevented. Increasing blood circulation and fat burning results in lowering cholesterol.

- *Diabetes.* Yoga stimulates insulin production and reduces glucose to prevent diabetes.

- *Gastrointestinal.* Yoga improves the gastrointestinal functions effectively.

- *Metabolism.* Yoga balances metabolism results and controls hunger and weight.

- *Pain prevention.* Increased flexibility and strength can help prevent the various instances of back and chronic pain. Neck pain can also be lessened with yoga practice.

- *Blood circulation.* Yoga postures can help improve circulation and eliminate toxic waste substances from the body.

Psychological

- *Mental calmness.* Yogasana practice is intensely physical. Concentrating so intently on what the body is doing brings calmness to the mind.

- *Stress reduction.* Physical activity is good for relieving stress, and this is particularly true of yoga. Yoga provides a much-needed

17 *Pranayama* is a Sanskrit word that literally translates to "extension of the prana or breath." *Prana* means "life force," and it is the life force or vital energy that pervades the body. Prana is the link between mind and consciousness. The physical manifestation of *prana* is breath, and *ayama* means to extend or draw out the breath. Pranayama is a part of a yoga system that teaches the art of extending breath in many different ways. When practicing pranayama, the breath is skillfully inhaled, exhaled, and retained. It helps in changing the depth, rate, and pattern of breathing.

break from stressors as well as helps put things into perspective. Yoga controls breathing, which reduces anxiety. It also clears all the negative feelings and thoughts from the mind, leading to the reduction of depression.

- *Concentration.* Yoga increases concentration and motivation quickly. This is why people from all aspects of life practice yoga, since better concentration can result in better focus on one's life and profession.

- *Memory.* Yoga stimulates better blood circulation, especially to the brain, which reduces stress and improves concentration and leads to better memory.

- *Body awareness.* Doing yoga will give an increased awareness of one's own body. It increases one's level of comfort in their body. This can lead to improved posture and greater self-confidence.

- Meditation as an ayurvedic technique can be defined as a practice where an individual uses a technique—such as focusing their mind on a particular object, thought, or activity—to achieve a mentally clear and emotionally calm state. It restores the body to a calm state, helping the body repair itself and preventing new damage from the physical effects of stress. It can calm the mind and body by quieting the stress-induced thoughts that keep the body's stress response triggered. There is an element of more direct physical relaxation involved in meditation as well, obviously, so this double dose of relaxation can really be helpful for shrugging off stress.

- A greater gain that meditation can bring is the long-term resilience that can come with regular practice. Research has shown that those who practice meditation regularly begin to experience changes in their response to stress that allow them to recover from stressful situations more easily and experience less stress from the challenges they face in their everyday lives. Some of this is thought to be the result of the increase in positive moods that can come from meditation; research shows that those who experience positive moods more often are more resilient toward stress. Other research has found changes in the brains of regular meditation practitioners that are linked with a decreased reactivity toward stress.

- The practice of learning to refocus on thoughts can also help in redirecting a person when they fall into negative thinking patterns. This can help relieve stress. Meditation offers several solutions in one simple activity.

- Deep diaphragmatic breathing in pranayama clears the lungs of carbon dioxide and increases oxygen intake, providing the body with more vital energy. Deep belly breathing also massages internal organs and promotes digestion by stimulating metabolism and encouraging peristalsis.

- *Kapalabhati* is a breathing technique that uses abdominal muscles to pull in the belly along with repeated forceful exhalations. This is said to strengthen the agni, or digestive fire, and can actually give the abdomen a nice workout.

Spiritual

- *Inner connection.* Yoga can help create a bond, a relationship between body and mind apart from all other benefits.

- *Inner peace.* Yoga is the only method known for better and quicker inner peace. The inner peace generated increases and improves the capability in making effective decisions even during serious circumstances.

- *Purpose of life.* Yoga is a simple exercise method that has numerous benefits psychologically and physically apart from allowing to attain inner purification. It helps find the purpose of life and secrets to a healthy, longer life.

Scientific studies have shown that the practice of yoga has curative abilities and can prevent disease by promoting energy and health. That is why more and more professionals have started using yoga techniques in patients with different mental and physical symptoms, such as psychosomatic stresses and different diseases. Our bodies have a tendency to build up and accumulate poisons like uric acid and calcium crystals. The accumulation of these poisons manifests in diseases and makes human bodies stiff. A regular yoga practice can cleanse the tissues through muscle stretching and massaging of the internal organs and brings the waste back into circulation so that the lungs, intestines, kidneys, and skin are able to remove toxins in a natural way.

Practicing yoga has many benefits in improving health. It keeps people away from ailments like headaches, fevers, the flu, asthma, and so on and helps in making them fit, flexible, and fresh for the whole day. In their daily life, people are busy working the whole day and forget all about health. As a result, they always feel pain and stress and have many chances to fall ill. But practicing yoga just once as a daily routine helps in reducing and overcoming the problems that even medicines are unable to cure. Many people have jobs that entail sitting in offices throughout the day. Neither practicing yoga nor doing any kind of physical exercise can thereby affect their body, making it obese and stiff. Practicing twelve posture series called *Surya Namaskar* (sun salutation), *Pranayama* (breathing exercise), and some joint movements can help overcome this problem.

Many people around the world have a breathing problem called asthma due to the increased pollution from vehicles and for many other reasons. Just by practicing some of the techniques of Shatkarma called *Jala neti* (water cleansing) and *pranayama* called *Anuloma-Viloma Pranayama* (alternative breathing) can help them cure asthma. Many people have skin allergies over their entire body. Just doing the practice of *Shankprachalna* (mouth-to-anus cleansing by water), *Jala Neti* (water cleansing), and *Pranayama* (alternative breathing) can help them cure skin allergies naturally. Deep breathing can also help lower blood pressure. Mind-calming meditation, another key part of yoga, quiets the nervous system and eases stress. All these improvements may help prevent heart disease and can definitely help people with cardiovascular problems (Corliss 2015).

4. Ayurveda and Health Justice

Historically, Ayurveda, which is an ancient, five-thousand-year-old Vedic system of medicine known as the "science of life" (Frawley 1997; Jones and Ryan 2007), placed an emphasis on the pure self (*Atman*) and true consciousness and its relation to the universe (*Brahman*). Essentially, the Ayurveda gave Hinduism a guide for medical and spiritual healing and enlightenment (Frawley 1997; Jones and Ryan 2007). Ayurveda, described as the fifth Veda in Indian texts, is the traditional Hindu science of medicine of long life that is practiced in one form or another by 80 percent of people of Indian descent. Around the Pacific Rim, peoples from Fiji, Indonesia, Malaysia, and Singapore use Ayurveda when seeking help for physical and mental disorders. Ayurveda, like other forms of medicine, is the reliance on past practices and continues to be updated as more knowledge is revealed. The term *Ayurveda* is a combination of *dyus*, meaning "life, vitality, health, longevity" (Crawford 1989, 3), and *veda*, meaning science or knowledge (Crawford 1989, 3). Ayurveda is the spine of Hinduism and a health-care system, which has made an environment of well-being in this country since long ago. Even after the advent of Western medicine in India, Ayurveda has not been diluted to date.

"Health is wealth" not only is a proverb in Hinduism but also finds a place in Ayurveda—an advanced branch of medicine. Ayurveda is based on the early teachings in the Vedas, which are the core of Hindu scriptures. Thus Ayurveda is strongly influenced by the religious doctrines of Charaka and Susruta. The philosophy of Ayurveda depends on nature (*prakriti*). An aspect of Prakriti is the ego, or "mineness," which generates three types of nature: *sattva* (purity), *rajas* (passion), and *tamas* (darkness). These natures stand on their own, yet when working together, they produce enlightenment. The example of a lamp epitomizes this dynamic interaction, because it contains fire, the wick, and oil, but combined these things form light. Yet each is separate and stand by themselves. The goal of integrating the spirit, soul, and body is the only way to bring about healing. An Ayurveda healer considers all these factors when dealing with a client. Individuals are a microcosm of the universe and contain the basic elements of space, air, fire, water, and earth. The relationship between individuals and nature underlies Ayurveda.

The earliest classical Sanskrit works on Ayurveda describe medicine as being divided into eight components (Skt. *aṅga*). This characterization of the physicians' art, "the medicine that has eight components" (Skt. *cikitsāyām aṣṭāṅgāyāṃ* चकित्सायामष्टाङ्गायाम्), is first found in the Sanskrit epic the *Mahabharata*,[18] circa fourth century BCE. The components are the following:

- *Kāyacikitsā*: general medicine, medicine of the body

- *Kaumāra-bhṛtya*: the treatment of children, pediatrics

- *Śalyatantra*: surgical techniques and the extraction of foreign objects

---

18 *Mahābhārata*, pronounced *Mahābhāratam*, is one of the major Sanskrit epics of ancient India. The title may be translated as "the great tale of the Bhārata (India) dynasty."

- *Śālākyatantra*: treatment of ailments affecting eyes, ears, nose, or throat

- *Bhūtavidyā*: pacification of possessing spirits and the people whose minds are affected by such possession

- *Agadatantra*: toxicology

- *Rasāyanatantra*: rejuvenation and tonics for increasing life span, intellect, and strength

- *Vājīkaraṇatantra*: aphrodisiacs and treatments for increasing the volume and viability of semen and sexual pleasure

The life energy is called Prana, which activates the body and mind, and it manifests itself in the body as five elements: ether, air, fire, water, and earth. These elements are arranged according to three basic principles: *vata, pitta,* and *kapha.* Each of these principles and elements affects different parts of the body as *kapha* (water and earth) in the lungs area, *pitta* (fire and water) in the stomach area, and *vata* (air and ether) in the intestines. However, the body also is affected by the *nutrients prana* and *vital prana.* There is a cycle of interaction in all these elements: body functions, environment, unconsciousness, and spiritual forces. Accordingly, there are different types of people: *Vata* types are thin, dry, cold, and quick moving and tend toward fear and anxiety. *Pitta* types are of moderate build and hot in body temperature. *Kapha* types are calm and solid, and their systems tend to be cold, oily, and sluggish. These types are the three *doshas* (movement, metabolism, and structure). Some people are a mix of all these types. What they do, eat, and think of reflect on how they interact with their world.

Ayurveda also contains *Dhanvantari Mantra.* Dhanvantari is in ancient Hinduism considered to be the father of medicine and health and the founder of what is known as Ayurvedic medicine. He is also said to be the first physician and surgeon. The Dhanvantari mantra is recited to remove fears and diseases; those wishing to improve their health and eradicate diseases recite this mantra:

Dhanvantari Mantra
Om Namo Bhagavate
Maha Sudarshana
Vasudevaya Dhanvantaraye;
Amrutha Kalasa Hasthaaya

Sarva Bhaya Vinasaya
Sarva Roka Nivaranaya
Thri Lokya Pathaye
Thri Lokya Nithaye
Sri Maha Vishnu Swarupa
Sri Dhanvantari Swarupa
Sri Sri Sri
Aoushata Chakra Narayana Swaha

The translation of this is, "We pray to the God who is known as Sudarshana Vasudev Dhanvantari. He holds the Kalasha full of nectar of immortality. Lord Dhanvantari removes all fears and removes all diseases. He is the well-wisher and the preserver of the three worlds. Dhanvantari is like Lord Vishnu, empowered to heal the Jiva souls. We bow to the Lord of Ayurveda (Mantra-Book)."

5. Spiritual Healing in Hinduism

The ultimate goal of Hindu philosophy is to free oneself from the cyclical nature of existence. This liberation is termed *moksa*—which is essentially the same ultimate goal in the practice of yoga, termed *kaivalya*. Techniques such as mantras and meditations used in yoga, which have been adopted from the Ayurveda, attempt to spiritually link the self and consciousness to the natural world that surrounds it (Frawley 1997). This broad look at the spiritual focus of Hindu philosophies to maintain the well-being of the self is linked to the spiritual healing that accompanies anomalies in one's spirit, such as spiritual possession.

The mind or brain is taken into account under neurology in the era of modern medical treatment, but in the ambit of Hinduism, it is considered a possession of the mind by some types of spirit that make an individual unhealthy. Hinduism takes such an unhealthy individual as a victim of spirit and permits them to sustain a normal life by some healing practices.

Possession can be understood as an altered, unusual, or extraordinary state of mind due to the controlling power of a spirit, god, goddess, or demon over an individual's consciousness (Crapanzano 1987). Spirit possession can be distinguished into two broad categories: positive possession and negative possession (Crapanzano 1987; Sax 2009, 2011). Positive possession is when the individual is spiritually possessed by a deity, a god, or a goddess (Crapanzano 1987; Sax 2011). Negative possession, on the other hand, is when an individual is spiritually possessed by a devil, a demon, or a ghost-like figure (Crapanzano 1987; Sax 2011). When an individual's spirit is possessed, the individual will display behaviors that are uncharacteristic of it; this is due to the fact that the body is possessed by some other entity—one that is no longer the normal self (Sax 2011). The possessed body may actually experience pain and various symptoms of disease and illness while under possession (Crapanzano 1987). In the Hindu tradition, spiritual healing (with regard to curing these aversive mental and physical symptoms) comes in many practices, objects, and materials, including but not limited to exorcisms, temples, healing amulets (*tabiz*), healing ash (*vibhuti*), gemstones, and soma (Crapanzano 1987; Jones and Ryan 2007; Sax 2009, 2011).

Exorcisms have always played a fundamental role in cleansing and ridding the soul of unwanted negative possession. Healing, in the form of an exorcism, can be a one-on-one ritual (*puja*, or worship) between the patient and the exorcist, or it can be a public affair, involving the whole community (Crapanzano 1987; Sax 2011). Exorcisms can take place privately or may be performed publicly—sometimes at a shrine (Crapanzano 1987).

Essentially, the goal of spiritual healing in Hindu philosophy seeks to protect the soul from demonic spiritual powers; the influence of this negative spiritual energy can be, and should be, warded off. Negative spiritual possession can be counteracted by the use of soma, which is an intoxicating, mind-altering, hallucinogenic drink that is perceived as divine and therefore connects the spirit of the ingesting person to a higher understanding and consciousness (Crapanzano 1987). Negative influences on the mind and spirit in general have been understood as celestially caused; the inauspiciousness that is associated with the universe at certain times is counteracted by the wearing of specific gemstones that repel negative spirits from interacting with the body (Sax 2009).

Along the same lines as the wearing of gemstones, the protection from evil spirits is also sought in other objects such as sacred healing ash (*vibhuti/bhasman/bhabhut*)[19] and healing amulets (*tabiz*).[20] The sacred ash is seen not only as protection from evil spirits but also as rejuvenation and

---

19 *Vibhuti* is ash derived from the cremation of humans or from the excretion of a sacred animal in the Hindu tradition—the cow.
20 *Tabiz*, on the other hand, are lockets in which sacred Vedic or other Hindu textual verses are held. They are usually made of copper, brass, or iron.

revitalization of the material and spiritual aspects of one's life (Sax 2009). Rituals that invoke the use of *vibhuti* essentially serve as a purification of the mind and the spirit. Similar to the ta'wiz in the Islamic tradition (Sax 2009; Dwyer 2003), the sacred healing ash (*vibhuti*) is placed inside the amulet for spiritual protection purposes (Dwyer 2003). The amulets serve as a force that diverts evil, malevolent, and harmful spiritual entities (Sax 2009). *Tabiz* and *vibhuti* are both ritual symbols that are commonly used in exorcisms (Sax 2009; Dwyer 2003).

There are many shrines in India that are dedicated solely to the curing of the spirit and the mind. A famous symbolic site that is renowned for spiritual healing in the Hindu tradition is the Balaji Mandir—a temple located in Rajasthan, a North Indian state near the village of Mehandipur (Sax 2009). The shrine is dedicated to the Hindu god Hanuman, who is a mythical destroyer of demons, and Pretraj, who is the "King of Ghosts" (Sax 2009; Dwyer 2003). Demonic and ghostly possession, trances, and exorcisms are all commonplace at the Balaji temple—the temple is famous for the healing of mental illness (Sax 2009). Daily, thousands of pilgrims, devotees, and spiritually suffering persons visit the shrine in the hope of having their soul cured of any negative spiritual possession (Sax 2009).

Contemporarily, yoga, Ayurveda, exorcisms, gemstones, and intoxicating substances still play important spiritual healing roles not only in India but in the West as well. Mindfulness, spiritual awareness, and yoga are implicated in contemporary Western conceptions of spiritual well-being (Srivastava and Barmola 2013). The present psychological healing that Hindu rituals have on positive thinking and spirituality worldwide shows that spiritual healing should not be underestimated as a powerful tool in curing mental illness (Srivastava and Barmola 2013). The most vital aspect of understanding our own consciousness is to understand how the spirit can be healed and refurbished with guidance from the spiritual healing practices of the Hindu tradition.

Hinduism works on the principle of live and let live, and it gives importance to the philosophy of benevolence, which admits the equality of men and considers the earth as a family (Vasudhav Kutumbkam). Hinduism connects human life with the metaphysical world and never takes human beings as merely biological. The human body is considered the abode of the soul, which should be free from all types of ailments. Yoga and Ayurveda are significant in this account. It is also significant to note that while other branches of medicine are expensive and have side effects, yoga and Ayurveda are economical and free from all types of side effects. In the era of globalization, Hinduism, with its health practices as enshrined in Veda and Ayurveda, is the key to health justice for all mankind.

References

Ācārya, Yādava Trivikramātmaja, ed. 1941. "Sūtrasthāna 30.28." In *The Carakasaṃhitā of Caraka, with the Commentary by Cakrapāṇidatta*, 189. Bombay: Nirṇayasāgara.

———, ed. 1945. "Sūtrasthāna 1.7–9." In *Suśrutasaṃhitā*, 2–3. Bombay: Nirṇayasāgara.

Bhishagratna, Kaviraj Kunjalal. 1907. *An English Translation of the Sushruta Samhita Based on Original Sanskrit Text*. Vol. 1. Kolkata, India: K. K. Bhishagratna.

Corliss, Julie. 2015. *More Than a Stretch: Yoga's Benefits May Extend to the Heart*. New York: Harvard Health.

Crapanzano, Vincent. 1987. "Spirit Possession: An Overview." In *Encyclopedia of Religion*, edited by Lindsay Jones, 8688–8694. United States: Thomas Gale.

Crawford, C. 1989. "Ayurveda: The Science of Long Life in Contemporary Perspective." In *Eastern and Western Approaches to Healing*, edited by A. Sheikh and K. Sheikh. New York: John Wiley & Sons.

Dwyer, Graham. 2003. *The Divine and the Demonic: Supernatural Affliction and Its Treatment in North India*. London: Routledge.

Encyclopædia Britannica. n.d. "Dhanvantari." Accessed August 4, 2010. https://tinyurl.com/y5fqruje.

Frawley, David. 1997. *Ayurveda and the Mind: The Healing of Consciousness*. Twin Lakes, WI: Lotus.

Jones, Constance A., and James D. Ryan. 2007. "Ayurveda." In *Encyclopedia of Hinduism*, edited by J. Gordon Melton, 58. New York: Facts on File.

Kiichiro, Tsutani, and Asako Kusama. 2000. "A Spiritual Dimension of Health in WHO's 'View of Health'—National Delegates' Statements." *Toyou Medical* 8 (6): 90–92.

Sax, William. 2009. "Healers." In *Brill's Encyclopedia of Hinduism*, edited by Knut A. Jacobsen. Leiden: Brill.

———. 2011. "A Himalayan Exorcism." In *Studying Hinduism in Practice*, edited by Hillary P. Rodrigues, 146–157. New York: Routledge.

"Services, Queensland Health Multicultural." 2013. In *Health Care Providers' Handbook on Hindu Patients*. Accessed October 11, 2019. https://tinyurl.com/yxaj5dcd.

Sharma, Priya Vrat. 1999. *Suśruta-Samhitā: With English Translation of Text*. Vol. 1. Varanasi: Chaukhambha Visvabharati.

Srivastava, Kailash Chandra, and K. C. Barmola. 2013. "Rituals in Hinduism as Related to Spirituality." *Indian Journal of Positive Psychology* 4 (1): 87–95.

World Health Organization (WHO). 2019. "Frequently Asked Questions." Accessed October 11, 2019. http://www.who.int/suggestions/faq/en.

Wujastyk, Dominik. 2003a. "Indian Medicine." In *The Blackwell Companion to Hinduism*, edited by Gavin Flood, 394. Oxford: Blackwell.

———. 2003b. *The Roots of Ayurveda: Selections from Sanskrit Medical Writings*. 3rd ed. London: Penguin Books.

Zysk, Kenneth G. 1999. "Mythology and the Brāhmaṇization of Indian Medicine: Transforming Heterodoxy into Orthodoxy." In *Categorisation and Interpretation*, edited by Folke Josephson, 125–145. Meijerbergs institut för svensk etymologisk forskning, Göteborgs universitet.

Additional Internet Sources

http://www.yogaabhyas.com; https://tinyurl.com/y4anw52s; https://tinyurl.com/y5nshvvy; http://www.yahooyoga.com/; https://tinyurl.com/6u3snj7; http://nccam.nih.gov/health/yoga/introduction.htm; http://www.scribd.com/doc/2941542/Mantra-Book.

6
___

Christian Organizations for Basic Health Justice in India in the Twenty-First Century

S. N. Among Jamir and Ronald Lalthanmawia

ABSTRACT

Background: India today possesses as never before technologies and knowledge required for providing health care to her people. Yet the gaps in health outcomes continue to widen. Over sixty-three million persons are faced with poverty every year due to health-care costs alone. *Role of Christian health care in India*: 80 percent of outpatient care and about 60 percent of inpatient care are provided by the private health-care facilities in India, including the Christian network. *Mandate of Christian health-care network*: Christian health care has reached where no public health facilities are available in India. It has served the country for over one hundred years in providing holistic quality health care particularly to the poor and the marginalized. *Models of Christian engaging in basic health justice in India*: (1) *Christian hospitals*: Reach, commitment, spiritual mandate, and technical expertise have been well recognized and are important contributions toward health justice and equity; (2) *Congregation-based health services*: Some exemplary initiatives of the churches in reaching out to disadvantaged groups—those requiring palliative care, people suffering from HIV and AIDS, those with substance abuse, orphans, and other vulnerable people—for basic health support and services; (3) *Church social action*: Addressing health and social justice issues in churches through sermons, bible studies, and outreach works; (4) *Mobilizing resources*: Within the churches and its congregations for financial and other resources. *Conclusion*: Churches play a vital role in healing ministry in India and the rethinking of the ministry will ensure basic health justice for all.

1. Background

India today possesses as never before technologies and knowledge required for providing health care to her people. Yet the gaps in health outcomes continue to widen. The "Draft National Health Policy of India 2015" (Ministry of Health and Family Welfare 2015) commits to leverage economic growth to achieve health outcomes and acknowledges that better health contributes immensely to improved productivity as well as equity in the country. In the past thirty years, the government has come out with two national health policies in India, one in 1983 and the latest one in 2002. India aims to attain the Millennium Development Goals (MDGs) but has not been able to reach the target until 2014. Maternal mortality now accounts for 0.55 percent of all deaths and 4 percent of all female deaths between the fifteen- to forty-nine-year age group. These still account for 46,500 maternal deaths and require further strengthening maternal and child health services.

Over the last decade or so, we have seen a robust growth of the health-care industry by a 15 percent compound annual growth rate (CAGR), which is twice the rate of growth in all services and thrice the national economic growth rate. However, we have witnessed that the growing expenditure due to health-care costs is one of the factors that leads to poverty. We have also witnessed the previous health policy responding to the contextual changes with universal access to affordable health-care services in an assured mode. The almost exclusive focus of policy and implementation often masks the fact that all the disease conditions for which national programs provide universal coverage account for less than 10 percent of all mortalities and only for about 15 percent of all morbidities. Over 75 percent of communicable diseases are not part of existing national programs. Overall, communicable diseases contribute to 24.4 percent of the entire disease burden, while maternal and neonatal ailments contribute to 13.8 percent. Noncommunicable diseases (39.1 percent) and injuries (11.8 percent) now constitute the bulk of the country's disease burden.

Over sixty-three million persons are faced with poverty every year due to health-care costs alone. In 2011–12, the share of out-of-pocket expenditures on health care in proportion to total household monthly per capita expenditure was 6.9 percent in rural and 5.5 percent in urban areas (Ministry of Health and Family Welfare 2015).

2. Role of Private Health Care in India

The role of the private sector in health has been significant. It should be understood that the private sector includes corporate hospitals (who cater to a relatively small number of people in the scheme of things), the not-for-profit hospitals, the small private clinics, and the quacks. Eighty percent of outpatient care and about 60 percent of inpatient care are provided by the private health-care facilities in India, including the Christian network (Ministry of Health and Family Welfare 2015). They also contribute immensely to health-care education with premier institutions like Christian medical colleges. The contribution to nursing education is widely acknowledged by the Indian Nursing Council and has approved boards of nursing education to Christian organizations. The Allied Health Science Education has been widely contributed to by the Church institutions for fifty years (Christian Medical Association of India [CMAI] 2014).

A small but high-profile group of corporate hospitals are catering to health-care tourism. There has also been a spurt in the Indian Systems of Medicine and Homeopathy (AYUSH), which are experiencing a major push by the present government. There has been a significant involvement of

Table 6.1. Achievement of the Millennium Development Goals

Indicators	Target	1990	2012	2015 (estimate)
Maternal mortality ratio	140	560	178	141
Under-five mortality rate	42	126	52	42

Table 6.2. Inequities in health outcomes

| Indicators | India | | | % differential |
	Total	Rural	Urban	
Total fertility rate (2012)	2.4	2.6	1.8	44
Infant mortality rate (2012)	40	44	27	63

the private sector to assist the government in the implementation of its various schemes under the National Rural Health Mission (NRHM) like the Janani Suraksha Yojana (Maternity benefits), Janani Shishu Suraksha Karyakaram (Newborn and infant care), and various disease control programs like Revised National Tuberculosis Control Programme (RNTCP), malaria control, and so on. The Rashtriya Swasthya Bima Yojana (RSBY; health insurance coverage for below-poverty-line [BPL] families) have improved the utilization of hospital services, especially in the private sector and among the poorest (20 percent of households and scheduled caste / scheduled tribe households); however, the problem of the low awareness about the entitlement and how and when to use an RSBY card has been observed. The problem of perverse incentives like the denial of services by private hospitals for many categories of illnesses and an oversupply of some services has been a grave issue with the scheme.

3. Role of Christian Health Care in India

Christian medical missions existed for hundreds of years and were formalized with the establishment of the Medical Missionary Association for South Asia in 1905. Renamed as the Christian Medical Association of India (CMAI) in 1926, the organization continues to serve the churches in India in its ministry of healing to create a just and healthy society. Since the beginning of the ministry of the Christian medical mission, they have contributed immensely toward health care in the country:

- Existence of Christian health care institutions all over the country especially in the rural and difficult-to-reach areas of the country. There were more than 750 hospitals during independence, and 70 percent of them were in rural areas.

- Contributing to medical education for the country.

- Centers of excellence for health care in the country.

Over the years, with the strengthening of the public health system, the role of mission hospitals changes toward its relevance in the government system. The government has a structure to reach the remote areas through subcenters, primary health centers, and community health centers to support the smaller health facilities. But the challenge remains in the system to appropriately provide human resources within this public health structure.

Some of the mission hospitals have become less relevant to the areas they served, and and some have closed for various reasons. In spite of that, they continue to serve the rural and hard-to-reach areas. Christian health-care institutions have been at the cutting edge of research, innovations, community health, alternative health care, and medical education. In the prevailing culture of commercialization of health care, it was felt that it is important for Christian health-care networks to come together to make sure that our institutions continue to advocate strongly for universal health care as a resource for poor people (irrespective of religion, caste, culture, or gender), especially in difficult-to-reach areas of India, where the majority of the Christian institutions remain.

The Christian health-care movement in India has always strived for the medical needs of the marginalized, the voiceless, and those located in the remote areas of India. It has also been the torchbearer for pioneering works in public health, health education, nursing care, and education and in areas related to communicable diseases. With the advent of globalization and the profit motive that has insidiously influenced the health-care industry in India, the members felt that the Christian health-care movement has not been immune to the profit motive either.

Currently there are more than 330 Protestant Christian health-care institutions in the country and over thirty-five hundred Catholic health-care institutions, including the nurse-run clinic across the country. All the Christian institutions, including Christian Medical Association of India (CMAI), Catholic Health Association of India (CHAI), and Emmanuel Hospital Association of India (EHA), constitute about four thousand in number, and together they have about seventy-five thousand inpatient beds.

4. Mandate of Christian Health-Care Network

Christian health care has reached where no public health facilities are available in India. It has served the country for over one hundred years in providing holistic quality health care, particularly to the poor and the marginalized (CMAI Annual Report 2014). Many of these institutions exist with a mandate to provide an abundance of life through Jesus Christ. It is important to provide theological perspectives for the work and witness of the Christian health-care network. This is in order to help Christian individuals and institutions grow strong in their faith and their understanding of and commitment to the healing ministry.

The WHO clearly defined "health" not as an entirely physical phenomenon or the mere absence of disease but as a state of complete physical, mental, and social well-being. In a broader sense, a state of complete well-being would include a spiritual dimension when we look at health from a Christian point of view. The Christian understanding of health and healing is intrinsically related to the Christian understanding of salvation.

5. Theological Perspectives on Health and Healing

In the Old Testament, health is regarded as a state of the well-being of the whole person, considering all aspects together as a complete and undivided entity. The Hebrew word that expresses this concept of health is *shalom*. It expresses the ideas of completeness, wholeness, well-being, harmony, peace, salvation, and justice. It entails complete obedience to God's law (Exod 15:26) and righteousness through a relationship with God (Isa 32:17). In the New Testament, health is understood as life, blessedness, holiness, and maturity (John 10:10; 1 Thess 5:23; Eph 4:13). In the Gospels, the Greek verb *sōzō* is used to mean both the healing of the body and the saving of the soul (Wilkinson 1984, 3–9).

The understanding of health corresponds with the Christian understanding of anthropology, in which there is a multidimensional unity of body, soul, and mind. When there is harmony and a balance of body, soul, and mind, it complements the goodness of God's creation of human beings as *imago Dei*, where the whole person reveals something about God, and the unity of body, soul, and mind teaches us about God (Williams 2008, 366). In Christian anthropological parlance, health is the purpose of God for all humankind where a human being is created to have fellowship with God and to live in a true relationship to God, to themself, to their neighbors, and to the environment. In this sense, shalom (well-being) is what God wills and desires for all people that describes an ultimate state of reconciled and healed relationships between creation and God, between humanity and God, between humanity and creation, and between humans as individuals and as groups or societies. Health, in Christian understanding, is a gift from God to humanity with a responsibility to maintain and develop it.

However, a state of shalom cannot be equated with health because people with poor health or deformities can still experience and testify to God's shalom in their lives. Basic health care and universal access to health are essential means to initiate a state of well-being, but realizing shalom is more than just good health. In Mary McDonough's view, "health is an essential part of life but not the goal of life" (McDonough 2007, 213). In an age of economic liberalization and privatization of medical health care driven by high-profit motifs, there is the danger of idolizing the body and its health solely on commercial terms. This contradicts the Christian notion of personal and corporate shalom that incorporates human relationships and qualities of justice, respect, concern, compassion, and support that surround those relationships and qualities (McDonough 2007, 211).

A comprehensive understanding of health is thus reiterated in the definition of health by the Christian Medical Commission (CMC), a subunit of the Unit on Justice and Service of the World Council of Churches (WCC) central committee of 1989 that defines health as a dynamic state of well-being of the individual and society, of physical, mental, spiritual, economic, political, and social well-being—of being in harmony with each other, with the material environment, and with God. The CMC definition thus provides a concept of wholeness that reflects the biblical vision of shalom, which characterizes the kingdom of God and includes all dimensions of life.

6. Called to Be a Healing Community

According to Scripture, God desires shalom for all people. And as such, when some people are deprived of their basic health care, it threatens communal shalom. William M. Swartley affirms that health, healing, and health care are all part of one whole (Swartley 2012, 19). The word *salvation* comes from the root word *salvas*, which means "healed," and it is only in the mending and healing that an abundant life of wholeness is achieved. Thus medical knowledge and skill, with its ability to cure, and the praying and caring church contribute toward God's healing work that enables shalom both personally and communally (Swartley 2012, 126–27). In the light of this broader Christian view of health care, Christian professional health-care providers, Christian health-care agencies, and faith-based organizations can all be regarded as part of the Christian calling of holistic healing. They are agents with both medical skills and nonmedical healing practices that can complement largely the healing ministry of the church and contribute immensely in providing basic health care to all people. Health-care personnel are thus called to be proactive partners in God's gift of healing. Understanding healing from a Christian perspective would thus incorporate the original intention of God for creation, the gift of abundant life in Jesus Christ, and the establishment of a new heaven and a new earth at the end of time (Rev 21).

The biblical concept of justice describes the moral nature of God that corresponds with the biblical concept of shalom. Justice in a biblical view involves tending to the need of the poor, widows, orphans, and those in the margins, to which James also endorses: "Religion that is pure and undefiled before God, the Father, is this: to care for orphans and widows in their distress, and to keep oneself unstained by the world" (Jas 1:27). Jesus in his earthly ministry worked relentlessly to bring justice especially to those who were socially ostracized and marginalized, like the lepers, the Gentiles, the prostitutes, and the so-called sinners. It is through his unconditional love and indiscriminating acceptance that Jesus modeled health care for all, including the poor and the marginalized. In his entire ministry, Jesus's compassion was always accompanied by a rapid and practical action of curing the human soul and attending to its body. He was concerned with the shalom of the whole person, which reflects the image of God.

In order for Christian organizations to adequately cater to the basic health justice in India, a responsible acceptance and conscious obedience to Jesus's model of health care need to be reaffirmed and practiced. According to Stephen Parsons, "A theology and practice of Christian healing does not begin with answers to the many questions about the mechanics of what makes it work, but with the obedient response to Christ to heal the sick as part of proclaiming the Gospel" (1986, viii). Richard Stearns puts it figuratively that unless the church and its related agencies and organizations own these ministries, it will choose "the hole in our gospel" instead of the whole gospel (Stearns 2009). Therefore, in the light of Christianity's long history of providing health-care services in India and in the face of the current challenges in providing basic health justice, Christian organizations must creatively confront the current issues at hand, discerning its role in health care and health education. Regardless of who provides it, basic health justice is an integral component of shalom, compassion, mission, and service, whether it is provided through religious bodies, private institutions, health companies, or state-run institutions. In a pluralistic country like India with a rich heritage of religious and cultural diversity, basic health care becomes a moral necessity for every citizen for which Christian organizations should strive relentlessly to reach out and provide God's gift of shalom for all humanity.

7. Models of Christian Engagement in Basic Health Justice in India

7.1. Christian Hospitals

Description: Christian hospitals are health-care institutions with developed infrastructure for medical, surgical, gynecological, obstetrics, and other streams of services. They started as twenty-bedded hospitals and developed to more than two-thousand-bedded multispeciality hospitals across the country.

Contributions: The contribution of Christian hospitals in India has been in existence for a long period of time. Currently, there are more than 330 Protestant Christian hospitals in the country and a large number of Catholic health centers, including bigger hospitals. Most of these hospitals are situated in rural and hard-to-reach areas. These hospitals provide health care to all irrespective of religion, caste, and economic background. Reaching out to the community's commitment, spiritual mandate, and technical expertise has been well recognized and is an important contribution toward health justice and equity.

The Christian hospitals in India have been in existence for more than one hundred years. They have been instrumental in serving the poor and the marginalized, especially in rural places. These hospitals not only provide services but have been instrumental in transforming communities. Some of these hospitals have developed into medical colleges. They are responsible for developing medical professionals with high integrity, ethical services, and a propoor approach to health and development in the country.

Prospects: The Christian hospitals have been known to provide ethical, relevant, and compassionate health care. They have been the source of healing for any section of the society. Their presence in many parts of rural India is the sole health-care service for the community. Maintaining quality, relevance, ethics, and value is a sustainable factor for many of the institutions.

Challenges:

1. *Vision, mission, and mandate.* Many of the Christian health-care institutions started with a mandate to be an instrument of healing and to facilitate abundant life in Christ and the wholeness of life. With a strong commitment to serve the poor and the marginalized

populations, most of the institutions based their ethos on serving and the abundance of life. With the recent changes in health care and also the commercialization of health care, it is a challenge for many of the Christian hospitals to remain charitable, low-cost institutions. Survival and sustenance have been a challenge for many of the institutions.

2. *Quality in health care.* There has been a recent emphasis on quality health care through various regulations and laws, which are also applicable to Christian health-care institutions. According to the 2010 Clinical Establishment Act, each state will develop its own standards and pass laws and regulations toward this. The National Accreditation Boards for Hospitals (NABH), even though a voluntary accreditation system, has been highlighted in various government schemes and programs.

   Christian medical mission needs to focus on improving its services and to comply with the various rules and regulations that are implemented. Many times, health-care professionals compromise the quality with the excuse of affordability and accessibility. This puts everyone at risk.

3. *Financial and human resources.* Many hospitals have closed down since India's independence. Around 330 are currently in existence. Even though the closing of some of the institutions is justified, many hospitals are closed due to the lack of financial and human resources. It is a challenge for the churches in India to understand why these constraints should hinder the provision of care to the people, especially the poor and the marginalized. The migration of health-care professionals to more lucrative opportunities, changes in the perspective of and commitment toward the medical mission, inadequate medical equipment in the hospitals, the lack of adequate management support, and many other factors have led to challenges toward human resources in the medical mission.

It is important for Christian hospitals to ask why we exist and strengthen toward excellence in whatever level we are, and the churches should support them wholeheartedly to build a just and healthy society.

7.2. Congregation-Based Health Services

Description: Churches and congregations have contributed immensely toward basic health justice in India. Congregations have contributed toward financial and human resources. There have been initiatives by the congregations, such as projects or outreach programs. There have been some exemplary initiatives of the churches in reaching out to disadvantaged groups—those requiring palliative care, people suffering from HIV and AIDS, those with substance abuse, orphans, and other vulnerable people—for basic health support and services.

1. *Projects.* Some of the churches take up funded projects. They have formed project management committees (PMCs) made up of the pastor, key members of the congregations, and community members. The committee develops plans and reports regularly based on indicators they have developed. One example is the Health and Development Project in Purnea, Bihar, implemented by Brethren in Christ Church along with Christian Medical Association of India.

2. *Outreach programs.* Some of the churches have regular outreach programs to the community, hospitals, or care centers. There has been a regular program developed for HIV and AIDS care and support centers where the congregation members visit and interact with people living with HIV and AIDS. Similar outreach programs are also conducted with the community for those who are chronically ill and other patients. The Marthoma Church in Trivandrum, Kerala, India, has started a palliative care service involving their congregation members to reach out to the community. The churches in the northeastern part of the country, especially the Presbyterian Church in Mizoram, have supported the hospice care for HIV and AIDS financially. There are other churches in India that conduct medical clinics regularly for patients of various diseases and provide treatment and counseling services. The volunteerism and commitment of the members of the churches have enabled sustainable programs that can be replicated at a larger scale.

Contributions: The congregations play an important role in providing a continuum of care for the community. Most of the hospitals do not have outreach components due to a lack of resources. The congregation members play an important role in providing a link between the hospital and the community.

Prospects: Congregation-based health services can play an important role in building awareness among the community and identifying those requiring medical assistance through screening or medical camps, and they also link to hospitals for necessary care and support. They also play an important role in the follow-up of the patients within the community.

Challenges:

1. In most instances, due to the nature of volunteerism, having a sustained program may be challenging for many congregations.
2. Lack of technical expertise, especially financial management, may be a challenge when implementing a project. Staff has to be recruited for this kind of activity.

7.3. Churches' Social Action Initiatives

Description: Many churches in India have started social action initiatives toward health and development work in the communities around them. These social action groups usually function as units within the church.

Contributions: The churches' social action initiatives have been addressing various issues like HIV and AIDS, substance abuse, and other social concerns from the pulpit. These initiatives have led to greater concerns toward these social issues within the community, thereby reducing stigma and discrimination.

Prospects: The churches' social action initiatives play a very important role in sensitizing on various issues within the church. It not only reduces stigma and discrimination but also creates awareness on important issues and social inclusion within the church. They are able to build awareness, provide support, and ensure sustainable interventions on health issues within the church and the community at large.

Challenges: In many instances, the churches' social action initiatives become stand-alone programs, and there is minimal involvement of the congregations and church leadership. Some of the sensitive issues may become difficult to address through social actions.

7.4. Mobilizing Resources

Description: Churches have been contributing financial and other resources to various health and development initiatives. Some of the churches have contributed onetime support, while other churches continuously support these initiatives.

Contributions: There are many examples of churches contributing to health and development initiatives. Some support logistics like building, new beds, and the material requirements of the health centers or hospitals, and others support with cash toward maintenance. Some churches open on weekdays to host programs or initiatives for the disadvantaged groups.

Prospects: Contribution and mobilizing resources are one of the most sustainable interventions for health and development initiatives. Churches hosting events such as Healing Ministry Week, Hospital Sunday, Disabled Sunday, AIDS Sundays, and others have greatly impacted in generating financial support and mobilizing other resources.

Challenges: Due to the nature of support, some of the members may consider it charity work. This may hinder the inclusion of a marginalized community within the church. The general attitude toward giving should be strengthened as a form of sustainable involvement rather than labeling them as disadvantaged groups within the community.

8. Conclusion

Christian contribution has been recognized in a country where the need is enormous and the public health services are limited. The role of private health-care providers plays a major role in the health delivery of the country. The Christian contribution to public health services in India has been very significant in the past and has made a great difference to the health, education, and welfare of India.

The commitment of the church, the commitment of the health-care professionals, and the mandate of healing ministry have been the driving forces behind many of these initiatives. On the other hand, rebuilding the vision and mandate of the church is important to ensure that commitment is not compromised by the market and health industries.

Toward this, the churches can

- revisit the healing ministry of the church;

- guide institutions toward the vision and mission;

- encourage the younger generation toward health justice for all through the healing ministry;

- support the existing health-care institutions through various resources;

- become aware, react, and act toward the need; and

- influence and contribute toward the national policies of the country.

Churches play a vital role in the healing ministry and in reaching out to people with Jesus's model of health care, which incorporates the healing of both the body and the soul. The healing ministry of the church entails a realization of shalom and partaking in God's gift of abundant life. It is in this direction and in upholding the rich legacy of the Christian medical mission in India that the church needs to rekindle the enthusiasm, response, and commitment toward its healing ministry in India.

References

Christian Medical Association of India (CMAI). 2014. *Annual Report 2014*. India: CMAI.

McDonough, Mary. 2017. *Can a Health Care Market Be Moral? A Catholic Vision*. Washington, DC: Georgetown University Press.

Ministry of Health and Family Welfare. 2015. "Draft National Health Policy of India 2015." Accessed March 12, 2015. https://tinyurl.com/6u3snj7.

Parsons, Stephen. 1986. *The Challenge of Christian Healing*. London: SPCK.

Stearns, Richard. 2009. *The Hole in Our Gospel*. Nashville: Thomas Nelson.

Swartley, William M. 2012. *Health, Healing and the Church's Mission: Biblical Perspectives and Moral Priorities*. Downers Grove, IL: InterVarsity.

Wilkinson, John. 1984. *Healing and the Church*. Edinburgh, Scotland: Handel.

Williams, Thomas D. 2008. "Theology of the Body and Humane Vitae." *Alpha Omega* 11 (3): 365–386.

Witnessing to Christ Today: Promoting Health and Wholeness for All. Accessed March 27, 2015. https://tinyurl.com/y3dj8ndp.

PART 2

Faith Traditions for Health and Well-Being

THEME INTRODUCTION

Ville Päivänsalo

1. Healing Maladies, Aspiring for Wholeness

Religious issues are directly relevant to the promotion of health—for example, in the contexts of traditional medicine. In Africa, up to 80 percent of the population uses traditional medicine—or in Western terms, *alternative* or *complementary medicine*—already in primary health care. Traditional birth attendants are also common: in several African countries, they have been estimated to assist in the majority of births (WHO 2015). But thinking about health beyond the primary care, what kinds of well-being might faith organization often promote? Could there be any sort of a common response to such a question?

Merely understanding the very concept of "illness" across cultures can be tricky. In Tanzania, for instance, whereas the Kiswahili word *ogonjwa* is often translated as "illness" or "disease," Stacey A. Langwick (2011) suggests that "malady" serves as a better translation. Malady (cf. *male habitus* in Latin) has connotations of illness as well as a moral defect or corruption. Moreover, illness as a malady has its political and ontological dimensions. A Tanzanian healer (*mganga*) correspondingly endeavors to provide a sick person with a more holistic healing and truth than what is customary in Western medicine. In Tanzanian everyday discourse of health, accordingly, science and religion as well as family issues and politics are all closely intertwined (15).

Aspirations for health and holistic well-being are in no way extrinsic to the Abrahamic religious traditions either. The ancient Hebrew notion of shalom, indicating at the same time both peace and wholeness and both health and harmonious well-being, has often served as the key concept to further discussions. Also the Genesis narrative about the abundant goodness of Paradise, which was soon profoundly lost, has served as a hugely influential starting point for the subsequent health traditions of world religions. Such ancient religious insights—akin to the traditional Tanzanian life view—reach far beyond mere notions of bodily sickness to intriguing ideas about the distracted human condition and its restoration. A publication by the World Council of Churches (WCC) and the German Institute of Medical Mission (DIFAEM) even depicts "every single act of healing [as] a sign of the realization of shalom" (WCC and DIFAEM 2010, 9).

The world religions stemming from ancient Indian and Chinese roots likewise centrally include aspirations for health and wholeness. Whether expressed in terms of liberation from suffering or achieving a state of perfect harmony and peace, traditions headed by Hinduism, Buddhism, and Confucianism—although not the focus of this volume—have framed the health concerns of billions of people through millennia.

2. Christian Traditions Encountering Modernity

The founder of Christianity, Jesus of Nazareth, was himself a healer and an exorcist. Miraculous healing practices became thereafter an integral part of both Eastern and Western Christianity, albeit in the West, they were often also despised as magical manipulations of spiritual forces. Later on in the Lutheran and Calvinist traditions, it became common to see miracles as specific signs of God for the apostolic era only (Porterfield 2005, 23).

In medieval times, Western medicine benefited a lot from the comparatively advanced Islamic medicine. Empirical medicine, in turn, emerged in Europe within a broadly Christian or Deist framework (Eckart 2009). Religious traditions have thus shaped the Western ideas of medicine and health not only through their supernatural beliefs but also through their ability to inspire secular types of research and care. Yet spiritualistic care did not disappear. Pentecostal visions of the Holy Spirit have also been part of the Western culture for centuries. And nowadays, they attract people burdened by maladies especially in the Global South, not least in sub-Saharan Africa, frequently as mixtures of traditional and Christian forms of faith healing (Okure 1995, i; Pfeiffer 2011).

Sometimes the role of faith in healing is much more subtle. Protestant liberal theologian Paul Tillich (1961, 171) once rejected fanaticism, dogmatism, ritualism, and magical healing as instances of unhealthy religion. Nevertheless, he searched for a state of being grasped by a "Spirit" in the sense of "the presence of what concerns us ultimately, the ground of our being and meaning." Interestingly indeed, a recent study on two cases of indigenous healing—a Hindu and a Muslim—in India emphasizes the significance of religion similarly: religious perspectives provide personally and socially meaningful explanations to those who suffer (Lohokare and Bhargavi 2010, 171). Both to modern and more religious minds, thus, much of the relevance of faith in healing could be measured not primarily in quantitative but in existential and hermeneutical terms.

In addition to the hugely influential Roman Catholic missions and their charities, a good part of the current Christian engagement in global health derives from the rise of the Protestant diakonia movement in nineteenth-century Europe. Parallel developments occurred in North America, mobilizing vast numbers of volunteers, and the emergent medical mission movement globalized patterns of Christian health care (Grundmann 2005; Porterfield 2015, 141–58). Christian medical missionaries often confronted traditional healing from a vantage point of modern medicine. Actually, mainstream faith-based health organizations tend to find themselves in a similar position today, endeavoring to perform—as William Summerskill and Richard Horton (2015) put it—the "Faith-Based Delivery of Science-Based Care."

Modern Protestant faith encouraged Christians to live true to their religious callings and to care in secular terms and often also within secular institutions. From such a standpoint, characteristic to a Nordic Lutheran faith, it became possible to see the modern welfare state as God's instrument of social justice (Andersen 2010). But in the Global South, toward the end of the twentieth century, much of the church-related practical health work had become rather dissociated from any straightforward religious ideas. This approach, advocating the case of the poor, the ill, and the oppressed, has suited Christianity-rooted development organizations in the officially secular India (e.g., Lutheran World Service India Trust 2013). In several African countries, the prevalence of faith-based but in practice largely secular third-sector organizations has been extensive enough so that they have almost functioned as a surrogate of the state (Jennings 2008).

3. Developments in the Islamic Heritage

One of the five pillars of Islam is giving to charity (*zakat*). It actually resonates with the idea of justice, as it is an obligation for a Muslim and it is regulated further in the sharia law. But the overarching perspective on health in Islam is that it is a blessing from the almighty God. Indeed, the Qur'an itself is to provide a kind of healing advice to human beings—as stated in the tenth Surah of the book (10:57): "O mankind, there has to come to you instruction from your Lord [i.e., the Qur'an] and healing for what is in the breasts and guidance and mercy for the believers."

The hadith (the early collected sayings of the Prophet Muhammad) is an important source for understanding what the good deeds are to mean in Islam in each field of life, firmly including those related to health and well-being. For instance, in a hadith on health and healing, entitled "Medicine," Abu Huraira reports that the Prophet said, "There is no disease that Allah has created, except that He also has created its treatment" (Sahih al-Bukhari n.d., hadith 1). According to Huraira, a favorite companion to the Prophet, the latter also taught that in the Day of Judgment, God will say, "Oh son of Adam! I was sick but you did not visit me" (qtd. in Rahman 1998, 59). Clearly resembling Jesus's teaching of the last judgment as reported by Matthew (25:36), this hadith urges people of faith to take care of the sick as a matter of obligation.

At the time when Islam originated and began to expand, one of the leading centers of medical knowledge in the whole world was Jundishapur (or Gundeshapur) in the region of modern Iran. As the Muslims then took over this city in 638 CE, many Jewish and Christian physicians had already migrated there and established a hospital with a medical school (Koenig and Al Shohaib 2014, 6–7). Often following this model, hospitals were subsequently established all over the Islamic world. In the so-called Golden Age of Islam, approximately from the mid-eighteenth century to the fall of Baghdad at the hands of Mongols in 1258, Islamic medicine was indeed broadly recognized as being more advanced than that of the West. Whereas many of the leading physicians in its centers were Christians, its outstanding developers—most famously, physician and scholar in philosophy and theology Ibn Sina (980–1037)—clearly worked within the Islamic framework of faith (Koenig and Al Shohaib 2014, 11–15, 19).

Islamic contributions to health and medicine continued with an impressive profile in several centers of that cultural sphere also after its golden age. From the perspective of health justice in particular, it is intriguing that the largest hospital of the time, the Masnuri Hospital in Cairo, provided its treatment for free. This hospital, sponsored essentially by Mameluk sultan Mansur Qala'un and completed in 1284, provided costless services to all, whether coming from afar or near and whether the people in need were men or women, rich or poor, learned or illiterate. As a document of the hospital states, "The entire service is through the magnificence of God, the generous one" (qtd. in Rahman 1998, 70).

In the subsequent era dominated by the Ottoman Empire, Islamic medicine was not particularly progressive anymore in the Middle East. An interesting development, however, took place in India, where Islamic medicine was heavily influenced by the Ayurvedic tradition predominant in that subcontinent. It is illustrative that the great Muslim Mughal emperor Akbar (reign 1556–1605) maintained in his court a team of twenty-nine doctors from the Muslim as well the Hindu traditions (Rahman 1998, 75).

In our times, Muslim-majority countries have adopted paradigms of modern medicine, albeit not uniformly so. In a time when new medical and health-care innovations have been seen as a part of Western colonialism, opposition to them has quite understandably emerged. Yet the risen standards of health care in the wealthier centers of the Muslim world have unraveled many of such tensions.

4. Challenges for the Twenty-First Century

The diversity among faith-based agencies in most regions of the Global South is great, even to the degree that reliable estimates of its mere extent are hard to find. Whereas some sources suggest that solely Christian faith-based organizations provide more than half of the health services in sub-Saharan Africa (Nordstokke 2013, 237), most of the measures used by Jill Olivier et al. (2015) in their recent *Lancet* article indicate somewhat lower figures. Jill Olivier et al. indeed regret the very lack of systematic data on this sector's agencies and also the deficient understanding of their diverse functions. Somehow, they state, "faith-based providers of health have disappeared off the policy and evidence map" (1765).

Echoing this request for better research by Olivier et al. (2015), Jean F. Duff and Warren W. Buckingham III (2015, 1789–92) have come up with a practical agenda to enhance collaboration for global health with faith-based organizations. Yet the future of this sector is uncertain for various reasons. Some of these challenges are related to reduced international funding (Nordstokke 2013, 237) and others to directly faith-related problems like proselytism, a rather common phenomenon in this sector. Still other challenges stem from the turbulent overall situation of the African continent in particular: increased inequalities, persistent conflicts, and rampant business values have shaken the traditional patterns of healthy living.

In India, the challenges are partly different. Regional surveys indicate that, in rural India, more than 70 percent of health-care providers have no formal medical training. Even though they are not likely to treat diseases as correctly as qualified doctors, it has been found, to their merit, that they have been less likely to prescribe unnecessary antibiotics. Training these doctors has been suggested as a means to major improvements of health in India (Pulla 2016). Critical analyses of religious issues would certainly need to be included in such training programs.

Among the most salient fields of further attention in the faith-based sector are the rights of the disabled, enshrined in the *Convention on the Rights of Persons with Disabilities* adopted by the United Nations General Assembly in 2006 and in the post-2015 agenda for development. About one billion people—15 percent of the world's population—are burdened by some form of disability (World Bank 2015, "Context"). The problem is relatively worse in developing countries, where also poverty, communicable diseases, malnutrition, and conflicts tend to hit the life prospects of the disabled harder. How then do faith-based organizations, having a broad, long-term involvement in this field, conceptualize their foundational insights and practical involvement for the support of the disabled today?

Key topics in the health work of faith organizations definitely include the challenges of the marginalized, often refugees. In what kinds of ways have some of the more innovative faith organizations attempted to support health and well-being among such groups of people? What could the division of labor between the public and the voluntary sector be in this field?

As a more subtle but also profound challenge of global health, the long shadow of colonialism must still be mentioned. Have the collaborative initiatives in sub-Saharan Africa, India, or perhaps elsewhere in the Global South already managed to move to properly postcolonial mindsets and practices? Hardly so. However, studies over recent decades also suggest moving beyond images of a unified concept of colonialism. As colonialism previously came in various forms, so also in the twenty-first century there is no monolithic African postcolonialism (Sadowsky 2011, 215)—or an Indian or a Bangladeshi one, for that matter. Yet it is imperative for any faith-based initiative for health in the Global South to reach, in one way or another, beyond colonial patterns of mind, spirit, and practice alike.

References

Andersen, Svend. 2010. *Macht aus Liebe: Zur Reconstruktion einer lutherischen politischen Ethik*. Berlin: De Gruyter.

Duff, Jean F., and Warren W. Buckingham III. 2015. "Strengthening of Partnerships between the Public Sector and Faith-Based Groups." *Lancet* 386:1786–1794.

Eckart, Wolfgang U. 2009. *Geschichte der Medizin: Fakten, Konzepte, Haltungen*. 6th ed. Heidelberg: Springer.

Grundmann, Christoffer H. 2005. *Sent to Heal: Emergence and Development of Medical Missions*. Lanham, MD: University Press of America.

Jennings, Michael. 2008. *Surrogates of the State: NGOs, Development, and Ujamaa in Tanzania*. Bloomfield, CT: Kumarian.

Langwick, Stacey A. 2011. *Bodies, Politics, and African Healing: The Matter of Maladies in Tanzania*. Bloomington: Indiana University Press.

Lohokare, Madhura, and Davar V. Bhargavi. 2010. "The Community Role of Indigenous Healers: An Exploration of Healing Values in Maharashtra." In *Health Providers in India: On the Frontiers of Change*, edited by Kabir Sheikh and Asha George, 161–181. London: Routledge.

Lutheran World Service India Trust (LWSIT). 2013. "Lutheran World Service India: Since—1974." Kolkata, India: LWSIT.

Nordstokke, Kjell. 2013. "Faith-Based Organizations and Their Distinct Assets." In *Religion: Help of Hindrance for Development*, edited by Kenneth Mtata, 225–242. Leipzig: Evangelische Verlag.

Okure, Theresa. 1995. Preface to *Inculturation of the Christian Mission to Heal in the South African Context*, edited by Stuart Bate, i–vi. Lewiston, NY: Edwin Mellen.

Olivier, Jill, Clarence Tsimpo, Regina Gemignani, Mari Shojo, Harold Coulombe, Frank Dimmock, Minh Cong Nguyen et al. 2015. "Understanding the Roles of Faith-Based Health-Care Providers in Africa: Review of the Evidence with a Focus on Magnitude, Reach, Cost, and Satisfaction." *Lancet* 386:1765–1775.

Pfeiffer, James. 2011. "Commodity Fetichismo, the Holy Spirit, and the Turn to Pentecostal and African Independent Churches in Central Mozambique."

In *Medicine and Health in Africa: Multidisciplinary Perspectives*, edited by Paula Viterbo and Kalala Ngalamulume, 177–209. Münster: LIT.

Porterfield, Amanda. 2015. *Healing in the History of Christianity*. Oxford: Oxford University Press.

Pulla, Priyanka. 2016. "Are India's Quacks the Answer to Its Shortage of Doctors?" *British Medical Journal* 352:i291. Accessed January 27, 2016. http://www.bmj .com/content/352/bmj.i291.

Sadowsky, Jonathan. 2011. "The Long Shadow of Colonialism: Why We Study Medicine in Africa." In *Medicine and Health in Africa: Multidisciplinary Perspectives*, edited by Paula Viterbo and Kalala Ngalamulume, 210–217. Münster: LIT.

Bukhārī, Muḥammad ibn Ismāʿīl. n.d. *Book of Medicine*, book 76 of Sahih al-Bukhari. Accessed September 14, 2020. https://sunnah.com/bukhari/76.

Summerskill, William, and Richard Horton. 2015. "Faith-Based Delivery of Science-Based Care." *Lancet* 286:1709–1710.

Tillich, Paul. 1984. *The Meaning of Health: Essays in Existentialism, Psychoanalysis, and Religion*. Edited by Perry LeFevre. Chicago: Exploration.

World Bank. 2015. "Disability Inclusion." Accessed January 22, 2019. https:// www.worldbank.org/en/topic/disability.

World Council of Churches (WCC) and the German Institute of Medical Mission (DIFAEM). 2010. *Witnessing to Christ Today: Promoting Health and Wholeness for All*. Tübingen, Germany: DIFAEM.

World Health Organization (WHO). 2015. "Traditional Medicine." WHO Media Centre. Accessed December 3, 2015. https://tinyurl.com/y4xkkwee.

7

———

Islamic Faith for Health and Welfare in the Globalizing South Asia

THE CASE OF BANGLADESH

Abu Sayem

ABSTRACT

This chapter describes some exemplary Islamic teachings about public health issues and identifies certain Islamic health values. It briefly provides an account of the ongoing health problems of South Asia, focusing on the context of Bangladesh with special attention to a significant role of Islamic faith-based organizations in the promotion of health and well-being for the Bangladeshi people. Finally, it provides some suggestions on how faith-based organizations can contribute to public health more effectively if they are supported by the government and other donor agencies.

1. Introduction

Health is a very important fact for human life. Nobody can go forward without good health. Welfare is a kind of human value and is essential to the quality of life. Welfare is mostly related to a healthy life. So public health is an important issue in the discourse of health. Public agencies, donor countries, development partners, nongovernmental organizations, and faith-based institutions are all taking part in the health discourse around the globe.

South Asian countries contain about one-fifth of the population of the world, but most of these people are living in an inadequate health condition with very inadequate social welfare policies. Bangladesh, although its public health project seems somewhat improved, is going through many challenges. In this chapter, there will be an effort to present an Islamic view of public health and welfare, connected to Bangladesh as a case study. Bangladesh is predominantly a Muslim-majority country where Islam plays a vital role in everyday life. So the chapter attempts to show how Islamic faith can work as an alternative tool for the promotion of public health in Bangladesh.

2. Some Islamic Views of Health and Well-Being

Islamic beliefs and practices regarding health, healing, and well-being are based on the Holy Qur'an and authentic prophetic traditions. The religious and cultural traditions of Islam provide some guiding principles on birth, illness, and death, covering social, legal, and political regulations. In this regard, Omar Hasan Kasule's statements seem very comprehensive and inclusive. A short account of Islamic views of health and well-being is presented in the following section based mainly on Professor Kasule's[1] description.

2.1. Health in a Holistic Outlook

Kasule summarizes the Islamic concept of health as spiritually sound, physically capable, mentally fresh, and socially fit. Spiritual health refers to the connection of a person with God; physical health is understood as a physiological function of human beings; psychological health implies mental soundness of a person; and social fitness articulates a healthy environment where humans are to live. So health, as Kasule interprets it, is a harmonious function of these four basic components. It is commonly known that when any part of the body is sick, the whole body is affected. If one member of a family is sick, all other members of the family are affected. Any sickness in the community results in a negative impact on all the community members. A person who is spiritually sick may

---

1 Dr. Omar Hasan K. Kasule is professor of epidemiology and Islamic Medicine in the Institute of Medicine, University of Brunei. He has also worked as a visiting professor of epidemiology at the University of Malaya. He is considered an authority on Islamic health and medicine education in the contemporary world.

become physically sick. Thus human health is deeply intertwined with its physical, emotional, and spiritual aspects as well as the surrounding environment (Kasule 2006).

Put another way, the sustainability of health depends on some basic things. For example, nutrition, environment, lifestyle, and psychological and spiritual factors play a vital role in determining health (Kasule 2006). Required nutrition and a balanced diet are crucial for maintaining good health. On the other hand, imbalanced diet and malnutrition are primarily responsible for diseases. In this context, the advice of Prophet Muhammad seems very relevant. The Prophet taught his followers to control their appetite for overeating. Prophet Muhammad advises his followers not to eat more as they desire to fill their stomach; if they persist to do that, let them fill one-third of their stomachs with food, one-third with water, and one-third should be vacant for breathing.[2] The environment is the source of life-supporting materials including foods, water, and oxygen. "The elements of weather like heat and cold have direct effects on health as well. . . . The environment also harbors many pathogens that cause disease in a human body" (Kasule 2006, §2). So for keeping in good health, people have to create a healthy environment around them. It is worth mentioning that the teaching of Islam is always fit for a healthy environment. The lifestyle that people choose affects physical and mental health; that's why an ideal and balanced life is prescribed in Islam for human beings. Thus it is evident that health is related not only to any single determinant but rather with many factors that work to keep human beings healthy. So human health is viewed in Islamic religious traditions from a holistic outlook.

2.2. Health as a Relative and Subjective Matter

Kasule (2006) shows that usually health varies by age, place, norms, and gender. Similarly, the state of belief in God (iman) or dependence on God (tawakkul) matters in health. Those who have a strong faith in God may feel subjectively healthier than those who do not believe in God. Good health also varies from place to place. Even in the same place, it may

---

2 Miqdam bin Ma'dikarib said, "I heard the Messenger of Allah (S.a.w) saying: 'The human does not fill any container that is worse than his stomach. It is sufficient for the son of Adam to eat what will support his back. If this is not possible, then a third for food, a third for drink, and third for his breath'" (Abū 'Īsā Muḥammad 2007).

also vary from era to era. The subjective feeling of good health varies by gender. Females may feel more worried about diseases than males.

2.3. Health as a Matter of Responsibility

Muhammad Haytham Al-Khayat (2004, 18) notes that according to Islam, good health is attached with a responsibility (*amanah*). He argues that poor health not only deprives society of the contributions of an individual but also creates a burden for others. For Imam Ibn Qayyim Al-Jauziyah (2003), according to the prophetic tradition of Islam, negligence to health is a kind of sin, and it is a religious obligation to seek treatment for the sick. So it is a responsibility of a person to undertake disease-preventing measures such as dietary regulation, hygiene, violence avoidance, mental depression control, the promotion of spirituality, and the avoidance of anything that impairs good health (Al-Khayat 2004, 19–23).

2.4. Health as a Special Gift of God

For Islamic scholars, good health is a precious gift from God (*ni'mah*). Human beings must be grateful to God for such a special gift. They should express this gratitude by worshipping God and doing good deeds on earth (Kasule 2006). Even on the day of judgment, God will ask humans about this blessing (Al-Khayat 2004, 14).

2.5. Health and Family Life

A healthy family life works to promote the good health of all its members. A family is to cultivate "trust, loyalty, a sense of belonging, and rights and obligations." These values are "needed for a balanced psychological health." A good family life works as an essential source of "primary health care." A mature marital relationship supports "psychological and physical health" of all the family members (Kasule 2006, §3). According to the Qur'anic description, "A family is a source of calmness and tranquility" (7:189). Islam always advocates for a sustainable family life for all humans.

2.6. Community Health

Human beings are not isolated entities in society. Like their family life, humans are also involved with community life. If one member of the community is sick, other members are also affected in some ways. Islam always encourages keeping all the members of the community healthy and fit for work.

2.7. Preventive Health Care

It is a universally accepted maxim that "prevention is better than a cure." Islam always promotes prior prevention before being ill. For religious scholars, many diseases can be prevented by using spiritual approaches. That is why Islamic scholars like Ibn Sina regard spiritual beliefs ('aqiidah) and religious practices ('ibadah) as influential factors for good health. For the same reason, Ibn Sina suggests avoiding unapproved things (haram) and advocates for legal things (halaal). Al-Khayat rightly mentions that Islam encourages each and every person to take measures to protect the body from unapproved things by prevention (2004, 11). So in Muslim communities, immunization, good nutrition, personal hygiene, and disinfection should be considered preventive measures for the protection of health.

3. Islamic Guidelines to Public Health for Muslim Patients

True Muslims always try to lead their lives in accordance with the prescription of the Holy Qur'an and the prophetic tradition. Muslims view Islam as the only way and complete code of life. Islam is understood as a guide for all aspects of Muslim life, ranging from birth to death, including health care and medical treatment. This faith tradition indeed suggests that a minimum level of cultural awareness is a necessity for the delivery of care that is culturally sensitive, especially for Muslim patients. Accordingly, Islamic scholars advocate for maintaining an Islamic way of life when serving Muslim patients in health-care facilities. Ann McKennis (1999) and K. M. Hedayat and Roya Pirzadeh (2001) present some guidelines for nurses and medical doctors as to how Muslim patients should be served.

3.1. Providing an Opportunity for Prayer

It is important for nurses to ask the patients and their family members whether they perform any religious rituals. If the patient wants to perform Islamic obligatory prayers (five times a day), the hospital authorities should allow it. Such a prayer truly gives some relief to a patient practicing Islamic beliefs and rituals.

3.2. Considering Dietary Restrictions and Halal Foods

Muslims believe that dietary restrictions promote health. Eating meat (beef, mutton, chicken, and the meat of many other animals that are recognized by Islamic sharia to eat) is permitted if the animal is slaughtered properly (according to the sharia law). Pork, alcohol, or any other intoxicating foods or drinks are forbidden. Healthy eating is part of one's religious obligation. The nurses caring for Muslim patients should consult with the dietitian about the families' food preferences and allow accepted (*halal*) foods to be brought from home. Islam teaches that medications made with pork or alcohol are to be avoided if possible but may be used if it is thought to be the best alternative for health care. Health-care providers should take care of this.

3.3. Circumcising Male Children

Male children are usually circumcised. Traditionally, the procedure was performed between ages four and ten, but nowadays in many countries, it is usually done within a few days after birth. Although it is not an injunction of Islam for female children to be circumcised, it is unfortunately being held in some Muslim cultures and countries as a source and part of their own cultural pride. Circumcision of female children is a traditional practice with which Islam has no logical relation, and it is treated as invalid by Muslim scholars.

3.4. Taking Care of Women during Menstruation

Islam advocates for special consideration and taking care of teen girls and other women during menstruation. Sexual intercourse is forbidden with menstruating women, because at that time, they are considered sick and weak. A menstruating woman is given a waiver from participating in certain rituals in a religious household.

3.5. Same-Sex Priority in Health-Care Provision

Islamic teachings regulate relationships between men and women. Muslim patients usually prefer to get health-care services from same-sex health-care providers. In an emergency situation, however, the priority is given to saving lives and preventing injuries as the most essential things in Islam.

3.6. Life and Death Issues as Trials from God

Life is believed as a precious gift of God. It is God who determines the time of death. So suicide, euthanasia, and the denial of nutrition or hydration are generally prohibited in Islam. Hedayat and Pirzadeh (2001) as well as McKennis (1999) note that the majority of modern Islamic scholars are of the opinion that the discontinuation of some life-supporting treatments can be accepted if the family members take such a decision after consulting the doctors.

3.7. Showing Courtesy to a Dying Person

When a Muslim individual dies, several things should be done to the patient according to the prophetic traditions of Islam: (1) turning the patient on their right side in the direction of Mecca, (2) requesting the visitors to remember the holy names of God in front of the dying patient, (3) suggesting other people to pray for him, and (4) alleviating the fear of the dying person and making them optimistic to God's mercy.

3.8. Special Duties to the Dead Body

After death, the dead body must be kept covered. It is best if only health-care professionals of the same gender touch the body. The body is washed and perfumed. Then it should be wrapped with white sheets. After the ritual washing and wrapping, the body is buried with a simple prayer. The body is placed in a deep grave, and the face is turned in the direction of Mecca, which is concurrently kept on the right side of the dead body. The body, which has been wrapped in white sheets, can be put directly into the ground. Coffins are not usually used. The ritual washing, prayers, and burial should take place only within a few hours, if possible.

4. Islam in Globalized Health Discourse for the Promotion of Public Health

Islam always advocates the promotion of health, though in the modern world, public health promotion has often been regarded as a Western enterprise in particular. Indeed, in most cases, the Western initiatives for the promotion of health are supported by Islamic health values and objectives of life. In the modern period, *the Amman Declaration*[3] may serve as a present-day Islamic working guide to the promotion of good health and well-being. In it we see sixty components of lifestyle through which Islamic teachings can make an impact. These sixty items are deeply intertwined with public health. The declaration advocates for proper nutrition, healthy food, hygiene, regular disposal systems of waste, mental health, decent sexual relationships, and a nonviolent attitude in life. *The Amman Declaration* can be a supportive force in the promotion of public health. It is also very significant in the ongoing globalized health discourses.

Since its inception in 1948, the World Health Organization (WHO)[4] has been working to cope with different health issues from a global perspective. Among international health documents, *the Alma-Ata Declaration*,[5] the Ottawa Charter for Health Promotion,[6] and *the Jakarta Declaration*[7] are notably mentionable ones. *The Alma-Ata Declaration* was an international commitment to emphasize the necessity of primary health care. The main theme of the conference where it originated, in 1978, was "health for all by 2000." The declaration suggests economic and social development as a prerequisite to achieving its goal of "health for all." It urges all member states of the United Nations (UN) to play their active role in this regard.

---

3 It stemmed from a conference held in Amman, Jordan, in 1989, jointly organized and sponsored by the Islamic Education, Science and Cultural Organization (ISESCO), and the World Health Organization (WHO). The conference theme was "health promotion through Islamic lifestyle."

4 As the specialized agency of the United Nations (UN), the WHO was established in 1948 in Geneva, Switzerland, with a noble vision—that is, to take care of public health all over the world.

5 The WHO arranged an international conference at Alma-Ata, Kazakhstan, in 1978, which is known as *the Alma-Ata Declaration*.

6 The Ottawa Charter for Health Promotion came from the international conference held at Ottawa, Canada, in 1986.

7 In 1997, the WHO arranged an important conference in Jakarta, Indonesia, whose collective decisions are known as *the Jakarta Declaration*.

Like *the Alma-Ata Declaration*, the Ottawa Charter takes the same action plan to achieve health for all by 2000. It was a primary response to the growing expectations for a new public health movement around the world. The charter identifies health promotion as a process of enabling people to be healthy. It considers health as a resource for everyday life. In this charter, health is connected with physical, mental, and social well-being. Health is also articulated with such fundamental conditions and resources as peace, shelter, education, food, income, a stable ecosystem, sustainable resources, social justice, equity, and respect for human rights. In 1988, WHO organized an international conference at Adelaide, Australia, on healthy public policy. This conference recognized health as a fundamental social goal and assessed the value of health in terms of social well-being as a whole. In their 1991 international conference in Sundsvall, Sweden, they focused on supportive environments for health.

Then in 1997, *the Jakarta Declaration* took some important decisions for leading health promotion into the twenty-first century with the motto "New Players for a New Era." It was the first conference organized in a Muslim country—so it accepted some ideas from Islamic working guidelines on public health. All these international initiatives and declarations can be considered a legitimizing process of health principles in the modern world. These discussions emphasize both individual and societal responsibilities recognizing multidimensional factors of health. In this way, an innovative approach is seen to work for the promotion of public health. Both *the Amman Declaration* and *the Jakarta Declaration* add some religious and spiritual values to the public health issues from an Islamic point of view.

As the Ottawa Charter is seen as a guiding formulation for the promotion of public health and well-being until now (De Leeuw 1989; cited in De Leeuw and Hussein 1999, 347), it should be compared with Islamic guiding principles of public health. In "Islamic Health Promotion and Interculturalization," Evelyne De Leeuw and Abdelmoneim Hussein (1999) present a comparative study between the Ottawa Charter and Islamic principles of health promotion. They identify as the three basic communication modalities of the Ottawa Charter enabling, mediation, and advocacy, and then they compare these modalities to the three Islamic concepts *da'wah*, *shura*, and *waqf*.

The Arabic term *da'wah* literally means inviting people to know what is beneficial to them in terms of their own welfare and well-being. Although it is a central concept in the dissemination of Islam, it pertains to the promotion of health as well. The mosque, the congregational worshiping place for Muslims, is the center of this *da'wah* activity, so here enabling, mediating, and advocating health matters may easily take place (De Leeuw and Hussein 1999, 349).

To reorient health services in Muslim countries, the concept of *shura* plays a vital role (De Leeuw and Hussein 1999, 349). The Arabic word *shura* refers to a process of mutual consultation. So *shura* is about collective decisions and initiatives taken for the delivery of health care. In this regard, the government must take the necessary steps for the promotion of public health. Islamic religious institutions like mosque committees, religious scholars, and local public agencies should communicate and cooperate with the ministry of health.

Finally, the Arabic term *waqf* refers to the Islamic system of private initiatives to voluntarily work for the development of a society in terms of education, food security, and health services. *Waqf* is formed on the basis of the private donation of a wealthy Muslim. Governments should promote such religious initiatives among Muslim people considering their social needs. In the past, *waqf* became instrumental in conducting libraries, hospitals, educational institutions, and mosques (Fayzee 1991; cited in De Leeuw and Hussein 1999, 349). Still now, it will work basically like the earlier forms of eradicating poverty and reducing health problems.

Thus De Leeuw and Hussein relate these three Islamic modalities with the three corresponding words of the Ottawa Charter. It is high time to properly utilize such an opportunity for the promotion of public health care. They also move on to discuss how to interculturalize health promotion in Muslim countries. In this regard, they advocate for identifying the structural components of an Islamic Ottawa Charter. They suggest that Muslim governments should support other working agencies in public health to execute the imperatives of the envisaged Islamic Ottawa Charter. It may be considered the first attempt to clarify the value of modern health promotion insights for both Muslim countries and Muslim communities living in non-Muslim countries. As such, it may contribute worldwide to the further development of health promotion in Muslim countries through the adaptation of the Ottawa Charter. It also helps the process of interculturalization in the West in the complex field of health promotion.

5. Public Health Challenges in Globalized South Asia

The current territories of Bangladesh, India, and Pakistan form the core countries of South Asia, and Nepal, Bhutan, Sri Lanka, and Maldives are generally included in it as well. When health is concerned, South Asian countries face health challenges on a demographic and geographic scale (Haté and Gannon 2010, 1). The Center for Strategic and International Studies' (CSIS) report (2010) on public health in South Asia shows a low life expectancy rate of the South Asian people especially due to a high rate of malnutrition. The report notes the incidences of tuberculosis (TB) and HIV/AIDS involved in infant mortality next to the countries of sub-Saharan Africa. The report identifies some health-related problems like poor sanitation, poor maternal health, poor access to health-care services, and widespread malaria at emerging levels. The rural situation is found worse than usually imagined in these health issues. The average allocation for public health in the fiscal year's budget in South Asian countries is very unsatisfactory. The CSIS report (2010) shows that less than 4 percent of the fiscal budget is allocated for public health, which is insufficient to cope with health problems. Such uneven distribution in the national budgets for health-care facilities is harshly criticized in the report. Out of seven South Asian countries, only Sri Lanka seems to have achieved a comparatively satisfactory level in the provision of health facilities to its citizens.

According to the CSIS report (2010), significant growth has occurred in health expenditure on a per capita basis, but it has simultaneously declined in comparison in terms of a share of gross domestic product (GDP). The World Health Statistics report shows that from 2000 to 2006, annual per capita health spending grew from US$26.5 to $31.8 in Bangladesh, from US$21.8 to $25.00 in India, from US$24.9 to $30.5 in Nepal, from US$20.6 to $16.4 in Pakistan, and from US$47.9 to $47.5 in Sri Lanka (WHO 2009). The report appreciates these increasing rates as impressive, but it criticizes the inefficient management of South Asian countries in handling the distribution of allocated funds. These countries are not free from corruption and mismanagement. Perhaps, for this reason, all these countries except Sri Lanka have failed to improve their public health sector effectively.

The region's health outcome has thus improved a bit in recent years but remains far below a satisfactory level. Though all seven countries have experienced a kind of progress in life expectancy, infant survival, and childhood immunization, still now the situation remains alarming.

With just a single example, it becomes clear to us that out of a total of twenty-seven million unimmunized children around the globe, approximately ten million live in India. Diarrhea, acute respiratory infections, and diseases preventable by vaccines make childhood mortality a continuing public health challenge, particularly in Pakistan, where ninety children of every one thousand die at the age of five (WHO 2006).

The report also shows a puzzling situation of maternal health in the region due to the absence of basic health systems and facilities. According to WHO's "Global Health Observatory" report, approximately 185,000 (one lakh eighty-five thousand) women in the region die during childbirth every year, though skilled professionals attended nearly 50 percent of births. Unfortunately, unattended home delivery remains a cultural tradition in many rural parts of Bangladesh, India, Nepal, and Pakistan (WHO 2006).

The report mentions HIV/AIDS as a big health challenge for South Asian countries. According to the National AIDS Control Organization (NACO), nearly 2.3 million HIV-positive patients are in India, and its prevalence rate is 0.29 percent (NACO 2010; cited in Haté and Gannon 2010, 1). In Pakistan, the HIV-positive prevalence rate is about 0.10 percent. In Nepal, 0.50 percent of its population has HIV (Population Reference Bureau 2009; cited in Haté and Gannon 2010, 4). In South Asian countries, the HIV/AIDS epidemic promotes a resurgence of TB, which is the leading cause of the deaths of HIV-positive people (Haté and Gannon 2010). India alone contains more TB patients than any other nation (Donald and Helden 2009). Noncommunicable diseases also create some challenges for public health. For instance, cardiovascular disease, respiratory disease, digestive disease, cancer, and diabetes cause more than 50 percent of deaths. India alone carries more than 80 percent of the region's chronic disease deaths (WHO 2005; cited in Haté and Gannon 2010).

Malnutrition is a very common phenomenon in South Asian countries. According to the same report, 20 to 25 percent of South Asian people suffer from malnutrition. Women suffer more than their male counterparts. Many children are found underweight because of malnutrition. In this region, drinking water and the sanitation situation remain risky (WHO and UNICEF 2008; cited in Haté and Gannon 2010). A joint report by WHO and UNICEF (2010) shows that 74 percent of the people in South Asia are deprived of standard sanitation facilities. In India, the problem is higher than in other South Asian countries. The majority of rural people in some states of India still prefer to defecate in open places.

As a result, some fatal illnesses—diarrhea, for example—are commonly perceived in those areas. In India, 386,000 people die from diarrhea every year; in Pakistan, 53,300; and in Bangladesh, 50,800 (WHO and UNICEF 2009; cited in Haté and Gannon 2010).

It is evident that the South Asian health-care system, as a whole, is just a nominal health-care system. There are not enough hospitals, doctors, medical staff, medicines, or ambulance services available in the system. Quality of care and accessibility to health-care facilities seem very poor. Many people depend on private hospitals for health care—except the poor, who depend on government hospitals because they cannot afford the costs of private hospitals and medication. Both public and private hospitals—and health-care agencies in general—have many limitations in terms of management and the delivery of services to the patient. All these countries rank at the bottom of the list on health-care facilities, especially when compared to Organization for Economic Co-operation and Development (OECD) or Brazil, Russia, India, China, and South Africa (BRICS) countries. Therefore, the governments of South Asian countries are bound to face a lot of criticism on their limited understanding of what universal health care really means and, on their failure, to increase public expenditure on health-care facilities.

6. The Role of Islamic Faith-Based Organizations in the Promotion of Health-Care Facilities in Bangladesh

Bangladesh is a poor country with a small area containing a huge number of people. With that, the country's inefficient administration, and the amount of mugging that occurs, people cannot effectively manage to solve the country's problems. However, as a member country of the UN, the Bangladesh government is morally committed to take care of the people in terms of health-care facilities, despite its relative poverty and the present inefficiency of its public health-care service. Many health-care agencies, government-owned organizations, private organizations, and nongovernment organizations are indeed working in the public health promotion, but they do so rather separately. Some faith-based organizations—for example, Christian Medical Association, Association of Bangladesh Catholic Doctors, Ayachak Ashrama Medical Service, Anjuman Mufidul Islam, Islamic Relief Bangladesh, Islami Bank Foundation, and Ibn Sina Trust—are also contributing to meet the challenges of health acuity. Of Islamic faith-based organizations in particular, we should have a look at Anjuman Mufidul Islam, Islamic Relief Bangladesh, and Masjid Council for Community Advancement (MACCA), trying to get some ideas on how these organizations work for the promotion of public health.

Anjuman Mufidul Islam is the oldest charity organization in the undivided Bengal. It was established in Kolkata, West Bengal, India, in 1905. Then it was transferred to Dhaka in 1947, after the country became independent of British India. At the outset, the organization has been undertaking humanitarian activities with the spirit of Islamic religious beliefs and practices. Of its objectives, three (7–9) are directly related to health care and health-servicing activities. These are (7) to provide medical assistance to patients irrespective of their religious beliefs, (8) to carry and bury unclaimed corpses, and (9) to provide free ambulance service to the poor patients (Dey 2003). Notably, its most important activity, for which it is famous in the country, is to bury unclaimed Muslim dead bodies. Anjuman Mufidul Islam works across the whole country through its affiliated branches in forty-three districts (Kashem 2014). The organization got the Independence Day Award in 1996 and Islamic Foundation Award in 1984 as a recognition of its outstanding service to the people in distress. Its sources of income mostly come from public and private donations.

Since 1991, Islamic Relief[8] has been working in Bangladesh with emergency reliefs, essential medicines, and primary health care. It works in thirty-seven districts of the country, providing access to health-care facilities and medication. Its programs deal with livelihoods, food security, health and nutrition, water and sanitation, education, disaster risk reduction, climate change adaptation, and so on. Thus Islamic Relief aims to improve public health and the nutritional status of the poor through increasing access to health-care services, nutritional facilities, and improving knowledge on health and hygiene awareness. Its health and nutrition programs include providing supplementary nutrition, medication, and mobile health care (health and eye clinics) and carrying out health and hygiene training. The program mainly extends preventive awareness interventions among the community.

8 Islamic Relief is a worldwide humanitarian and development organization. Being founded in 1984 in Birmingham, UK, it is working now in forty-four countries for most vulnerable people. Inspired by Islamic values in terms of health, it supports suffering people. For details, see Islamic Relief Bangladesh (2018, "About Us").

For a medical emergency case, it has formed a medical emergency team, which it sends to the affected areas to provide emergency medical support. It also provides fortified blended food items to the vulnerable community people to enable them to meet sufficient nutrition. Since the delivery of these programs, particular attention has been paid to vulnerable women and children (Islamic Relief Bangladesh 2018, "Health and Nutrition").

MACCA[9] is a faith-based development, humanitarian, and campaigning organization. It works for human health, food security, sustainable development, and communal harmony. It aims to overcome people's vulnerability and sufferings in terms of health. Since its inception in 1999, MACCA has been working to make an egalitarian society true by reducing malnutrition and major health problems.

7. Conclusion and Recommending Remarks

The preceding discussion shows that Islamic faith is a supporting factor for health and welfare. Many verses of the Holy Qur'an and the prophetic tradition emphasize the importance of public health and health-care services. In Islam, health is seen as one of the fundamental human rights: accordingly, Muslim people are advised to keep their health good, and at the same time, the rich and responsible Muslims, when they are in state power or individually capable, are encouraged to take care of the people who are not able to bear the cost of their own treatments. Such a combined approach is always highly encouraged in Islam. To some extent, when the health-care service is essential for the needy, Islam imposes an obligation upon the capable people and rulers to provide the minimum required service to those ones.

In this present world, international organizations like WHO and UNICEF are working for the promotion of public health across the world. For this noble purpose, these organizations are allocating huge funds to the developing, underdeveloped, and poor countries to improve their public health sectors. But in spite of these initiatives, public health has not achieved the kind of satisfactory improvement as it should. Where South Asian countries are concerned, there has been a slight improvement in public health. Among these countries, Bangladesh is not at a

---

9 MACCA was established in 1999 in Dhaka as a local faith-based organization. For details, see Macca (2018).

satisfactory level either. With the limited wealth of the country and insufficient support from donor agencies, the government of Bangladesh cannot manage to improve its public health sector. On the other hand, the country's dishonest and corrupt administration and inefficient system are misusing and abusing the amount allocated for public health. Therefore, the public health agencies, government hospitals, and government-sponsored health-service institutes are failing to play their proper role in this essential sector. In addition, there is a tremendous demand for health service in Bangladesh; consequently, taking this opportunity as a profitable business, many private entrepreneurs are on the timeline to run highly specialized and equipped hospitals for earning money from the rich patients, while the poor and middle-class patients cannot afford to go there. However, due to the failure of public health agencies and the untouchable costs of privately owned hospitals and health services, some faith-based organizations have gone ahead with their serving mentality, benefiting people of all classes through offering some basic categories of health services at reasonable prices and sometimes free of cost.

For the greater interest of health care and the well-being of the common people, however, there is an urgent need for holistic initiatives to ensure affordable health service for the poor in Bangladesh. At the very least, all the ongoing health-service agencies should keep "service to humanity" before any other things. The privately owned hospitals and health-care providers should lower their price and extend their helping hands to the poor patients. In this regard, the ministry of health of this country should monitor all these highly costed private hospitals regularly and bring the hospitals and diagnosis centers under control by a regulatory system. Presently, people with low income and the poor are deprived of the access to health-care facilities at a reasonable price. Public health agencies should thus provide fairness and transparency in terms of financial affairs, and physicians should prefer the quality of health service—and should prefer it over their expected earned income. At the same time, those faith-based hospitals and health-service-providing organizations that are already involved in the promotion of public health should be provided subsidiary and other financial supports from both the government and donor organizations to quickly improve the unpleasant situation that de facto prevails in the public health in Bangladesh. If all such considerations are taken properly into account, this country may be able to meet the acute health problems of its people and thereby to provide the other South Asian countries a truly impressive example.

References

Al-Hilali, Muhammad Taqi-ud-Din, and Muhammad Muhsin Khan. AH 1420. *The Noble Qur'an* (English Translation of the Meanings and Commentary). Madinah, Kingdom of Saudi Arabia: King Fahd Complex for the Printing of the Holy Qur'an.

Al-Jauziyah, Imam Ibn Qayyim. 2003. *Healing with the Medicine of the Prophet.* Translated by Jalal Abaul Rub. Edited by Abdul Rahman Abdullah and Raymond J. Manderola. Al-Mansoura, Egypt: Dar al-Ghadd Al-Gadeed.

Al-Khayat, Muhammad Haytham. 2004. *Health as a Human Right in Islam.* Cairo, Egypt: World Health Organization, Regional Office for the Eastern Mediterranean.

at-Tirmidhī, Abū 'Isā Muḥammad ibn 'Isā as-Sulamī aḍ-Ḍarīr al-Būghī. 2007. *Jami' at-Tirmidhi.* Translated by Abu Khaliyl. Edited by Hafiz Abu Tahir Zubair Ali Zai. Riyadh, Kingdom of Saudi Arabia: Darussalam. https://sunnah .com/tirmidhi/36/77.

De Leeuw, Evelyne. 1989. *Health Policy: An Exploratory Inquiry into the Development of Policy for the New Public Health in the Netherlands.* Maastricht: Savannah-Datawys.

De Leeuw, Evelyne, and Abdelmoneim Hussein. 1999. "Islamic Health Promotion and Interculturalization." *Health Promotion International* 14 (4): 347–353.

Dey, Sunil Kanti. 2003. "Anjuman-i-Mufidul Islam." In *Banglapedia: National Encyclopedia of Bangladesh*, edited by the board of editors (with Sirajul Islam as the chief editor). Dhaka: Asiatic Society of Bangladesh.

Donald, Peter, and V. P. Helden. 2009. "The Global Burden of Tuberculosis-Combating Drug Resistance in Different Times." *New England Journal of Medicine* 360:2393–2395. https://doi.org/10.1056/nejmp0903806.8.

Grad, Frank P. 2002. "The Preamble of the Constitution of the World Health Organization." *Bulletin of the World Health Organization* 80 (12): 981–982. https://tinyurl.com/y67483ue.

Haté, Vibhuti, and Seth Gannon. 2010. *Public Health in South Asia: A Report of the CSIS Global Health.* Washington, DC: Center for Strategic and International Studies (CSIS). Accessed October 28, 2019. https://tinyurl.com/y6e6m55e.

Hedayat, K. M., and Roya Pirzadeh. 2001. "Issues in Islamic Biomedical Ethics: A Primer for the Pediatrician." *Pediatrics.* https://doi.org/10.1542/peds .108.4.965.

Islamic Relief Bangladesh. 2018. Accessed March 27, 2018. http://islamicrelief
.org.bd.

Kashem, Kazi Abul. 2014. "Anjuman Mufidul Islam." In *Banglapedia: National Encyclopedia of Bangladesh*. Dhaka: Asiatic Society of Bangladesh.

Kasule, Omar Hasan K. 2008. "The Concept of Health: An Islamic Perspective." *Islamic Medical Education Resources* 5. http://omarkasule-05.tripod.com/id291.html.

Koenig, Harold G., and Saad Al Shohaib. 2014. *Health and Well-Being in Islamic Societies: Background, Research and Application*. Cham, Switzerland: Springer International.

Logghe, K. L. R. 1998. *De Verschillen Kun Je Neit Wegpoetsen* [You cannot eradicate the differences]. Tilburg, Netherlands: BOZ en Palet.

MacDonald, T. 1998. *Rethinking Health Promotion: A Global Approach*. London: Routledge.

Masjid Council for Community Advancement (MACCA). 2018. "About." Accessed October 12, 2018. http://www.masjidcouncil.bd.org.

McKennis, Ann T. 1999. "Caring for the Islamic Patient." *AORN Journal* 69 (6). http://dx.doi.org/10.1016/S0001-2092(06)61885-1.

National Aids Control Organization (NACC), Department of AIDS Control, Ministry of Health and Family Welfare, Government of India. 2010. *Annual Report, 2009–10*. https://tinyurl.com/y3t2amt9.

Population Reference Bureau. 2009. "HIV/AIDS Among Adult Population, Ages 15–49, 2007/2008 (%)." https://tinyurl.com/y6hvf3am.

Roberts, Dorothy. 2002. *Shattered Bonds: The Color of Child Welfare*. New York: Basic Boards.

Seedhouse, D. F. 1995. "The Way around Health Economics' Dead End." *Health Care Analysis* 3 (3): 205–220. https://doi.org/10.1007/BF02197670.

World Bank. 2012. "Feature Story on HIV/AIDS in Pakistan." https://tinyurl.com/y2fpe466.

World Health Organization (WHO). 1996. *Health Promotion through Islamic Lifestyles: The Amman Declaration*. Alexandria: WHO Regional Office for the Eastern Mediterranean. http://apps.who.int/iris/handle/10665/119558.

———. 2005. "Improving Maternal, Newborn and Child Health in South East Asia." http://apps.searo.who.int/pds_docs/b0263.pdf.

———. 2006. "Implemented GIVS Activities." May 12, 2006. https://tinyurl.com/yxbpuody.

———. n.d. "Regional and Country Specific Information Sheets: Impact of Chronic Disease in Countries." https://tinyurl.com/y42kyfvv.

World Health Organization (WHO) and UNICEF. 2008. "A Snapshot of Sanitation in SACOSAN Countries." https://tinyurl.com/yylnd5mj.

———. 2009. "Diarrhea: Why Children Are Still Dying and What Can Be Done."
https://tinyurl.com/y675wq3p.

———. 2010. "Progress on Sanitation and Drinking Water." http://www.unicef
.org/eapro/JMP-2010Final.pdf.

World Health Statistics. 2009. "General Government Expenditure on Health as %
of Total: Expenditure on Health." https://tinyurl.com/r6hq5c.

8

Healing and Salvation

THE RELATION OF HEALTH AND RELIGION
IN THE CONTEXT OF CHRISTIANITY

Thomas Renkert

ABSTRACT

Health and religion exist in multiple dimensions. They are, at the same time, global as well as local contextual phenomena impacting societies on various levels. They are matters of cultural norms, policies, and markets. They are institutionally organized yet at the same time associated with profoundly personal, existential experiences. Moreover, both concepts share common historical as well as linguistic or even anthropological determinants, which make it necessary to explore their relationship. However, the link between health and religion cannot simply be understood as a static concept: health only becomes noticeable within and through the dynamics of its loss and recovery, and the continuity or volatility of practiced religiosity is often fundamentally connected to personal well-being. Thus in the case of Christianity, the question is how the dynamic relationship between processes of healing and salvation is to be understood. I give an overview of the biblical account on this question and try to sketch a preliminary typology of possible interpretations against this background. In a final step, I draw some conclusions for a systematic-theological approach to health and its global implications.

1. Introduction

It is easier to talk about illness and disease than about health. The reason for this lies in our intuition to use and understand these words as diametrical opposites in everyday language. The terms *health* and *disease* seem to mutually exclude each other in an ontological sense. Yet semantically, they both appear to be located on the same plane of discourse: being healthy means not being ill and vice versa. If we look, however, at the different experiences associated with these concepts, a striking qualitative difference occurs. Whereas a sick person consciously experiences their body and its individual organs as fragile and finite, a sound person, ordinarily, does not experience their body in the same way. In fact, usually they do not experience their body in a conscious way at all. We only become aware of our bodies when and where they fail to function normally, where we are suddenly (i.e., through an accident or a disease) or slowly (i.e., by the natural process of aging) unable to live our lives without having to dedicate a fair amount of time to our growing list of physical or mental limitations or frailties.

The philosopher Hans-Georg Gadamer (1996) called this the "enigmatic character of health" (103–16). Health as an existential phenomenon is hidden from consciousness and only ever becomes visible and manifest in contrast to sickness. Conversely, individual beliefs, forms of personal or communal religiosity, as well as socioreligious macrocontexts form an "invisible determinant" (Eidler 2014) of health.[1]

In this chapter, I want to trace some of the vague and concrete, closer or looser ties between health and religion. This chapter is divided into three parts: I will start by discussing the multiple dimensions of health (1) and its similarities to and common history with religion, especially Christianity (2). Here, I will look at possible systematic and biblical reconstructions of the relationship between healing and salvation. A brief glance at the current challenges of health on a global scale will conclude this chapter (3).

2. Dimensions of Health

We begin with the question of how health should be defined. Starting from the definition of health proposed by the World Health Organization

---

1 For a deeper discourse on the theories of health, I would like to recommend the already somewhat classic works by Boorse (1977), Nordenfelt (2007), and Whitbeck (1981).

(WHO) in 1946, we focus on three different dimensions of the concept of health: the scientific, the existential, and the sociocultural.

2.1. The WHO Definition

The often criticized (cf., for instance, Jadad and O'Grady [2008], Larson [1999], and Moltmann [1985]) WHO definition of health as "a state of complete physical, mental and social well-being and not merely the absence of disease or infirmity"[2] introduces a central element into the debate on health and illness.[3] Instead of viewing health as an isolated, purely medical or physical/somatic state, it emphasizes the broader context of health, including its mental, social, and—by extension—even economical, political, ecological, and cultural dimensions. This correlates with the fact that a person's experience of health and well-being or disease and infirmity is in large part shaped by factors that lie beyond the limits of their own body or their sphere of influence. But this experience depends, at the same time, on the internal perspective of the (self-)observer. Specific diseases are usually and primarily described and defined as biological and thereby ontological statements (e.g., the description of pathogenic causal pathways or the probabilistic expectations of any therapy), which does not necessarily correspond to the (self-)experience of the patient. This perception gap also exists in the concept of health. And it also does not apply only to individuals: the perception and self-perception of health and illness across different nations and cultures are empirically measurable and show enormous differences, which correlate only marginally with the "objective" or biological de facto health status of members of these societies.[4]

But as the WHO definition implies, this argument can also be inverted. The direct ontological antithesis of "disease or infirmity" is, in fact, the absence of any disease, which is not identical with the existential experience of "complete ... well-being." Diseases or disabilities are similarly not just "the absence of" such well-being but much more manifest, concrete,

---

2 Preamble to the Constitution of the World Health Organization as adopted by the International Health Conference, New York, June 19–22, 1946; signed on July 22, 1946, by the representatives of sixty-one states (Official Records of the World Health Organization, no. 2, 100) and entered into force on April 7, 1948.

3 For a more nuanced discussion, see Callahan (1973).

4 Cf. McCracken and Philipps (2012) on the implications of cultural contexts for health surveys.

and consequence-laden phenomena, yet again not necessarily directly correlated with perceived states of well-being or "unwell-being."[5]

The WHO definition of health, therefore, reveals the—in various ways—complex asymmetrical relationship of the terms *health* and *disease* as well as the interdependence of subjective, intersubjective, and contextual factors, either within or beyond the control of the individual person. It encompasses the multitude of dimensions in which health exists as a biological, existential, and social phenomenon.

2.2. The Scientific Dimension

The WHO definition of health states that health is *more* than the "absence of disease." This, however, implies that health is *also* exactly this: the absence of illness. Within the scientific-biological model, health can be viewed as the normal state of any functioning organism, whereas disease constitutes a deviation from this norm, an anomaly. It is debatable as to what constitutes this biologically normal state of a healthy organism and what counts as possible aberrations, as one can arrive at different definitions depending on the methodology used. Statistical average values, specified standards of performance, and the use of indicators for the quality of life all lead to different definitions of health norms and, consequently, to profound variations of our understanding of disease, some of which may even be incompatible with each other (cf. Schockenhoff 2013, 302).[6]

Already within the scientific-biological dimension, where we would most likely expect a higher level of objectivity, health and disease are not fixed antithetic values but points on a continuum with complex dynamics of transitions between both states. There exists, for instance, a genetic variation that causes sickle cell anemia while—at the same time—making the carrier less susceptible to malaria. This genetic infirmity is especially common in malaria-endemic areas around the globe.[7]

---

5 There are, of course, a large number of psychological or neurological cases where the distinction between the objective and the subjective seems to stop working altogether. One stark but illustrative example is body integrity identity disorder (BIID), where fully functional limbs are subjectively perceived as irritations and threats to the integrity of the body as a whole. People affected by BIID experience themselves as ill or disabled despite being objectively healthy. Cf. Smith (2004).

6 This problem becomes even more prevalent if we look at health on the level of populations. Here, complex empirical indicators are needed to make observation data from vastly different settings comparable. For an overview, cf. Gold et al. (2002).

7 Cf., for instance, Aidoo et al. (2002).

There are similar cases illustrating the notion of health as a negotiation between advantageous and detrimental properties that influences the scientific definition of "ill" and "healthy." Other factors for possible consideration are, for example, whether or not a deviation from the biological norm (Boyd 2000, 10) is temporary or permanent, whether or not the organism is able to tolerate the irritation and restore a healthy balance on its own, and so on. What all these approaches have in common is the underlying notion of a "dynamic equilibrium" (Schockenhoff 2013, 303–4) of beneficial and detrimental factors in which organisms exist. Depending on the chosen frame of reference, organisms can be viewed as more or less able to achieve or maintain this balance between positive and negative factors. But this notion of health as a dynamic equilibrium also implies that an organism is never either *completely* healthy or *completely* ill; rather, these labels are used once certain limit values are exceeded or the context of observation changes. When an organism can no longer sustain this equilibrium on its own and within a certain context, when it loses the ability to adapt to change and cope with negative influences, the need for medical intervention rises.

2.3. The Existential[8] Dimension

Time and again during the nineteenth and twentieth centuries, more holistic notions of health and medicine that overcome the mechanical-somatic perspective of established science have been demanded from different alternative schools of thought. Although the commonalities between these different concepts of alternative medicine are rather small, they all—unlike conventional medicine—share the notion that the focus of therapeutic attention has to lie on the individual patient as a whole, instead of the deficiency-oriented approach of curative therapy, in order to get to the most fundamental causes of a disease and to restore health and well-being in a more comprehensive sense.[9]

---

8 We could also call this the "anthropological" or "biographical" dimension. For a number of reasons, I think that "existential" fits here best.

9 It is important to note that the different approaches grouped under the heading "alternative medicine" are respectively based on very different levels of scientific evidence. And while some can probably be taken seriously, a large number of them should be classified either as empirically unsubstantiated pseudomedicine or as (quasi-)religious ideologies. Sometimes, these "alternatives" also entail political dimensions. Some people within the growing group of "Reichsbürger" ("sovereign citizens") in Germany, for instance, practice a form of "Germanic medicine," a mixture of cultural myths with pseudoscience, pseudoreligion, and political demands. Cf. Hardinghaus (2016).

These models rely on anthropological-existential premises that assert that diseases have to be viewed as effects of more fundamental causes of underlying factors (e.g., somatic, psychological, social, and biographical), which cannot be treated independently from each other and, therefore, necessitate a holistic approach of the individual person in its totality.[10]

From this point of view, health is the ability to successfully cope with irritations as part of one's life, to act independently despite sickness, disability, and frailty. The goal here is to preserve a sense of existential coherence and to reestablish your own experiences of health and sickness as meaningful. Of course, this experience of meaning cannot be isolated from the social and cultural context in which it is embedded.

2.4. The Sociocultural Dimension

From a sociological perspective, the health status of the individual can be understood as the person's ability to adequately fulfill her role within society (e.g., as an employee, parent, volunteer, and so on). Immanuel Kant thus defined health as the ability to "transact certain public business" (Kant 1996, 326)—that is, to live a "civil existence" (326) within a public setting determined by economic, political, and religious processes and roles. In turn, the subjectively experienced well-being of a person strongly correlates with her social status and the quality of her relationships—her "social capital"—in the form of family ties and romantic relationships, employment and workplace satisfaction, and friends and neighborhood ties as well as social engagement, religious affiliations, and worldviews (Helliwell and Putnam 2004, 1444). It is no wonder, then, that health—similar to societies where public and practiced religiosity is a vital concept—directly and indirectly denotes social status and thus can promote social stratification (Lahelma 2001).

The social dimension of health also extends to health as a collective phenomenon located on the social level—for instance, as the public health of a population or a certain subgroup. A healthy population is, in turn, a prerequisite for functioning institutions, political representation,

---

10 Another major difference to established medicine is that many holistic perspectives do not focus on therapeutic interventions once the patient themself experiences their sickness but begin at a much earlier stage. To move the focus away from the established medical paradigm of searching for the cause of an illness (pathogenesis), Aaron Antonovsky has developed the theory of *salutogenesis* (Antonovsky 1987), an approach concerned with promoting health independent of manifest diseases, which has gained some traction over recent decades.

and social systems, as Talcott Parsons (1964, 274) defines health "as the state of optimum capacity of an individual for the effective performance of the roles and tasks for which he has been socialized."[11]

And Stella Quah (2014) points out that even these roles are socially coded on a spectrum of "healthy," "sick," and "ill" according to the specific sociocultural context in which they are being performed. In this perspective, the notions of individual as well as public health become more and more politically charged.[12]

Moreover, health and disease as concepts, apart from their implications for functioning social roles, depend strongly on their respective cultural contexts and are shaped by a culture's norms and values. To give just one example from the area of dietary differences, certain phenomena of substance abuse and addiction seem to correlate with the majority religion of a given country.[13] Similarly, the cultural salient images of youth and old age, or masculinity and femininity, can influence the health-related behavior of these social groups. But fashion can also play a role: there have even been instances where the cultural settings rendered illnesses as something worthwhile.[14] Thus health is a socially normative concept that depends on and shapes the culture it exists in.

For the present cultural situation, some thinkers argue that Western culture has replaced religious values (at least in some instances) with a veneration of health as the supreme value of human life. This shift from health as a means for a meaningful life to health as an end in itself becomes manifest in current trends of medicalization (Conrad 2008), self-tracking, and a paradigm where health has become ideologically charged. This development has been coined "healthism" (Crawford 1980). With the advent of medical big-data research and constant (self-)monitoring of human behavior, we are in the midst of a significant paradigm shift. The latent and manifest medicalization of up to now nonpathological, everyday phenomena will become our "new normal" in the near future. And as Yuval Harari (2017) and others claim, this trend will result in a maximized longevity or virtual immortality, which are goals of obvious quasi-religious character.

---

11 In this perspective, the existential and, perhaps, even the scientific dimensions are largely ignored in favor of a purely functional argument.

12 Cf. Schramme (2017).

13 As with many aspects of the empirical study of religion, it is difficult to get good quantitative data. As Kalema et al. (2016) show, premature conclusions might be unwarranted.

14 In her book *Illness as Metaphor*, Susan Sontag (2002) argues that within literary circles in the nineteenth century, tuberculosis as a disease had positive connotations (26–36). She writes, "It was glamorous to look sickly" (28).

The three dimensions of health outlined here primarily demonstrate their incompleteness. Health as a comprehensive conception only seems to come into focus one aspect at a time—our definition thus has to remain fragmentary for the time being.

3. Health and Religion

A growing number of recent studies suggest multiple correlations between well-being and personal religiosity as well as the overall health of a population. And although this scientific interest in the relationship between religion and health is not a new development,[15] a majority of the causal factors are still not well understood. Research in this area focuses on the underlying somatic or psychological functions of religiosity or spirituality for the health of the individual person and has lately become more important, as L. M. Chatters (2000, 336) asserts: "Whereas religion and health were once considered marginal to serious scientific inquiry, they are currently enjoying an unprecedented level of research interest and prominence."[16]

In the *Handbook of Religion and Health*, after evaluating more than twelve hundred studies, Koenig, King, and Carson (2012, 591) draw the conclusion that "in the vast majority of the [studies], religious beliefs and practices rooted within established religious traditions were found to be consistently associated with better health and predicted better health over time," but more modest perspectives exist as well (63–77, esp. 74).[17] Nevertheless, it is imperative to emphasize that the possible negative effects of religion on health issues have been researched less extensively compared to its positive effects.[18]

It is possible that we are dealing with forms of bias caused by our intuitive associations of "health" and "religion" with individual and personal phenomena. The effects of religions within social contexts—for example, on norms and policies regarding reproductive health and

---

15 Cf. the excellent overview provided by Chatters (2000).
16 Cf. also Utsch and Klein (2011, 25–26).
17 Cf. also Zwingmann et al. (2011).
18 Measuring religiosity and the content of beliefs is in itself highly debated; see Hall et al. (2008).

bioethics,[19] hygiene customs, fasting, and burial[20] rites, as well as the social acceptance of mental health issues or the faith-based provision of health services—as a determinant of public health are much less researched in comparison to the individual dimension.

Focusing on the dynamic notions of healing and salvation rather than the static terms *health* and *religion*, I want to explore their interrelations within the context of Christianity.

3.1. Healing and Salvation in Christianity

The Role of Language

The close historical linkage between health and religion is already tangible when we compare the respective semantic fields. In German, the nouns *Heilung* ("healing") and *Heiligung* ("sanctification") are both related to the noun *Heil* ("wholeness," "hail") and the verb *heilen* ("to heal, cure"), which all come from a proto-Germanic adjective *haila-* ("whole, sound"; Kroonen 2013). These terms are related to the possible proto-Indo-European root **slH-u-*, which is also present in the Greek ὅλος ("whole, perfect, complete"), and the Latin *salus* ("health, salvation"), *salvus* ("save, sound, healthy"), and *salvatio*, from which of course the English words *salvation* and *salubrious* ("wholesome") but also *solid* and others can be derived.[21] This is only a very small sample of the manifold interrelations that exist already on an etymological level that point back at a much closer historical connection between two concepts that have grown apart over time.

The underlying idea connecting health and religion on a linguistic level is the notion of wholeness, soundness, completeness, and thus harmony. The restoration or preservation of this wholeness seems to be the common denominator of both "coping strategies": therapeutic intervention and spiritual sensemaking.[22] The theologian Paul Tillich

---

19 The fundamental changes in the public opinion on prostitution, the status of unborn life, and the rights of children and the duties of fathers were the reasons for the appeal of Christianity to the society of the Roman Empire, as Markschies (2016, 245–46) points out.

20 K. Marshall and S. Smith (2015), for instance, point out the necessity to adapt religious funeral customs to prevent future Ebola outbreaks.

21 For further reading on the etymological roots within the context of health in Indo-European languages, cf. Mallory and Adams (1997, 262, 357–77).

22 Cf. also Sharf and Vanderford (2003) and Luhmann (2013).

(1984, 17) writes, "Salvation is basically and essentially healing, the re-establishment of a whole that was broken, disrupted, disintegrated."

If salvation is "essentially healing," can Christianity as a whole be called a "religion of healing" or just "health spiritualized"?

Healing and Salvation in the Early Church

Church historian Adolf von Harnack ascribed the success of early Christianity to its characteristics as a "religion of healing" or a "medical religion," which set it apart from competing cults, religions, or worldviews and subsequently promoted its expansion in antiquity. The promise of wholeness and well-being in a somatic and psychological but also spiritual sense was the reason Christianity appealed to a "world addicted to healing."[23] Christianity decoupled the prospect of health and healing from purely functional cultic rites and normative traditions and put it in the much larger context of its individual and collective framework of eschatological hope. The main difference between ancient medical cults and Christianity thus lies in the way the latter viewed those that were superficially healthy: in the Christian worldview, no human being is completely free of sin, and therefore no one is totally sound and whole in a holistic sense of physical and spiritual health. What early Christianity had to offer besides rituals and rudimentary institutional care was the person of a *soter*, a savior, together with his work and sermon, which culminated in a new concept of life, promising immortality (Harnack 1892, 96).

The view on Christ as a healer or "heavenly physician"[24] (Origen 1990, 153) was clearly the predominant one in the early church. But over time, notions of spiritual "healing" became more and more dominant and understood as the deliverance from sin. Together with the development of rational medicine in Greek philosophy and the prevalence of Platonist ideas, this marks the beginning of a fundamental paradigm of European thought where physical health and spiritual salvation are seen as increasingly separate concepts. This dualism was reinforced by (for instance) Descartes's distinction between body and mind and became consolidated during the Enlightenment and by the rise of the natural sciences.

---

23 I refer to Harnack primarily as an illustration. For a more differentiated discussion of the reasons for Christianity's success in antiquity, see Markschies (2016, 215–50).
24 Homily on Leviticus 8.

And although organized care for the sick has always been a part of Christianity, a more exhaustive, comprehensive, and professional provision of health care and social services only takes shape during the nineteenth century in the development of diakonia and caritas in progressively industrialized Europe and the delegation of the first specifically medical missionaries to India, China, and Africa. Within the nineteenth and twentieth centuries, the emergence of Pentecostalism and the charismatic movement reintroduced the idea of supernatural healing as a form of divine intervention as a more prominent belief and practice (cf. Williams 2013). But the established churches also increased their theological and practical work on global issues of health and healing, starting—on the Protestant side—with the Tübingen consultations and the resulting Tübingen I declaration in 1964 as well as the founding of the Christian Medical Commission (CMC) in 1968 (cf. McGilvray 1981, 60–76).

To which degree can these different developments of the association between healing and salvation be traced back to the biblical traditions? And could a systematic reconstruction provide further insights?

Healing and Salvation: The Biblical Account

The Bible is sympathetic toward those who suffer from sickness. And although the biblical authors discuss the interdependencies between religious practice and personal or collective well-being, they have quite an integrated view on healing and salvation. Even where the Bible distinguishes between physical healing and spiritual salvation, both concepts are interrelated in complex ways.

In the Old Testament, sickness is seen as a deprivation of vitality and entails a possible isolation from social contexts. Laments of sickness and the experience of recovery are common themes in the prayers of the Old Testament (cf. Psalms 30, 38, 41, 116). It is important to note that healing and salvation (or redemption, deliverance) as well as sickness are viewed as God's actions (Deut 32:39; Job 5:18; 1 Sam 2:6).

A too-narrow causative interpretation of this concept is famously problematized in the book of Job, where a virtuous man suffers from a devastating sickness for apparently no reason.

The New Testament emphasizes the problems of any simple identification of salvation and healing (cf. John 9:2–3). Miraculous healings are instead viewed as *signs* of the near salvation of mankind and the whole of creation in God's kingdom. Jesus of Nazareth's healing ministry is a sign of the closeness of God's kingdom (cf. Luke 11:20), and the disciples are as witnesses explicitly instructed to follow this example (Matt 10:8), which was taken seriously by the early congregations (Jas 5:14).

Within the New Testament, the meaning of wholeness is not the absence of illness, frailty, or disability but being an integral part, a member, of the community of Christ's disciples in spite of sickness or infirmity (Luke 4:17–19; John 9:1–3; Rom 15:7). Because of their communion with God, this community is *able* rather than *obligated* to follow the example of Jesus and show solidarity toward those who suffer in life.

Models of Healing and Salvation: A First Attempt at a Typology

Despite—or because of—the increasing secularization in many of the more prosperous parts of the world, a close connection between health and religious or spiritual ideas is anything but gone. Health has the status of an ultimate value, thereby influencing everyday decision-making, lifestyles, and worldviews as a whole. Through this development, the idea of healing has gained salvific functions.

Is it possible to draft a uniform typology of the relationship of healing and salvation, combining these different models? P. Dabrock (2006) has suggested such a preliminary typology that operates with four possible relations: (1) healing through salvation, (2) salvation through healing, (3) healing as salvation, and (4) salvation as healing. These models are located on the same spectrum: its end points are marked by the concepts of 3 and 4, while the concepts of 1 and 2 describe more centered, moderate forms of this relationship.

1. Healing through salvation

    Healing through salvation means that religion is seen as a vehicle for well-being. The theurgic work of faith healers or congregations praying for their sick members are possible forms of this model, where health status and spiritual/religious status are inextricably linked.

    In a more pronounced interpretation, the notion of healing through salvation implies a direct causal chain between a person's religious "capital" and his biological or financial well-being.

2. Salvation through healing

    Salvation through healing is Dabrock's inversion of the first model. A moderate form of salvation through healing exists in the form of religious engagement for society as a whole—for example, in the provision of health services or in communities where care for a healthy body is viewed as a form of divine service. Here, the idea of salvation accompanies the healing practices or constitutes their foundation.

The ends of the spectrum for this type can be formulated as *healing instead of salvation* (model 3), where health is an end in itself and can provide quasi-religious meaning.[25]

3, 4. Healing as salvation; salvation as healing

In their most extreme forms, models 1 (*healing through salvation*) and 2 (*salvation through healing*) take the form of models 3 (*healing as salvation*) and 4 (*salvation as healing*). In both cases, the existential tension between the physical and the spiritual dimensions is eliminated by the adoption of a dichotomous worldview. For model 3, physical healing is already "salvation," which it therefore replaces or conflates. For model 4, the reliance on secular medicine is viewed as lack of faith.

Though his typology represents a good starting point, it remains unclear what Dabrock actually means by the phrasing "through" and "as"—for example, in "healing through salvation" or "salvation as healing." In what follows, I will modify and broaden Dabrock's four models.

Nine Models

We can imagine a number of possible interpretations, but in my opinion, the most important ones would be causal and epistemological interpretations, where health "causes" salvation (or vice versa) and health "indicates" salvation (or vice versa). Similarly, it seems logical to interpret the word "as" as denoting equivalence: health "is identical with" salvation. This identification promotes the view of one concept superseding or replacing the other because they are seen as identical, which is also a possible interpretation implied in Dabrock's typology.

This means that we now have doubled our scope of possible interpretations, opening up the space for further differentiation. If we add the more cautious biblical perspectives of an unclear, complex, or mostly nonexistent link between healing and salvation, we can distinguish at least nine fundamental models.

To outline these models, I will use the following abbreviations: model (M), healing (H), salvation (S), "causes" ($\Rightarrow$), "indicates" ($\rightarrow$), "is equivalent to" ($\equiv$, where both concepts are identical), and "replaces/

25 Cf. "healthism," mentioned earlier.

supersedes" ($\Leftrightarrow$, where one concept replaces the other). This set is extended by the abbreviations "are (somehow) correlated" ($\approx$) and "are not correlated at all" ($\parallel$).[26]

These nine models are only a preliminary draft of how possible relationships between healing and salvation can be understood. Especially M1, M2, and M5 should be broken down further to elucidate the possible interpretations of the epistemological arrow. This provisional typology primarily tries to clarify Dabrock's suggestion by using M1–M4 and

Basic models on the relationship between healing and salvation.

Model		Interpretation
M1	$S \Rightarrow H$; therefore, $H \rightarrow S$	Salvation causes healing, healing indicates religious status, "syllogismus practicus," "health and wealth gospel"
M2	$H \Rightarrow S$; therefore, $S \rightarrow H$	Healing causes salvation, salvation indicates healing, "healthism," individual well-being as an indicator of social status
M3	$H \equiv S$; *but not* therefore, $H \Leftrightarrow S$	Holistic view on healing and salvation, but no replacement of one concept with the other
M4	$H \equiv S$; therefore, $H \Leftrightarrow S$	Scientist or fundamentalist view: one concept replaces the other completely
M5	$\neg S \Rightarrow \neg H$; therefore, $\neg H \rightarrow \neg S$	Sin and punishment, bad health indicates a low religious status, inversion of M1
M6	$\neg H \Rightarrow S$	Suffering leads to God / enhances the spiritual status
M7	$H \approx S$; M1–M6	Healing and salvation are related; M1–M6 are possible options
M8	$H \approx S$; not reducible to M1–M6	Healing and salvation are related, but in more complex ways than M1–M6 suggest
M9	$H \parallel S$	Healing and salvation are not related at all, neither in an ontological sense nor in an existential one

26 Please note that these shortcuts are not meant to be understood as logical operators in the way they are being used in symbolic logic.

extending them with M5 and M6, which have been falling out of favor in Western religiosity but have had great impact historically and globally. M7 and M8 try to capture aspects of the biblical perspectives, which seem to run perpendicular to the idea of simple causative or epistemological pathways. Model M9 is also an important addition, capturing the modern sense that somatic health and spirituality either are located in completely different realms of reality or should be kept separate in order to avoid that patients overinterpret their disease in negative ways.

To get a fuller picture, we now turn to the metalevel abstractions from M1–M9. Because of the lack of space, we will (partly) explore only one possible abstraction, the individual dimension.

For our purposes, it is useful to extend this typology a little more and introduce two new abbreviations: "belief" (B) and "patient" (p). With these additions, we should be able to construct two hypotheses, H1 and H2, with a possible conclusion, or H3, that refers to M1–M9.

These three hypotheses make the point that M1–M9 are never to be viewed isolated from a person's own convictions, values, and worldviews. Of course, this is far from the whole picture. And one could easily imagine adding possible H4–Hn to H1–H3 in order to capture other contextual

Hypotheses

Hypothesis		Interpretation
H1	$B\,p(M1–M9) \approx B\,p(Hp \vee Sp)$	A patient's (p) personal belief about the general relation of health and salvation influences p's belief about his own health and religious status.
H2	$B\,p(Hp \vee Sp) \approx (Hp)$	A patient's (p) personal belief about p's health status influences p's observable health.
Conclusion: H3	$B\,p(M1–M9) \approx (Hp)$	A patient's (p) personal belief about the general relation of health and salvation influences p's observable health. This view combines epistemic, ontological, and causal aspects.[*]

* There are some similarities to the proposal of a "sobjectivist" model by A. K. MacLeod (2015).

factors like social ties, cultural values, administrative institutions, and other determinants that not only inform p's B but also have direct and indirect influence on p's health status (e.g., religiously motivated social inclusion, health services, care ethos, empathy,[27] and so on). Due to the constraints of space and time, we cannot present a fully developed typology here, but I'd like to at least emphasize the importance of extending and modifying these sets of factors within contexts of disability and mental health.

Nonetheless, these relationships between individual convictions and cultural norms should be taken seriously, especially from a theological point of view.[28]

And another important distinction should be introduced, which is also only implicitly mentioned in Dabrock's proposal: my/our own perceived health/healing and salvation and that of others. If we want to be able to talk about beneficial and detrimental forms of relationships between healing and salvation, we'll have to make clear *whose* health and salvation we are talking about and how they are linked. While I might not be able to see my own illness in relation to my beliefs, the doctors who cure me might see my health as their religious responsibility and so on.

Already the models M1 and M2, for instance, are only intelligible when we distinguish between at least two actor-centric perspectives. Without this differentiation, (transnational and intercultural) health care in a public, social setting cannot be grasped by our typology. However, it is also important to note that these socio-cultural frameworks are constantly shifting. With the COVID-19 pandemic we are currently experiencing massive and rapid shifts on a global scale ranging from individual behaviour to global policy making that also tremendously effect faith communities and religious institutions.

3.2. A Systematic-Theological Interpretation of Healing and Salvation

With these fields of tension in mind, we are now able to draw further conclusions from our typology:

---

27 These factors play a big role for the structure and function of welfare regimes and the implementation of health-care services, despite or because of their invisibility. Just to give one example, U. Körtner (2010) discusses the benefits and disadvantages of the Christian concept of mercy within the modern health-care sector—a discussion that we will need to have again very soon, but adapted to a global perspective.

28 With regard to disability, cf. especially Eiesland 1994, Bach 2006, and Betcher 2007.

Any theological approach toward the relationship of healing and salvation should start with the hypotheses H1–H3 and their cultural embeddedness. Since the biblical traditions are cautiously hinting at models of the complex interrelatedness of healing and salvation, theological interpretations in line with models M8 and M9 should be taken seriously. Also, any such theology should be careful not to depart into the territory of M1–M6 all too quickly. Otherwise, theology runs the risk of offering naive and potentially cruel explanations for obviously complex phenomena, which can have profoundly problematic implications for the concepts of God and man. However, within contexts of counseling, it is unjustified to, for example, play off M7 against M9, because this would go against the potential coping strategies as expressed in H1–H3.

Theology has to take seriously the fact that a large number of biblical authors see a close connection between salvation and healing without, at least most of the time, further specifying the nature of this relationship (M8). The debate as such among the biblical texts explicitly suggests the lesson that we should abstain from reading a direct and simple causal chain into this untransparent relation. Sin does not necessarily lead to sickness, and salvation does not necessarily lead to healing in a physical sense. At the same time, the biblical evidence prevents us from favoring or retreating to only one of the models mentioned. This also applies to the use of M9 and every complete dissociation of both categories. For the bible, the relationship between healing and salvation cannot simply be defined in terms of implication, identification, or cause and effect—a fortiori, if we take the eschatological, and cosmological, perspective into account.

3.3. God, Community, and the Responsibility for Health

Our existence is limited, mortal, and therefore fragile. The ontological chances of illness, disability, suffering, and the fact of death apply to all life, which, in turn, poses enormous difficulties for Christian theology to speak of God as the benevolent and omnipotent creator. This problem of theodicy designates the need for God to prove that his creation is truly good (Gen 1:31) at the end of time, as Lutheran theologian Wolfhart Pannenberg (2004, 645) writes.[29] But other approaches exist as well.

---

29 "The kingdom of God will be actualized and the justification of God in the face of the sufferings of the world will be achieved but also universally acknowledged" (Pannenberg 2004, 645).

G. Thomas (2009), for instance, sees sickness and health as analogous to God's nature as a living God, which becomes manifest in the risk he takes with his creation and incarnation as well as in the nuanced work of the Holy Spirit. In Thomas's view, on the one hand, the very existence of creation poses a profound risk for its creatures and for God himself. On the other hand, the limitation and finitude of life are necessary risks to take in order for the chance of true freedom, autonomy, and development within creation. But as W. Pannenberg (1980, 151) points out, the need for finitude should not simply be identified with the need for death. For Pannenberg, sickness and death are not essential parts of human nature (Pannenberg 1980, 153), which is similar to Karl Barth's (2009) perspective on disease as "an element in the rebellion of chaos against God's creation" (363). If we read Barth's definition of health as the "strength for human life" (356) in combination with the idea of health as dynamic (healing), it becomes clear that this strength is not just a personal possession: it is the strength for the life of others, the strength of communities to care for those inside and outside. The notion of cocreativity of human beings in cooperation with God's will to overcome chaos (Gen 1:28) and to reduce the negative effects of the fundamental risk of creation points at the responsibility for humans to reduce suffering and enhance well-being in all domains. Therefore, the event of healing, not just static health, signifies the hope of the salvation and transformation of the whole cosmos, the eschatological overcoming of death.

The capability to influence seemingly natural processes is part of human cocreativity and autonomy and has become the defining characteristic of the Anthropocene in which we live. Ethically speaking, a person's capabilities correlate with her responsibility to help those who are less capable: strength for life is (also) strength for the life of others. This applies to and necessitates looking at the capabilities of social groups, communities, or societies[30] but also at the special responsibilities[31] of religious authorities.

---

30 It is disputable what kind of moral duties can follow from this approach. Do collectives, groups, nations, or humanity as a whole have ethical responsibilities for the health and well-being of others? With the inevitable shift of the topic of health to a more global perspective, this question becomes more and more pressing. Religious communities, churches, and the WCC are in the unique position to act according to their capabilities, but does that mean that they are morally obligated to do so? See Schwenkenbecher (2013) for an introduction to the debate.

31 For instance, C. Grundmann (2009) argues for a special responsibility of religious leaders in the context of HIV/AIDS, which is a view that gets adopted very hesitantly.

4. Outlook: The Task of Global Health

The picture the Bible paints of the relationship between healing and salvation is perpendicular to (1) our Western, scientistic approach, where healing and salvation are either completely separate or more or less identical concepts, and (2) our human intuition of a clear way in which one part affects the other and how religious or ersatz religious practices can be seen as methods to influence, shape, and control this connection.

The Bible, however, neither severs the link between healing and salvation nor views them as identical. Instead, the biblical traditions hint at the nonreducible complexity of this relationship, which is founded in creation as a fundamentally risky endeavor.

This complexity has no present solution but—as Christians hope—will have a future, eschatological one. In this future, the creator will (have to) reveal that the risks of harm, infirmity, frailty, and suffering are still outweighed by the benefits and opportunities of freedom, development, and life in a final, holistic, all-encompassing sense. Until then, the promotion of health within a fragile world lies at the core of the Christian mission because events of healing are early signs of this ultimate redemption, deliverance, and the hint at the kingdom of God coming to the poor, sick, and marginalized. Biblical theology thus views the community of the redeemed themselves as part of this ostensive movement, pointing at the eschatological state of peace and the victory of life.

In this sense, even the WHO definition of health is—at its core—an expression of eschatological hope, at least implicitly. The eschatological concept of a new creation implies a vision of wholeness and perfection of physical existence free from mortality and frailty. In this ultimate perspective, the categories of physical and spiritual coincide once again. To follow and modify P. Tillich, salvation *will be* healing and *healing will be* salvation.

But this hope is not an invitation to inaction. On the contrary, the capabilities of humans to transform their fate, their strength for life, implies a serious responsibility. This responsibility grows with every technological,[32] scientific, political, and theological advancement and has long reached the global scale. "Health" in all its dimensions is a more and more global issue with global implications for all religions.[33] Health

---

32 Cf., for instance, Jonas (1985) as an early example of ethics addressing global and future perspectives.
33 Cf. Brown (2014).

is also a dynamic act of sociopolitical and communal intentionality, a call to action, a practical negotiation between life and death, between contingency and capability. This global and dynamic nature of health has implications for our conceptions of health, as they, too, have to become much more dynamic, adaptable to an ever-changing present[34] but also aware of the wider context of globalization.

Recently, different proposals to promote global health justice and reduce inequality in global health have been made. Thomas Pogge's (2009) concept of a "Health Impact Fund" and Jennifer Ruger's (2009) idea of a "provincial cosmopolitanism"[35] as a way of linking national consensuses to moral responsibility on a global level are among the best known. The fact that the WHO takes on more and more responsibilities as an actor with regard to epidemics and public health (Hanrieder 2015) is also an apt example of how much health has become a global task. Cultures, markets, moral values, policies, and religions are all affected by this global dimension of health.

But in stark contrast to this development, the medical engagement of the World Council of Churches (WCC) has declined drastically since the 1990s. To address health and just health care on the global level, a sensitivity for and understanding of the ethical, cultural, and religious factors involved are indispensable. It is no coincidence that the health sciences work on these issues in increasingly interdisciplinary modes, since they have long realized that a purely medical approach does not suffice. With regard to recent global developments, S. H. E. Harmon (2015, 369–70) sees specific foundational social values as a central requirement for the just implementation of global health because medical progress and governance structures alone cannot guarantee the ethical commitment to global health justice. The churches, diakonia, and caritas as well as academic theology could contribute substantial insights and promote the discussion on global values and human rights, as they have in the past.[36] They are the institutions with the capacity to take H3 into account—especially within settings of interreligious encounters and discourse—and to point out the pitfalls of any overeager sensemaking or scientistic dismissals, which would only provide simplistic views on the complex links between healing and salvation.

---

34 Cf. Frenk (2014).
35 But there are other proposals as well. Cf., for example, Gostin (2014) and Harmon (2015).
36 Cf. Hanrieder (2017) and Weindling (1995).

Churches and theology should work with the "fragile signs of the salvation of a risky creation." Without utopian expectations but with a "hopeful lamenting pragmatism of love" (Thomas 2009, 525), they can promote activities toward global healing in the light of the coming kingdom of God. Any concept of healing on a global scale is inconceivable without the simultaneous propagation of justice and peace, and thus, salvation.

References

Aidoo, M., D. W. Terlouw, M. S. Kolczak, P. D. McElroy, F. O. ter Kuile, S. Kariuki … and V. Udhayakumar. 2002. "Protective Effects of the Sickle Cell Gene against Malaria Morbidity and Mortality." *Lancet* 359 (9314): 1311–1312.

Antonovsky, A. 1987. *Unraveling the Mystery of Health: How People Manage Stress and Stay Well*. San Francisco: Jossey-Bass.

Bach, U. 2006. *Ohne die Schwächsten ist die Kirche nicht ganz: Bausteine einer Theologie nach Hadamar*. Neukirchen-Vluyn: Neukirchener.

Barth, K. 2009. *The Command of God and the Creator*. Edited by G. W. Bromiley. London: T & T Clark.

Betcher, S. V. 2007. *Spirit and the Politics of Disablement*. Minneapolis: Fortress.

Boorse, C. 1977. "Health as a Theoretical Concept." *Philosophy of Science* 44 (4): 542–573.

Boyd, K. M. 2000. "Disease, Illness, Sickness, Health, Healing and Wholeness: Exploring Some Elusive Concepts." *Medical Humanities* 26 (1): 9–17.

Brown, P. J. 2014. "Religion and Global Health." In *Religion as a Social Determinant of Public Health*, edited by E. L. Idler, 274–297. Oxford: Oxford University Press.

Callahan, D. 1973. "The WHO Definition of 'Health.'" *Hastings Center Studies* 1 (3): 77–87.

Chatters, L. M. 2000. "Religion and Health: Public Health Research and Practice." *Annual Review of Public Health* 21 (1): 335–367.

Conrad, P. 2008. *The Medicalization of Society: On the Transformation of Human Conditions into Treatable Disorders*. Baltimore: JHU.

Crawford, R. 1980. "Healthism and the Medicalization of Everyday Life." *International Journal of Health Services* 10 (3): 365–388.

Dabrock, P. 2006. "Heil und Heilung. Theologisch-identitätsethische Unterscheidungen und ökumenische Herausforderungen im Verständnis von und im Umgang mit Gesundheit." *Una Sancta* 61:129–139.

Eiesland, N. L. 1994. *The Disabled God: Toward a Liberatory Theology of Disability*. Nashville: Abingdon.

Frenk, J., and O. Gómez-Dantés. 2014. "Designing a Framework for the Concept of Health." *Journal of Public Health Policy* 35 (3): 401–406.

Gadamer, H.-G. 1996. "On the Enigmatic Character of Health." In *The Enigma of Health: The Art of Healing in a Scientific Age*, 103–116. Stanford: Stanford University Press.

Gold, M. R., D. Stevenson, and D. G. Fryback. 2002. "HALYS and QALYS and DALYS, Oh My: Similarities and Differences in Summary Measures of Population Health." *Annual Review of Public Health* 23 (1): 115–134.

Gostin, J. 2014. *Global Health Law*. Cambridge: Cambridge University Press.

Grundmann, C. 2009. "Die Verantwortung religiöser Amts- und Würdenträger angesichts der globalen HIV/AIDS Pandemie: Eine christliche Perspektive." *Wege zum Menschen* 61 (5): 423–432.

Hall, D. E., K. G. Meador, and H. G. Koenig. 2008. "Measuring Religiousness in Health Research: Review and Critique." *Journal of Religion and Health* 47 (2): 134–163.

Hanrieder, T. 2015. "Globale Seuchenbekämpfung: Kooperation zwischen Ungleichen." *Aus Politik und Zeitgeschichte* 65 (20/21): 19–24.

———. 2017. "The Public Valuation of Religion in Global Health Governance: Spiritual Health and the Faith Factor." *Contemporary Politics* 23 (1): 81–99.

Harari, Y. N. 2017. *Homo Deus: A Brief History of Tomorrow*. New York: Harper.

Hardinghaus, W. 2016. "Reichsbürger und Germanische Medizin." *Der Klinikarzt* 45 (12): 579.

Harmon, S. H. E. 2015. "In Search of Global Health Justice: A Need to Reinvigorate Institutions and Make International Law." *Health Care Analysis* 23:352–375.

Harnack, A. 1892. *Medicinisches aus der Ältesten Kirchengeschichte*. Leipzig: J.C. Hinrichs'sche Buchhandlung.

Helliwell, J. F., and R. D. Putnam. 2004. "The Social Context of Well-Being." *Philosophical Transactions of the Royal Society of London Series B: Biological Sciences* 359:1435–1446.

Idler, E. L. 2014. "Religion, the Invisible Social Determinant." In *Religion as a Social Determinant of Public Health*, edited by E. L. Idler, 1–23. Oxford: Oxford University Press.

Jadad, A. R., and L. O'Grady. 2008. "How Should Health Be Defined?" *British Medical Journal* 337:1363–1364.

Kalema, D., W. Vanderplasschen, S. Vindevogel, and I. Derluyn. 2016. "The Role of Religion in Alcohol Consumption and Demand Reduction in Muslim Majority Countries (MMC)." *Addiction* 111 (10): 1716–1718.

Kant, I. 1992. *The Conflict of the Faculties*. Lincoln: University of Nebraska Press.

Koenig, H. G., D. E. King, and V. B. Carson. 2012. *Handbook of Religion and Health*. Oxford: Oxford University Press.

Körtner, U. H. J. 2010. "Is Mercy a Category of the Modern Health Care Sector?" *Diaconia* 1 (2): 214–229.

Kroonen, G. 2013. *Etymological Dictionary of Proto-Germanic*. Leiden: Brill.

Lahelma, E. 2001. "Health and Social Stratification." In *The Blackwell Companion to Medical Sociology*, 64–93. Oxford: Blackwell.

Larson, J. S. 1999. "The Conceptualization of Health." *Medical Care Research and Review* 56:123–136.

Luhmann, N. 2013. *A Systems Theory of Religion*. Stanford: Stanford University Press.

MacLeod, A. K. 2015. "Well-Being: Objectivism, Subjectivism or Sobjectivism?" *Journal of Happiness Studies* 16 (4): 1073–1089.

Mallory, J. P., and D. Q. Adams. 1997. *Encyclopedia of Indo-European Culture*. London: Fitzroy Dearborn.

Markschies, C. 2016. *Das antike Christentum: Frömmigkeit, Lebensformen, Institutionen*. Munich: C. H. Beck.

Marshall, K., and S. Smith. 2015. "Religion and Ebola: Learning from Experience." *Lancet* 386 (10005): e24–e25.

McCracken, K., and D. R. Philipps. 2012. *Global Health: An Introduction to Current and Future Trends*. London: Routledge.

McGilvray, James C. 1981. *The Quest for Health and Wholeness*. Tübingen, Germany: German Institute for Medical Mission (DIFAEM).

Moltmann, J. 1985. *God in Creation: A New Theology of Creation and the Spirit of God*. London: SCM.

Nordenfelt, L. 2007. "The Concepts of Health and Illness Revisited." *Medicine, Health Care and Philosophy* 10 (1): 5.

Origen. 1990. *Homilies on Leviticus 1–16*. Translated by G. Barkley. Washington, DC: Catholic University of America Press.

Pannenberg, W. 1971. *Basic Questions in Theology: Collected Essays*. Michigan: SCM.

———. 1980. "Tod und Auferstehung in der Sicht christlicher Dogmatik." In *Grundfragen systematischer Theologie: Gesammelte Aufsätze*, vol. 2, 146–159. Göttingen: Vandenhoeck & Ruprecht.

———. 2004. *Systematic Theology*. Vol. 3. London: T & T Clark International.

Parsons, T. 1964. *Social Structure and Personality*. New York: Free Press.

Pogge, T. 2009. "The Health Impact Fund: Boosting Pharmaceutical Innovation without Obstructing Free Access." *Cambridge Quarterly of Healthcare Ethics* 18:78–86.

Quah, S. R. 2014. "Health and Culture." In *The Wiley Blackwell Encyclopedia of Health, Illness, Behavior, and Society*, 926–934. Chichester, UK: John Wiley & Sons.

Ruger, J. P. 2009. "Global Health Justice." *Public Health Ethics* 2:261–275.

Schockenhoff, E. 2013. *Ethik des Lebens: Grundlagen und neue Herausforderungen.* Freiburg: Herder.

Schramme, T. 2017. "Health as Notion in Public Health." In *Handbook of the Philosophy of Medicine,* edited by T. Schramme and S. Edwards, 975–984. Dordrecht: Springer Netherlands.

Schwenkenbecher, A. 2013. "Joint Duties and Global Moral Obligations: Joint Duties and Global Moral Obligations." *Ratio* 26 (3): 310–328.

Sharf, B. F., and M. L. Vanderford. 2003. "Illness Narratives and the Social Construction of Health." In *Handbook of Health Communication,* edited by T. L. Thompson, A. M. Dorsey, K. I. Miller, and R. Parrott, 9–34. Mahwah, NJ: Erlbaum.

Smith, R. C. 2004. "Amputee Identity Disorder and Related Paraphilias." *Psychiatry* 3:27–30.

Sontag, S. 2002. *Illness as Metaphor.* London: Penguin.

Thomas, G. 2009. "Krankheit im Horizont der Lebendigkeit Gottes." In *Krankheitsdeutung in der postsäkularen Gesellschaft,* edited by G. Thomas and I. Karle, 503–525. Stuttgart, Berlin, Cologne: Kolhammer Verlag.

Tillich, P. 1984. *The Meaning of Health.* Edited by Perry LeFever. Chicago: Exploration.

Utsch, M., and C. Klein. 2011. "Religion, Religiosität, Spiritualität: Bestimmungsversuche für komplexe Begriffe." In *Gesundheit—Religion—Spiritualität: Konzepte, Befunde und Erklärungsansätze,* edited by C. Klein, H. Berth, and F. Balck, 25–45. Weinheim: Juventa.

Weindling, P. 1995. "The Role of International Organizations in Setting Nutritional Standards in the 1920s and 1930s." *Clio Medica* (Amsterdam) 32:319–332.

Whitbeck, C. 1981. "A Theory of Health." In *Concepts of Health and Disease: Interdisciplinary Perspectives,* edited by A. L. Caplan, H. T. Engelhardt, and J. J. McCartney, 611–626. Reading, MA: Addison-Wesley, Advanced Book Program/World Science Division. Reading, Massachussets: Addison-Wesley.

Williams, J. W. 2013. *Spirit Cure: A History of Pentecostal Healing.* Oxford: Oxford University Press.

Zwingmann, C., C. Klein, and A. Büssing. 2011. "Measuring Religiosity/Spirituality: Theoretical Differentiations and Categorization of Instruments." *Religions* 2:345–357.

9

The Role and Impact of Christian Medical College, Vellore, in the Promotion of Health Justice in India

Arul Dhas T.

ABSTRACT

Health is an expensive proposition in today's India: the access, investigations, treatments, and medications are costly. Only the rich or those with medical insurance can access quality health care. The public health system is not comprehensive enough in all places. Private hospitals are keen to make profits, and the pharmacological industry has its own agenda. One unique success model significantly contributing to the health care in India is the 120-year-old Christian Medical College, Vellore (CMC). Training, service, and research are its thrust areas. Right from the selection of training candidates until the choice of whom to treat at the most critical treatment, CMC has a heritage of enhancing justice in health care. CMC has its roots in the Christian faith. Its founder, Dr. Ida Sophia Scudder, understood the health care as an outworking of her faith in her Lord Christ Jesus. With an analysis of the foundations of its services in Christian faith, this chapter will concentrate on the role and impact of CMC, Vellore, in the promotion of health justice in India.

1. Introduction

Health is a state of total well-being. India aims to spend 2.5 percent of its gross domestic product (GDP) on governmental health-care expenditures. However, the health index in this large land is not uniform. Even though 74 percent of Indians live in villages, the cities get more access to health care than villages. Christian health-care institutions along with their educational institutions have played a major role in making people experience shalom and peace. A preoccupation with health has been a heritage of Christian faith since the Lord Jesus Christ himself undertook healing as part of his threefold ministry (along with preaching and teaching).

Christian faith understands God as a healing God. Healing is the curing not just of illness but of a person's whole being. It includes the wellness of body, mind, and spirit. It is not just an individual experience but a community experience. This dimension of healing is demonstrated by Lord Jesus Christ when he did his earthly ministry by teaching, preaching, and healing. Many of his miracles are miracles of healing.

2. Historical Background of the Origins

Dr. Ida Sophia Scudder, the founder of the CMC, came to visit her missionary parents in the 1890s (George 2018, 54). She was confronted with the situation where men were not willing to take the help of a male doctor to attend to their wives during their labor pain. Their culture and practice did not allow them to make that happen. Saddened by the existing reality of rural Tamil Nadu, India, she was moved with compassion to dedicate her life to health-care ministry. She went back to the United States and graduated from Cornell University and started the one-bedded hospital in Vellore in 1900.

Health-care facilities were very minimal in those days in rural India. However, Dr. Ida S. Scudder decided to come to a remote village like Vellore and settled here for her ministry. She trained women to be doctors, and subsequently, the training encompassed different dimensions of health care such as nursing and allied health-care professions. Men were included for training only after 1947 in the CMC.

3. Christian Medical College to Build the Kingdom of God

When Dr. Scudder built CMC, she was very clearly dedicated to building not just a medical school but rather the kingdom of God. All those who were trained in this place had a little bit of that broad understanding about whatever they were doing either in Vellore or in any remote part of India. Most of its graduates are working in mission hospitals in this country.

It is illuminating to look at some of the practices during the time of Dr. Scudder. She used to hold Bible studies every week to inspire the staff members and faculty in spiritual affairs. She normally took 1 Corinthians 13 as the text for the reflections to the extent that that chapter is known as the favorite Scripture passage of Dr. Ida Scudder. CMC even today considers Bible studies as a very important aspect of its existence. Staff and students from different religious backgrounds form part of the study groups in the institution. In fact, the chaplaincy of CMC produces every year the study materials that are based on the Christian Scriptures and applicable for people of all faiths. The departments and batches are provided with earmarked times for this exercise.

Dr. Ida Scudder used an ancient Irish hymn, "Be Thou My Vision, O Lord of My Heart," often. Today this hymn is considered Aunt Ida's favorite hymn. In the CMC, weekly and daily community worship is very common. All are encouraged to participate in these worship times. Singing and prayer seem to direct the lifestyle of people that eventually dictates the actions.[1]

CMC understands God as the healing God. In addition to the founder, many leaders in CMC later also promoted health as an expression of their commitment to Christ and an expression of faith. Their focus has been mainly training health-care professionals. In the mission statement of CMC, service, teaching, and research are considered the integral parts of the existence of CMC.

4. Context of Health Care in India

The twelfth five-year plan of the government of India (2012–17) has envisioned providing cashless in-patient treatment to the population below poverty line (BPL) through an insurance-based system. It is also hoped (Wikipedia 2015) that by the end of the twelfth five-year plan, the governmental expenditure on health will increase from the present 1.04 percent of GDP to 2.5 percent of GDP.

In India, it is understood that it is the state's responsibility to provide public health, nutrition, and standard of living. Malnutrition, high infant

---

1 For more on Dr. Scudder, see Jeffrey (2014) and Wilson ([1959] 1990).

mortality, lack of safe drinking water, and various communicable and noncommunicable diseases are real issues in today's India.

The need for the public and private players in the health-care arena is indisputable. Especially, the faith-based organizations and charity organizations can play a major role to make sure that health-care-related justice is shown toward the common people.

5. Training and Nurture of Health-Care Professionals

Justice and fairness in health care take the conceptual framework in the minds of the health-care professionals during their undergraduate training. It is understandable that CMC has invested heavily in the training and mentoring of the individuals. Justice is one of the foundational principles of bioethics. How distributive justice operates in the area of scarce health-care resources is an important aspect of their ethical training in CMC.

Many former trainees of CMC have made significant contributions in many rural parts of the country to facilitate the marginalized access to health care.

6. Healing and Wholeness through the Ministry of CMC

CMC has an infrastructure to provide health care for about 2,500 inpatients and about 8,000 outpatients daily. From primary care to specialized care, CMC is equipped with personnel and equipment. In addition to this intensive care, there are about 150,000 people covered through the community health programs.

This health care is provided in a comprehensive manner. Most of the staff members here understand health as a holistic phenomenon. Physical healing is only one of the different dimensions. Sufficient attention is given to emotional, social, and spiritual dimensions of healing.

7. Health-Care Advocacy through CMC

CMC is part of a national network called the Christian Medical Association of India (CMAI). Due to its long-standing witness in the ethical and compassionate health care, there is a great respect in the nation for what CMC has to say on health-care issues.

CMC has been training personnel from the churches to be effective health-care ministers, and after their training, they have an obligation to work among the needy areas on whose behalf they came to CMC initially. This has been an effective model, and now we see the government of India promoting this pattern for all their medical graduates so that villages will be covered by health care. Otherwise, there is a general tendency to move to cities and other countries where facilities and benefits are better.

Making the medicines accessible to the poor is one of the main concerns of CMC and the Christian mission hospitals. The promotion of generic medicines is to promote this idea so that ordinary people will get access to medicines.

CMC makes a special effort to keep its fee minimal for the health-care trainees with the hope to inspire them to work among the needy areas. This system definitely is a rewarding one.

8. Community Empowerment through Health-Care Service

Both in the training and in the service, health-care orientation as well as community health take priority to shape the minds of the trainees in this place. Even in the mission statement of the CMC, this concern is powerfully articulated as follows: "CMC reaffirms its commitment to the promotion of health and wholeness in individuals and communities and its special concern for the disabled, disadvantaged, marginalized and vulnerable" (Chaplaincy, CMC 2015, 5).

More than 20 percent of the annual budget goes for charity-related work in the institution to facilitate health care to the poor and the marginalized.

CMC in its annual graduation celebrates individuals' contributions to the health of villages. The Paul Harrison Award is one such to recognize such men and women. This functions as an inspiration to others in CMC and also those in the country. There is another award, College Motto Award, that is given to someone who demonstrated the college motto "Not to be ministered unto but to minister." This is another way of holding the "service" motive at the highest in the minds of people.

9. Conclusion

The CMC brings out hundreds of trained personnel every year to be instruments of healing and go out as "compassionate, professionally excellent, ethically sound ... servant-leaders of health teams and healing communities" (Chaplaincy, CMC 2015, 5). It has created a brand name of its own in achieving this purpose. This has significantly contributed to actualize the manifesto of the Lord Jesus himself.

"The Spirit of the Lord *is* upon Me,
Because He has anointed Me
To preach the gospel to *the* poor;
He has sent Me to heal the brokenhearted,
To proclaim liberty to *the* captives
And recovery of sight to *the* blind,
To set at liberty those who are oppressed;
To proclaim the acceptable year of the Lord." (Luke 4:18–19 NKJV)

In the midst of commercialization and profit orientation, CMC stands firm to demonstrate that a faith-based organization can make a difference in the health scenario of the region. Together, it is possible to materialize health justice on earth.

References

Chaplaincy, Christian Medical College. 2015. *Maitri: In Pursuit of Maturity in Christ.* Vellore, India: CMC.

George, Reena. 2018. *One Step at a Time: The Birth of the Christian Medical College, Vellore.* Delhi: Showcase Roli Books.

Jeffrey, Pauline. 2014. *Ida S. Scudder.* Chennai: Word of Christ.

Wikipedia. 2015. "Health in India." Accessed February 10, 2015. https://en .wikipedia.org/wiki/Health_in_India.

Wilson, Dorothy Clarke. (1959) 1990. *Dr. Ida: Passing on the Torch of Life.* Chennai: Evangelical Literature Service.

World Council of Churches and the German Institute for Medical Mission Witnessing (DIFAEM). 2010. *Witnessing to Christ Today: Promoting Health and Wholeness for All.* Tübingen, Germany: DIFAEM.

10

Empirical Perspectives on Religion and Health Justice

THE CASE IN FINLAND AND ACROSS CULTURES

Henrietta Grönlund

ABSTRACT

The role of religion has been crucial in compassion and social engagement throughout human history. Although religion has also intertwined with violence and injustice, advocacy and work for health and social justice can be seen throughout organized religions, and religions have had a central role in addressing perceived injustices in different contexts. This chapter studies the connections between religion and religious agencies and health justice. I understand the term *health justice* broadly, adopting a social understanding of health, and cover themes related to social justice, social work, and social engagement. I include different forms of social engagement and prosocial behavior as components of work for health justice. My focus is on the connections of religion with these subject matters. I will introduce the rationale explaining these connections and demonstrate empirical findings on them. Through this, I discuss the particular role of religious agents in the promotion of social justice in today's post-secular, high-income societies, focusing especially on northern European countries and particularly on the case of Finland.

1. Introduction

The role of religion has been central in the history of human compassion and social engagement (Cnaan et al. 2016; Grönlund and Pessi 2015). Advocacy and work for health and social justice can be seen throughout organized religions, and organized religions have been central in addressing perceived injustices in different contexts (Judd 2013; Lee and Barret 2007). The foundation for helping those in need can be found in all world religions and their texts. Almost all faith traditions have tenets that ask the adherents of these traditions to behave ethically, not to harm others, and to exhibit charitable behavior. Helping the needy and seeking out justice are essential tenets of most religions, and they encourage prosocial behavior among their members with their values, norms, practices, and social pressure (Cnaan et al. 2016; Putnam and Campbell 2010). Judaism, Islam, and various Asian religions share a strong obligation to help. Also, the traditions of the Middle East, ancient Greek culture, and Christian doctrines echo the universal principle of compassion, to treat all others as we wish to be treated ourselves (Neusner and Chilton 2005).

Religions have in different times motivated individual acts of caring, and religious communities and organizations have helped, served, and provided asylums for those in need. In many countries, welfare and health services have been or are still provided by religious or religiously motivated actors and bodies. Religious organizations have been and still are central in providing assistance for nations and people suffering from crises, poverty, and injustice also abroad. In addition to providing for those in need, religious actors have been central in seeking justice and equality—in health and other issues—for different marginalized and discriminated groups (Cnaan et al. 2016; Neusner and Chilton 2005; Pessi and Grönlund 2012). However, religions have also intertwined with violence and injustice through human history and also today, which must not be overlooked.

This chapter studies the connections between religion and religious agencies and health justice. I understand the term *health justice* broadly, referring among others to the World Health Organization (WHO) Commission on the Social Determinants of Health, which has underlined the way in which differences in health and social disadvantage intertwine (2008). Thus I adopt a social understanding of health and include themes of social justice, social work, and social engagement in this chapter, covering different forms of social engagement and prosocial behavior as components of work for health justice. My focus is on the connections of religion with these subject matters. I will in the following introduce the rationale for explaining the connections between religion and different forms of social work and social engagement affecting health justice. Furthermore, I will demonstrate empirical findings on these connections. I will especially focus on high-income countries and northern Europe, and in particular on the case of Finland, which demonstrates the changing role of religious agents in health justice in today's postsecular society.

2. Religion Promoting Health Justice: Rationale and Empirical Findings

Religion intertwines with works for health justice at the level of an individual, the level of communities, and the level of societies. These three levels also intertwine with each other. Religion can affect the choices and actions of an individual that influence their health, and religion can affect the choices and actions of an individual that influence the health of others. This chapter focuses on the latter: the ways in which religion intertwines with action for justice and well-being of others at the level of individuals, communities, and societies.

Looking at the empirical connections between individuals' social engagement and religion, several positive correlations can be found. Different indicators of religion are connected with social engagement and prosocial behavior such as blood donation, volunteering, and philanthropic giving (Grönlund and Pessi 2015; Putnam and Campbell 2010). Religious individuals donate more not only to religious organizations but to all charitable organizations. For example, in a recent study on individuals' philanthropic giving (Grönlund and Pessi 2015), all countries that tested connections between religion and philanthropic giving (donations) found that religion, religious affiliation, religious attendance, and/or religious belief had an impact on giving. These countries included Austria, Canada, China, Indonesia, Israel, South Korea, Switzerland, Taiwan, and the United States. Individuals with a religious affiliation had a higher probability of giving, and religious affiliation also influenced incidences of giving and amounts donated in several countries. Donating to religious communities or causes explained a part of these results, but not all of them. Similarly, religious individuals volunteer more than nonreligious, and this connection holds also in volunteering in the wider community in addition to volunteering within religious communities (Cnaan et al. 2016).

The specific mechanisms driving the connections between religion and prosocial behavior or social engagement have been and continue to be examined (for outlining explanations on the mechanisms, see, for example, Cnaan et al. 2016; Hustinx et al. 2014; Luria, Cnaan, and Boehm 2017; Wiepking and Bekkers 2012). At the psychological level, an individual's religion is considered to be linked with their prosocial motives and values (see Cnaan et al. 2012; Grönlund 2012). Acting according to one's values is central to the self-image of the individual; thus, philanthropic giving, volunteering, and other prosocial behavior can help the individual act in accordance with their religious self-image. Several studies (such as Cnaan et al. 2012; Wiepking and Bekkers 2012) show connections between religious beliefs, prosocial values, and action.

The previously introduced individual connections between religion and social engagement are often mediated by religious activity and social ties. Prosocial behavior is especially connected with religious activities such as attending places of worship and active membership in religious community, according to several studies. In their study of 145 countries, Buster G. Smith and Rodney Stark (2009) found that religious attendance was statistically significantly connected with philanthropic giving and volunteering in 90 percent and 87 percent of the countries, respectively. Robert D. Putnam and David E. Campbell (2010) have found that the influence of social ties spreads also outside the religious community. For example, the more friends an individual has within a religious congregation, the more likely they are to donate money or volunteer.

Similar influences can also be discerned at the societal level in different contexts in terms of values, norms, and cultures alike. A national religious culture can affect cultural values and increase the opportunities and expectations for prosocial behavior. Thus the influences of a religious culture can even extend to nonreligious citizens (Lim and MacGregor 2012; Ruiter and De Graaf 2006). Making choices and valuing choices as meaningful are always cultural productions, and religion as a central cultural feature influences them in manifold ways (in relation to philanthropy; e.g., Grönlund 2019). Furthermore, cultural contexts moderate the connections between religion and social engagement in different countries. For example, Luria, Cnaan, and Boehm (2017) found that individualism and cultural values moderated the effect of religion on volunteering. The relationship between religious attendance and volunteering was stronger in contexts with self-expression values and low individualism.

A central impact of religion on health justice is the role of religious communities and organizations in providing health and welfare services throughout human history. They have been and continue to be central actors especially in countries with less comprehensive welfare services, where hospitals, orphanages, and social services have been and continue to be carried out by religious actors. Nevertheless, the role of religion and religious communities continues to be central also in many high-income countries and welfare states despite the different religious cultures and contexts (Grönlund and Pessi 2015). In Germany, the social functions of the majority of churches (both Protestant and Catholic) are part of the basic organization of the welfare system (Leis-Peters 2006). In the Nordic countries, the majority of churches offer complementary services to the public sector but also fill in the gaps of public welfare services and act as advocates for the rights of the disadvantaged (Pessi, Angell, and Pettersson 2009). In the US, several religious organizations provide substantial care through both informal partnerships and their own programs. Even in contexts where the official statuses of religions have weakened, their role in health, welfare, and philanthropy has reemerged and persevered (Grönlund and Pessi 2015).

It is noteworthy that religions and religious institutions actually have fundamentally affected the establishment and development of welfare states and systems of health justice all over the world (Bäckström and Davie 2010; Grönlund and Pessi 2015). In Europe and the United States, theologians had a profound impact on the public health movement in the nineteenth and early twentieth centuries (Cochrane 2008). In the 1960s, medical missionaries working in developing countries for primary health care created the Christian Medical Commission (CMC), a specialized organization of the World Council of Churches. The work of this organization made a global impact—for example, through its meetings with WHO—leading to the adoption of primary health care as a global strategy (Cochrane 2008).

The societal positions of religious organizations influence their role in health justice. As parts of civil society, religious organizations can act as voices of the people. They can act as political agents that try to influence society, the political system, and political decision-making—for instance, by criticizing political decisions related to health justice and also by motivating people to act politically (Wagner 2008). Religion and religious organizations can also work as partners of ruling authorities, complementing public services and working toward cohesion. Nevertheless, when religious bodies work closely with ruling authorities, they can maintain the status quo, a just or an unjust one. Religious bodies have in many cases enabled and allowed injustice and inequality instead of fighting for justice and increasing well-being. Religious beliefs and doctrines can be interpreted in ways that violate human rights and avert health justice and the well-being of individuals or groups of people. Although religion faces and opposes oppression, empowers people, fights for justice, and helps those who are suffering, it is also used to oppress people and violate human rights. Thus the link between religion and social engagement or health justice is not simple or unproblematic.

3. Religion and Health Justice in Postsecular Societies: The Case of Finland

Today the role of religion is particularly interesting in contexts of assumed secularization, such as in Europe. As described earlier, churches continue to be welfare agents and active in social policy dealing with social problems and health justice in many European countries, and these activities are appreciated by citizens. Europeans seem to support the idea of religious actors battling social problems and acting in times of crises (e.g., Bäckström and Davie 2010). I will next scrutinize the role of religion and one religious body in one specific context: Finland.

The Finnish majority church, the Evangelical Lutheran Church of Finland (69.7 percent of the population were members in the beginning of 2019), officially changed from a state church to national church in the nineteenth and twentieth centuries, and the responsibility for many health and welfare services previously provided by the church has been transferred to the state and the local authorities. The public sector has for decades provided a majority of health and social services. The nonprofit sector, private businesses, and the church have complemented the public sector, located unnoticed needs, and experimented with new working methods. This welfare state model has been rooted in a long tradition of political democracy, a history of social-democratic political values, a strong will for and an ability for social and national integration, and also the Lutheran version of Christianity. The values of individualism and gender equality and the aim of equal treatment for all citizens are intertwined with this welfare model (Grönlund 2019; Pessi and Grönlund 2012).

The mission of practicing the principle of loving one's neighbor is registered in the Church Act of the Evangelical Lutheran Church of Finland, chapter 1. The welfare activities of the church are instrumental in carrying out this mission. In all local parishes, employees are engaged in social work, and all parishes provide various kinds of aid. The central administration of the church coordinates this work and also organizes a variety of services at the national level, such as a national help line, a diaconal fund, and pastoral care for hospitals. Under the Church Act, the main duty of diaconal work is to help the most distressed who receive no other help.

In addition to helping the most distressed, the work of religious organizations in Finland includes also more holistic ideas of well-being. The Evangelical Lutheran Church provides help and support to different groups of people in a wide range of issues related to health and well-being at both local and national levels. For example, marital and relationship counseling, meeting places for parents with small children who are cared for at home, and group activities for the elderly and the unemployed are provided free of charge to church members and nonmembers alike all over Finland. This approach comes close to the Finnish welfare context, with an emphasis on universalism and equality; practically all households receive some form of income transfer or use social and health services at some point.

This range of approaches to well-being can also be seen in the work of other religious organizations and nonprofits with religious backgrounds, such as city missions, deaconess institutes, and the Salvation Army in different cities of Finland. For example, in Helsinki—the capital of Finland—the Salvation Army and Helsinki Deaconess Institute have focused on helping those who have the least, such as Romanian beggars, homeless, prisoners, and people with substance abuse problems (Helsinki Deaconess Institute 2015; Helsinkimissio 2015; Pelastusarmeija 2015). On the other hand, Helsinkimissio (formerly Helsinki City Mission) has adopted a more holistic approach and initiated a battle against loneliness over a decade ago (Helsinkimissio 2015). This work has included, in addition to concrete social work, visible campaigns reminding people to mind and take care of each other, especially their elderly parents and other relatives. Only later has Finnish society also more broadly identified loneliness as a central social-political problem and an established risk factor for mental and physical illnesses (see, e.g., Masi et al. 2011). Thus the Evangelical Lutheran Church as well as nonprofits with religious backgrounds influence societal debates and also work to improve the situation of those in need societally.

Thus the mission of the Evangelical Lutheran Church in health justice can be seen as twofold. On the one hand, it provides help and services for those in need; on the other hand, it fights for their rights societally. For example, during a severe economic recession and cutbacks in public services in Finland in the 1990s, the focus of diaconal work shifted from working among the elderly toward financial and mental health issues and people representing all age groups, as the public sector was unable to provide help for all those in need (Yeung 2003). In addition, the church issued statements that called for social solidarity, expressed its opposition to cutbacks in social and health services, and demanded improvements in the conditions of people in need (Hiilamo, Raunio, and Yeung 2007). Such a role has continued also after the recession of the 1990s. For example, in 2011 and 2015, the central administration of the church published goals of the church for government programs, the action plans agreed by the parties represented in newly elected governments (Evangelical Lutheran Church of Finland 2011, 2015, 2019). The goals highlighted the position of the weakest in Finland and abroad. They include themes such as child poverty and climate change. In 2015, the church council requested that the level of international aid should be raised to 0.7 percent in 2025 at the latest. In 2019, the church suggested improvements related to, for example, palliative care, human rights of asylum seekers, and the level of international aid.

Paul Avis (2000) has listed traits of national or state churches, which include, for instance, being territorially widespread to all of the population in all local communities, having a close relationship to the national culture, and having chaplaincy in national institutions (such as hospitals and penal institutions). Avis also states that "critical solidarity" is the hallmark of national churches. They can be critical and use their prophetic voice but usually look for consensus. The Finnish church has—in practice—accepted the gap-filling role to some extent but, as described earlier, not without criticism. The Finnish church is active in providing welfare services as a partner of the public sector but also acts as a critical voice that seeks justice for those in need.

Despite declining membership rates and claims of secularizations, church members and nonmembers alike appreciate this work and have high expectations toward the church to help and speak on behalf of those in need (Pessi and Grönlund 2012). Among the church members, this work is a significant reason for the membership (Haastettu kirkko 2012), and over 70 percent of the Finns think that the church should increasingly be an advocate for the disadvantaged in social debates (Haastettu kirkko 2012; Pessi and Grönlund 2012). Moreover, the expectations of the Finns toward the role of the church in welfare differ from the expectations people have toward the nonprofit sector in their scope and magnitude, making the role of the church distinct from other unofficial welfare providers. The church seems to have a uniquely strong and trusted position among citizens in a wide manner, regardless of their religious affiliation. Also, Finns seem to hope for the church to be both a welfare provider and a political agent.

4. Religion and Health Justice in Contemporary Societies

To conclude, the connections between different religions and health justice are manifold and central in human history. They are verified also today in a range of empirical studies examining this issue. The connections can be detected at the levels of individuals, communities, and cultures, making the processes explaining the influence of religion on health justice manifold and multidimensional. Psychological processes, dynamics of religious communities, religious cultures, and the societal roles and positions of religions and religious organizations in different contexts all influence the ways in which religion intertwines with health justice. A key connection is the role of religion in building and reinforcing the foundations for prosocial behavior, justice, and welfare. Religious traditions encourage individuals and initiate social missions and public welfare services. Religious organizations also provide services for communities and fight for justice in most contexts all over the world.

In the twenty-first century, the roles of religions and religious organizations are changing in many societies. In Western countries, especially, the public roles of religions are becoming challenged through religious diversity and increasing demands for nonreligious spaces and societies. In the process of modernization, different sectors of society have been presumed to increasingly differentiate their own spheres. Religion and religious organizations have been assumed to withdraw to the private sphere of individual life and religious practice (e.g., Beyer 1994; Dobbelaere 1989). Similarly, the world of welfare and health has in many ways been stripped of religion in these contexts. In addition, the increasing individualization as a dimension of modernization in many Western societies has resulted in believing religion to withdraw to the private sphere of individual lifestyles and worldviews.

The role of religion in welfare and health is also increasingly viewed as a question of equality in religiously diverse societies, as religious organizations are not neutral. Receiving services from religious organizations can make individuals feel uncomfortable or obliged to conform or respond to the ideology of the service provider. Such views have been demonstrated in the context of the United States (Cnaan et al. 2002). However, findings on Finland partially contradict this view at both the institutional and individual levels. People seem to view the church work as based on free will; as a middle-aged woman interviewed for a study stated, "The help is very easy to accept—They help me simply because they want to. They are not obliged" (Yeung 2008).

This may be explained by the differences in the American and Finnish welfare models. In Finland, the help from religious organizations is ideologically secondary, as the public sector is responsible for providing basic welfare. Thus the help from religious organizations can be viewed as voluntary to give and as a choice to accept (e.g., Salonen and Grönlund 2018). This is not the case in the United States, where the level of public services is low, and welfare and health services are extensively provided by voluntary organizations, religious and other. Also, the European system of national and state churches has resulted in a situation where religious organizations, especially churches, are institutionalized, often well established, and viewed as relatively neutral service providers. In contrast, in the United States, a variety of smaller religious organizations, individual choice of membership, and the dependency on individual donations constitute the religious landscape. The relationship of an individual with such a religious organization can be viewed to include more expectations of reciprocity or commitment compared to a more institutionalized organization, making it possibly more difficult to view their help as purely altruistic.

Despite the secularization claims and increasing claims for religious neutrality in many Western countries, religion—as described earlier—is not disappearing or withdrawing as previously suggested. Recent empirical studies in general strongly indicate that private and public as well as religious and secular cannot be separated but rather form continuums. Dichotomies in general are not accurate ways of describing the reality of religions (e.g., Collins 2008). Churches and religions continue to be publicly visible and have public roles and missions, also in relation to welfare and health. According to Jean-Paul Willaime (2006), the search for meaning and relationships and the uncertainty and privatization of values are central features of the ultramodern. Societies are incapable of intermediate collective meanings, which can make religions significant reference groups. They can provide meanings, trust, and ethical legitimacy as well as ideological and communal grounds for individual reflection (Dawson 2006). The strong role of religion in health justice in different contexts also today is one indicator of how multilocated religion in contemporary societies is. Modernized societies or the role and position of religion in them are not static but continually changing (Eisenstadt 2002).

Jose Casanova (2001) writes about the deprivatization of religion, meaning that religions refuse to adopt a detached and privatized role previously assumed to be a consequence of modernization (secularization). According to him, religions can use their position to remind societies and individuals of the need to become more responsive to human needs and to maintain the principle of the "common good" against the claims that reduce common good to an aggregated sum of individual rational choices. Religions can remind us that morality can only exist as interpersonal norms. This is central to the role of religions in health justice also today.

Contexts—and changes within them—influence the activities, roles, and positions of religion. However, the central role of religion in social engagement and in questions of justice seems to persevere in different times and different contexts at the levels of individuals, communities, and societies. This role should not be overlooked anywhere in debates or on practical measures for welfare and justice.

References

Avis, Paul. 2000. "Establishment and the Mission of a National Church." *Theology* 103:3–14.

Bäckström, Anders, and Grace Davie. 2010. *Welfare and Religion in 21st Century Europe: Volume 1.* Aldershot, UK: Ashgate.

Bekkers, R., and P. Wiepking. 2010. "A Literature Review of Empirical Studies of Philanthropy: Eight Mechanisms That Drive Charitable Giving." *Nonprofit and Voluntary Sector Quarterly* 40:924–973.

Beyer, Peter. 1994. *Religion and Globalization.* London: Sage.

Casanova, Jose. 2001. "Civil Society and Religion: Retrospective Reflections on Catholicism and Prospective Reflections on Islam." *Social Research* 68:1041–1080.

Cnaan, Ram A., with Stephanie C. Boddie, Femida Handy, Gaynor Yancey, and Richard Schneider. 2002. *The Invisible Caring Hand: American Congregations and the Provision of Welfare.* New York: New York University Press.

Cnaan, Ram A., Anne B. Pessi, Sinisa Zrinščak, Femida Handy, Jeffrey L. Brudney, Henrietta Grönlund, Debbie Haski-Leventhal, Kirsten Holmes, Lesley Hustinx, Chulhee Kang, Meenaz Kassam, Lucas C. P. M. Meijs, Bhagyashree Ranade, Karen Smith, and Naoto Yamauchi. 2012. "Student Values, Religious Values, and Pro-social Behaviour: A Cross-National Perspective." *Diaconia: Journal for the Study of Christian Social Practice* 3:2–25.

Cnaan, Ram A., Sinisa Zrinščak, David H. Smith, Henrietta Grönlund, Ming Hu, Meme D. Kinoti, Boris Knorré, Pradeep Kumar, and Anne B. Pessi. 2016. "Volunteering in Religious Congregations and Faith-Based Associations." In *Palgrave Handbook of Volunteering, Civic Participation, and Nonprofit Associations*, edited by David H. Smith and Robert A. Stebbins, with Jurgen Grotz, 472–494. Basingstoke, UK: Palgrave Macmillan.

Cochrane, James R. 2008. "Fire from Above, Fire from Below: Health, Justice and the Persistence of the Sacred." *Theoria: A Journal of Social & Political Theory* 55:67–96.

Collins, Peter. 2008. "Accommodating the Individual and the Social, the Religious and the Secular." In *Religion and the Individual: Belief, Practice, Identity*, edited by Abby Day, 143–156. Aldershot, UK: Ashgate.

Dawson, Lorne. 2006. "Privatization, Globalization, and Religious Innovation: Giddens' Theory of Modernity and the Refutation of Secularisation Theory: Classical and Contemporary Debates." In *Theorising Religion: Classical and Contemporary Debates*, edited by James Beckford and John Wallis, 105–119. Aldershot, UK: Ashgate.

Dobbelaere, Karel. 1989. "The Secularization of Society? Some Methodological Suggestions." In *Secularization and Fundamentalism Reconsidered: Religion and the Political Order*, edited by Jeffrey K. Hadden and Anson Shulpe, vol. 3, 27–44. New York: Paragon House.

Eisenstadt, S. N. 2002. "Multiple Modernities." *Daedalus* 129:1–29.

Evangelical Lutheran Church of Finland. 2011. *Kirkon hallitusohjelmatavoitteet 2011.* Kirkkohallituksen yleiskirje no. 5/2011. Accessed September 10, 2020. https://tinyurl.com/y4yzzhlp.

———. 2015. *Suomen Evankelis-Luterilaisen kirkon esitykset tulevaan hallitusohjelmaan.* Accessed September 10, 2020. https://tinyurl.com/y3vzhj4c.

———. 2019. *Kirkon hallitusohjelmatavoitteet.* Accessed September 10, 2020. https://tinyurl.com/y5o2jndz.

Grönlund, Henrietta. 2012. "Religiousness and Volunteering: Searching for Connections in Late Modernity." *Nordic Journal of Religion and Society* 25:47–66.

———. 2019. "Between Lutheran Legacy and Economy as Religion: The Contested Roles of Philanthropy in Finland Today." In *On the Legacy of Protestant Lutheranism in Finland: Societal Perspectives.* Studia Fennica Historica, edited by Kaius Sinnemäki, Anneli Portman, Jouni Tilli, and Robert Nelson. Helsinki: Finnish Literature Society.

Grönlund, Henrietta, and Anne B. Pessi. 2015. "The Influence of Religion on Philanthropy across Nations." In *The Palgrave Research Companion to Global Philanthropy*, edited by Pamala Wiepking and Femida Handy, 558–569. Basingstoke, UK: Palgrave Macmillan.

Helsinki Deaconess Institute. 2015. Accessed September 10, 2020. https://www.hdl.fi/en.

Helsinkimissio. 2015. Accessed September 10, 2020. http://www.helsinkimissio.fi.

Hiilamo, Heikki, Antti Raunio, and Anne B. Yeung. 2007. "Lähimmäinen hyvinvointivaltiossa." In *Oikeudenmukaisuus hyvinvointiossa*, edited by Juho Saari and Anne B. Yeung, 220–235. Helsinki, Finland: Gaudeamus.

Hustinx, Lesley, Johan von Essen, Jacques Haers, and Sara Mels, eds. 2014. *Religion and Volunteering: Complex, Contested and Ambiguous Relationships.* New York: Springer.

Judd, Rebecca G. 2013. "Social Justice: A Shared Paradigm for Social Work and Religion?" *Journal of Religion & Spirituality in Social Work: Social Thought* 32:177–193.

Lee, Eun-Kyoung O., and Callan Barrett. 2007. "Integrating Spirituality, Faith, and Social Justice in Social Work Practice and Education: A Pilot Study." *Journal of Religion & Spirituality in Social Work* 26:1–21.

Leis-Peters, Anette. 2006. "Protestant Agents of Welfare in Germany." In *Churches in Europe as Agents of Welfare.* Working Paper 2:1 and 2:2 from the Project Welfare and Religion in a European Perspective, edited by Anne B. Yeung, with Ninna Edgardh Beckman and Per Pettersson, 56–122. Uppsala, Sweden: Uppsala Institute for Diaconal and Social Studies.

Lim, Chaeyoon, and Ann MacGregor. 2012. "Religion and Volunteering in Context: Disentangling the Contextual Effects of Religion on Voluntary Behavior." *American Sociological Review* 77:744–779.

Luria, Gil, Ram Cnaan, and Amnon Boehm. 2017. "Religious Attendance and Volunteering: Testing National Culture as a Boundary Condition." *Journal for the Scientific Study of Religion* 56:577–599.

Masi, Christopher M., Chen His-Yuan, Louise C. Hawkley, and John T. Cacioppo. 2011. "A Meta-analysis of Interventions to Reduce Loneliness." *Personality and Social Psychology Review* 15:219–266.

Neusner, Jacob, and Bruce Chilton, eds. 2005. *Altruism in World Religions.* Washington, DC: Georgetown University Press.

Niemelä, Kati, Harri Palmu, Hanna Salomäki, and Kimmo Ketola. 2012. *Haastettu kirkko. Suomen evankelis-luterilainen kirkko vuosina 2008-2011*. Kirkon tutkimuskeskuksen julkaisuja 115. Tampere, Finland: Kirkon tutkimus keskus.

Pelastusarmeija. 2015. Accessed September 10, 2020. https://www.pelastusarmeija .fi.

Pessi, Anne B., Olav H. Angell, and Per Pettersson. 2009. "Nordic Majority Churches as Agents in Welfare State: Critical Voices and/or Complementary Providers?" *Temenos: Nordic Journal of Comparative Religion* 45:207–234.

Pessi, Anne B., and Henrietta Grönlund. 2012. "The Place of the Church: Public Sector or Civil Society? Welfare Provisions of the Evangelical Lutheran Church of Finland." *Journal of Church and State* 55:353–374.

Putnam, Robert D., and David E. Campbell. 2010. *American Grace: How Religion Divides and Unites Us*. New York: Simon & Schuster.

Ruiter, Stijn, and Nan D. De Graaf. 2006. "National Context, Religiosity, and Volunteering: Results from 53 Countries." *American Sociological Review* 71:191–210.

Salonen, Anna S., and Henrietta Grönlund. 2018. "Vastavuoroisuus ja vapaaehtoinen auttamistoiminta avun vastaanottajan näkökulmasta: Empiirisen tutkimuksen tulkinnallisia mahdollisuuksia ja haasteita." *Teologinen Aikakauskirja* 123:150–163.

Smith, Buster G., and Rodney Stark. 2009. "Religious Attendance Relates to Generosity Worldwide: Religious and the Secular More Charitable If They Attend Services." Gallup. https://tinyurl.com/cxookam.

Wagner, Anton. 2008. "Religion and Civil Society: A Critical Reappraisal of America's Civic Engagement Debate." *Nonprofit and Voluntary Sector Quarterly* 37:626–645.

Wiepking, Pamala, and Rene Bekkers. 2012. "Who Gives? A Literature Review of Predictors of Charitable Giving II: Gender, Marital Status, Income and Wealth." *Voluntary Sector Review* 3:217–246.

Willaime, Jean-Paul. 2006. "Religion in Ultramodernity." In *Theorising Religion: Classical and Contemporary Debates*, edited by James Beckford and John Wallis, 77–89. Aldershot, UK: Ashgate.

World Health Organization (WHO). 2008. *Closing the Gap in a Generation: Health Equity through Action on the Social Determinants of Health*. Geneva, Switzerland: World Health Organization. https://tinyurl.com/czbkhg.

Yeung, Anne B. 2003. "The Re-emergence of the Church in the Finnish Public Life? Christian Social Work as an Indicator of the Public Status of the Church." *Journal of Contemporary Religion* 18:197–211.

PART 3

Transforming Agendas of Faith Communities

THEME INTRODUCTION

Ayesha Ahmad and George Zachariah

1. Cultures, Institutions, Communities

Faith traditions and health justice serve as crucial weight bearers for the structural inequalities that shape the discourses around HIV/AIDS and women's rights and health to be discussed during this part of the volume. The advent of global health, whereby there are governmental, nongovernmental, and civil society organizations as well as activists, academics, researchers, and clinicians aligned to the goal of universal, good-quality, sustainable health care, has brought increased attention to the pluralism involved in conceptualizing health and illness. The degree of health inequalities and health injustices as well as stigmas, harmful beliefs, and forms of violence associated with topics covered in this section play an essential role in customizing health responses that address barriers to seeking and receiving treatment. The examination of cultural beliefs can have a strong religious rooting.

At the same time, the place and space of health-care institutions in addressing societal elements of health are increasingly instrumental in mediating harmful discourses. The agenda of faith communities can, then, both transcend and be transcended in terms of potentialities for reaching health justice. This thematic session details the transgression of key, fundamental health challenges in the different contexts of Bangladesh and Saudi Arabia. While these contexts are exclusively explored in terms of the issues they present in grappling with various concepts of health and illness inscribed, at times, with varying aspects of religious doctrine, they are not exhaustive examples. HIV/AIDS and rights-based discussions toward women's health have consistently been part of global health, and the need to steer the agendas of faith communities toward shared goals for health outcomes has been an essential focus. This section endeavors to provide a critical analysis of attempts in the respective countries and their national health systems.

Reaching such goals of transforming agendas in faith communities, however, is a significant challenge. Creating approaches to improving health is at times fraught with conflicts toward dominant religious viewpoints or ideologies that are embedded in the structural aspects of religion and health in a society. A trend throughout the subsequent chapters is the evolution of new hospitals to provide transformative care, the oscillation of ideologies that from the outside are often perceived as solid, and the historical variation of attitudes toward women that is often overlooked. These examples illustrate that agendas can be transformed and that faith communities play an important role in affecting health, with both having the potential for positive and negative impact. The analysis undertaken for this section further supports how transformative elements of the agendas of faith communities are shaped by national and international actors. The crucial part to remember when striving toward health justice is the need for critical analysis, open dialogue, pluralistic frameworks, and the understanding of the nuances of lived experiences of injustice—for example, the persecution and victimhood of sufferers from HIV/AIDS and the silenced existence of a woman due to sociocultural norms. Bringing these to light serves a purpose for faith communities to raise the standards of a society and, in turn, its health institutions.

2. Faith Communities Facing HIV and AIDS

Religion is a complex phenomenon. When its adherents perceive and practice religion as a private and personal faith, religiosity not only becomes a spiritual bliss of the heart but also provides legitimization to the prevailing order of the day. On the other hand, religion can also be manifested in the public witness of its adherents where religious traditions, scriptures, and rituals inspire faith communities to become testaments of love, justice, and solidarity in the public sphere. Said differently, religious traditions contain both prophetic and transformative and fanatic and constraining elements. In the context of tragic and evil realities that destroy the health and welfare of people and community, the need of the hour is to enable the prophetic and transformative potentials of our religious traditions so that these faith traditions can continue to inspire us to engage in the mission of bringing about healing and restoration in our communities.

HIV/AIDS is more than a medical condition; it is a social reality that exposes how an infected body can become the site of stigma, discrimination, exploitation, and demonization. The pandemic is also a litmus test to different civil society organizations, including religious traditions, to testify their commitment to practice solidarity by accompanying the infected in their journey toward healing and restoration. When it comes to religious traditions, in spite of their claims of love toward the vulnerable and the needy, there is ambiguity in their responses to the pandemic and interventions with the infected. This calls for genuine acts of introspection so that our faith communities can be transformed into sites of healing, acceptance, and restoration.

Right from the beginning of the outbreak of HIV/AIDS in the 1980s, there have been varied religious reflections on the pandemic, providing theological arguments related to HIV prevalence, treatment, and care. The dominant problematization of HIV/AIDS as caused by sexual immorality inspired religious communities to focus the attention of their interventions on awareness building and sexual morality so as to reduce the spread of the pandemic. Research done in different parts of the world testifies that HIV prevalence is minimal among religious communities that practice strict sexual morality compared to followers of religious traditions with a liberal understanding of sexual morality. At the same time, such moralistic problematizations of the pandemic have also been contested theologically, informed by the body-mediated experiences of women, people living with HIV and AIDS, and queer communities. Structures of patriarchy and economic and social injustice make women, the poor, and socially excluded communities more vulnerable to HIV and AIDS. Theological discourses continue to interrogate dominant problematizations of the pandemic and provide new insights privileging the perspectives of the infected.

Moralistic interpretations of the causes of HIV/AIDS by different religious traditions continue to influence and determine the faith responses to the pandemic. The dualistic religious worldview of pure/impure and sacred/profane provides theological legitimization to the stigmatization of the infected bodies and the demonization of the infected people. As a result, the sacred places and sanctuaries that are meant to welcome and offer comfort, healing, and solace have become inhospitable places for people living with HIV/AIDS. Religious discourses and rituals reinforce the myth that the infected are sexual perverts and thereby create a sense of guilt in the victims of the pandemic. Such distorted theological problematization of the pandemic not only prevents the faith communities from engaging in genuine acts of compassionate care and justice but also disables the moral agency of the infected. As a result, care and treatment are not adequately informed by the dreams and hopes of the infected.

At the same time, religious communities, which affirm compassionate justice as its vocation in an unjust world, are engaged in a different type of intervention in the context of HIV/AIDS. Privileging the voices and aspirations of the infected in the very perception of the problem and interventions, these communities use an intersectional approach in responding to the pandemic. For them, HIV/AIDS requires medical, ethical, economic, and social interventions. Care and treatment in a world controlled by transnational corporations demand a consistent struggle against neoliberal globalization to make medicine and treatment affordable to the people. Hospitals and other medical facilities should be reoriented to practice ethical values that respect the rights and dignity of the infected. Transformative religious communities consider stigma as an infectious disease and engage in the task of developing an immunity to this deadly disease. Such religious communities are also at the forefront of initiating alternative theological discourses on human sexuality, gender justice, and masculinity.

Religion is a great resource for the infected, even as they experience the feeling of utter Godforsakenness. Scriptures, religious symbols and teachings, sacraments and rituals, hymns and prayers, and the presence of religious people as caregivers provide them comfort, hope, and courage to face the future. Alternative reading practices help them reimagine scripture as a resource in their journey toward healing. They read their stories in the pages of the scripture and experience the mediation of grace in a special way in the sacraments and rituals.

In the context of HIV/AIDS, the challenge before the faith communities is to become aware of the possibility for religion to become an inhuman institution that perpetuates and aggravates the pain, stigma, and tragedy of the infected. With that awareness, faith communities can be transformed into sanctuaries that accompany the infected in the true spirit of solidarity toward healing and restoration.

11

The Contribution of Islamic Faith-Based Hospitals to the Promotion of Public Health in Bangladesh

A STUDY OF ISLAMI BANK AND IBN SINA HOSPITALS

Jibon Nesa and Ville Päivänsalo

ABSTRACT

This chapter aims to highlight how Islamic faith-based hospitals respond to health challenges in Bangladesh and contribute to the improvement of public health. Out of these faith-based hospitals, two groups of hospitals, the Islami Bank and Ibn Sina hospitals, have been selected to be discussed as case studies, focusing on their ongoing activities. To start with, this chapter shows that particular religious community-based hospitals can work to significantly reduce serious health problems. Following this observation, this chapter argues that the national and international bodies involved in public health, as mainstream agencies, should recognize the contribution of faith-based hospitals and accept such organizations as alternative agencies in the promotion of public health. This is not to say that international partners should turn a blind eye to any of the challenges that health organizations have been facing in Bangladesh, including the challenges of transparency. Instead, viable forms of partnership could help the health agencies in the country in the public, voluntary, and private sectors develop so as to better serve especially the less fortunate in Bangladesh.

1. Introduction: Responding to the Persisting Need

Bangladesh is a poor country with a small geographical area containing a huge number of people. The country faces numerous environmental and public health problems such as unhygienic and hazardous environmental conditions. The country's public health status has improved to a degree over the past three decades—but as in other South Asian countries, the level achieved is by no means satisfactory. As of 2015, the World Health Organization (2019, "Bangladesh") figures show that the country spent only 0.4 percent of its gross domestic product (GDP) on public health—compared with India's 1.0 percent ("India"), which is also a worryingly low figure. In terms of human development in general, Bangladesh ranked 136th on the list of 189 countries in 2017 on the United Nations Development Programme's (UNDP) Human Development Index (2019, table 1).

Following its Millennium Development Goals (MDGs) and, since 2015, Sustainable Development Goals (SDGs) approaches,[1] the United Nations (UN), along with the WHO and other international supporting bodies, has assigned priority to some basic health issues in Bangladesh, akin to other low-income countries of the world. However, despite their numerous efforts to reach the MDGs as a whole by 2015 and the SDGs thereafter, there still remain great and diverse development challenges for the people of Bangladesh. Indeed, in some health issues like maternal mortality, infant and child mortality, and malnutrition, the country has achieved somewhat satisfactory improvements. According to the *Millennium Development Goals: Bangladesh Country Report 2013* (General Economics Division of Bangladesh Planning Commission 2014), Bangladesh was on track to achieve its MDG for maternal and child health. The government's *Voluntary National Review* (Government of the People's Republic of Bangladesh 2017, 19) of the SDG program reported further significant progress—for example, in terms of infant and child mortality, under-five mortality, and maternal mortality rates in 2015. However, in practice, what is commonly seen everywhere in the country is that people are a

---

1 At the turn of the millennium, the 189 United Nations (UN 2015) member states at that time and at least 23 international organizations committed to help achieve the following eight goals by 2015: (1) eradicate extreme poverty and hunger; (2) achieve universal primary education; (3) promote gender equality and empower women; (4) reduce child mortality rates; (5) improve maternal health; (6) combat HIV/AIDS, malaria, and other diseases; (7) ensure environmental sustainability; and (8) develop a global partnership for development. About the seventeen SDGs, see, for example, UN (2019).

long way from achieving a good quality of life and from any international standard of health-care services.

As a member country of the UN, the Bangladeshi government is morally committed to taking care of the population in terms of their health. But with the nation's limited wealth and due to the inefficiency of its proper utilization, public health-care services remain seriously defective. Along with corruption in the administration, business interests are aggravating the problems. In the prevailing unideal circumstances, there are many sorts of health-care-supporting organizations and medical hospitals across the country endeavoring to meet the basic needs of the people. As recognized by senior British health activist Nigel Crisp (2010, 4–5), the voluntary sector has been very important to the progress of public health in Bangladesh. At least since the World Bank Study by Hassan Zaman et al. (2007), the patterns of governance in the Bangladeshi voluntary sector have been quite well known, and the concept of Islamic banking has also received attention (Salahuddin, Islam, and Islam 2014; Nabi, Islam, and Akter 2015), but the functioning of the faith-based voluntary sector has received less attention.

Apart from public hospitals, there are numerous privately owned medical hospitals, but only the wealthy can afford to access their services. The owners of these hospitals may claim that, being committed to the service of humanity, they are running the hospitals and medical services for ethical reasons. Unfortunately, however, their working policies imply that for them, the health challenges of the country primarily mean an opportunity to make money. Many of these hospitals, being technologically well-equipped and advanced, attract upper-middle-class and middle-class families to receive treatment and other medical services there. Expert medical doctors are also drawn by the attractive salary offers and other financial opportunities to work there. Thus these organizations have turned into health service providers for very specific classes of society.

Government hospitals are common in the country, but most of them are still old-fashioned and not equipped with up-to-date medical technology. In recent years, the government has spent a lot of money to improve public health services, particularly the medical treatment provided by public hospitals and other health-care agencies.[2] However,

2 The *Voluntary National Review* by the Government of the People's Republic of Bangladesh (2017, 20) particularly mentions "the US $14.71 billion mega programme called 4th

rampant mismanagement of the bureaucratic system in the whole of the health sector disturbs such efforts.

Although individual cases of corruption may be difficult to unveil, the ranking of the country as 143rd among the 180 countries listed in the "Corruption Perceptions Index 2017" by Transparency International (2018) definitely indicates major challenges in this respect. The organization's country report specifically mentions "the corruption and poor quality of public service delivery such as education, health, issuance of passport and infrastructure" (Salahuddin and Khair 2014, 27). Similarly, Mohammed Ameeruz Zaman (2011), with a long career both in science and in the development sector in Bangladesh and abroad, has called it a "standard plea, which is repeated with sickening frequency" in the country, "that the rule of law should be adhered to" (9). On the grass-roots level, such challenges tend to translate into shortcomings in treatment. In particular, people in need who come to public health agencies, especially to public hospitals, instead of receiving appropriate services, may face harassment and misbehavior by hospital administrators and doctors alike. Consequently, marginalized people tend to avoid seeking treatment at these hospitals. Thus while privately owned hospitals are focusing on profit more than service, public hospitals suffer from corruption, mismanagement, and misbehavior. Both kinds of hospitals thus fail to contribute to public health as they ought to.

Considering all these challenging circumstances and the crucial health needs of the people, religiously motivated groups have come forward to try to improve medical services and treatment. Inspired by the egalitarian and universal teachings of their religions, they have, both individually and collectively, worked quite extensively in the fields of health service and medical treatment. Many hospitals and medical services all over the world were established by such groups and continue to be maintained through their collaboration. The majority of these hospitals and medical services were and are charity-based organizations, so they are not able to become fully financially independent institutions or expand rapidly. In practice, in Bangladesh, their services are limited to the treatment of some common diseases—yet these institutions have continually provided services to disease-affected people.

Because of their financial dependence on the subscriptions of faith community members, these charity-based hospitals (e.g., Christian

---

Health, Population and Nutrition Sector Program (4th HPNSP) 2017/2022, [which] is guided by Bangladesh's Vision 2021, and is in line with the SDGs."

Medical Association, Association of Bangladesh Catholic Doctors, Ayachak Ashrama Medical Service, Anjuman Mufidul Islam, Islamic Relief Bangladesh, etc.) cannot flourish as financially stable, independent, large-scale hospitals in the same way as privately owned or public hospitals. With this point in mind, religiously inspired and motivated groups have thought a lot about how to manage health-care institutions stably and sustainably in conditions of scarcity.

In practice, such hospitals are therefore not being run as pure charity hospitals, providing health and medical services completely for free. Rather, they charge a reasonable fee from the patients in exchange for services. These institutions thus also have a commercial basis for their work. It is not the main purpose of their activities, though: they accept commercial benefits to ensure the sustainable running of the hospitals and diagnostic centers, aiming for complete independence from charity donations. Insofar as the faith-based institutions in question receive charitable donations from individuals or companies, this money is spent on treating the poor and needy, who cannot afford the cost of their treatment. These function as a new form of hospital in between the spirit of charity and the commercial benefit of their shareholders or owners. The main objective of these hospitals is to serve people suffering from diseases and to provide them with all kinds of health services. In Bangladesh, these types of faith-based hospitals include Islami Bank hospitals and Ibn Sina hospitals. They provide health-care services across the country at a reasonable price. People of all classes, regardless of their creed, color, gender, or ethnic identity, receive treatment under their auspices, and patients have generally been satisfied with their services.

The following section will discuss how these hospitals were established, how they are run, how they currently contribute to the improvement of public health, and finally, how they could contribute to it in the future. The potential contributions, indeed, could be considerable if they were to receive increased support from public health agencies and international health organizations.

The two Islamic faith-based hospitals in question are presently under government pressure, and their services are being rigorously monitored by the government—see, for instance, the *Economist*'s report on the intervention in the Islamic Bank in January 2017 (2017). Thus they cannot really produce printed books, journals, or published reports. Nor are their employers or employees particularly willing to share information with outsiders, notwithstanding the data available on the websites of these institutions. Hence this chapter also largely depends on the data available on the respective web pages, albeit complemented by the knowledge of the context and Jibon Nesa's communication with some of the employees.[3]

2. Islami Bank Foundation and Islami Bank Hospitals

With a bold mission and working plan, through the entrepreneurship of some religiously dedicated people, Islami Bank Bangladesh Limited (IBBL) was established in 1983 as the country's first faith-based bank for operating a banking system in accordance with the Islamic sharia laws.[4] Since its inception, it has undertaken charitable initiatives for the welfare of disadvantaged people alongside its main banking operations. As part of its Corporate Social Responsibility (CSR) scheme, the Islami Bank hospitals were established under a social welfare foundation called the Islami Bank Foundation (IBF; IBBL 2018; IBF 2018).

The aims and objectives of this foundation are to serve the needy and distressed through providing health care and medical facilities, along with other basic needs like employment and education. IBF has indeed launched many programs to improve the living conditions of the poor. Under its Health and Medicine Program, the foundation contributes to the realm of public health care through the establishment of medical centers, supporting charitable dispensaries, offering lump-sum help for the treatment of poor patients, and providing funding for the installation of plumbing and sanitary latrines. Across the country, the foundation (IBF 2018, "Institutions") has established eleven hospitals, including the Islami Bank Central Hospital, Kakrail, Dhaka; the Islami Bank Hospital, Motijeel, Dhaka; the Islami Bank Hospital, Mirpur, Dhaka; the Islami Bank Hospital, Khulna; the Islami Bank Hospital, Barisal; and the Islami Bank Hospital, Laxmipur, Rajshahi, among others, as well as one medical college, the Islami Bank Medical College Hospital, Rajshahi.

In these hospitals, patients are treated twenty-four hours a day by male and female emergency medical officers at a nominal cost. Patients suffering from more complicated conditions are referred to specialists. The fee payable to a specialist is comparatively reasonable. Whereas

---

3 During the process of writing this chapter, she communicated with the staff members of the hospitals several times on the available data and was told that the web pages indeed contain what has been made publicly available on behalf of these institutions.

4 IBBL (2018, "IBBL at a Glance") mentions "strict observance of Islamic Shari'ah" among its core values.

details may vary (please check IBF 2018, "Institutions"), generally the hospitals offer a specialist consultation service by the country's eminent doctors in a number of disciplines: neurology; nephrology; endocrinology and diabetology; gastroenterology; oncology; respiratory medicine; general surgery; neurosurgery; phacoemulsification surgery; orthopedics; spine surgery; plastic surgery; urology; ears, nose, and throat (ENT) services; gynecology and obstetrics; pediatrics; and so on. The hospitals have modern and well-equipped operating theaters. The hospitals provide a twenty-four-hour ambulance service. All pathological and imaging services are available at least in the larger of the hospitals. These include video endoscopy, video colonoscopy, bronchoscope, automatic biochemistry analyzer, blood culture auto analyzer, immunology auto analyzer, electrophoresis, latest CT scan, latest MRI, color Doppler, mammography, computed radiography, audiometry, uroflowmetry, biometry, 4D ultrasound, ECO cardiogram, spirometry, and so on. Medicines are available in the hospital drug stores at a reduced price, and a discount is given on locally produced medicines. An intensive care unit, a high-dependency unit, a diabetic center, and a dental unit are available, and dialysis, physiotherapy, and speech therapy are available. Therefore, due to their humanitarian ethos, reasonable pricing, and the availability of modern facilities, the Islami Bank hospitals can provide middle-class and upper-middle-class people as well as a considerable number of the poor an opportunity to access good-quality treatment.

The growing popularity of these hospitals offers further proof for this favorable view. In addition, the hospitals have stimulated other community service projects across the country. In particular, Islami Bank community hospitals are a unique venture of the Islami Bank Foundation (IBF), set up jointly with local sponsors. The number of Islami Bank community hospitals is increasing; as of 2018, nine community hospitals were in full operation (IBF 2018, "Institutions").

The Islami Bank Foundation also carries out many other important initiatives across the country with the help of Islami Bank hospitals and Islami Bank community hospitals. A midwifery training program is one such initiative. It is usual that in villages, traditional birth attendants (TBAs) assist with normal deliveries. They do not have any formal training in performing this crucial work; they base their services on traditional knowledge and experience. Therefore, a good number of mothers and babies die during delivery. Although the mortality rate has decreased and mother and child health care has slightly improved due to more investment by the government in this field, Bangladesh has not achieved satisfactory results. However, the Islami Bank Foundation runs thirty-day midwifery training programs where traditional birth attendants are trained by the medical doctors of Islami Bank hospitals and Islami Bank community hospitals. As a result of these training programs, TBAs have been capable of offering a safer and higher-quality service. Thus these training programs have helped significantly reduce the mother and child mortality rate.[5]

In Bangladesh, because of malnutrition and lack of awareness regarding eye health, eye-related diseases and problems are common. In order to increase awareness about how to take care of the eyes and to treat problems of the eyes, Islami Bank Foundation, with the participation of Islami Bank hospitals' and Islami Bank community hospitals' medical doctors specializing in ophthalmology, has arranged eye camps across the whole country. At such eye camps, people are educated about eye health.

For religious reasons, it is obligatory for Muslim male children to be circumcised. This practice is usually performed by a traditional village practitioner who has no formal medical training or knowledge. In urban areas, though, circumcisions are more often carried out by a physician. Islami Bank Foundation occasionally organizes special training programs across the country in order to train traditional village practitioners to improve the safety of these procedures. Without a doubt, this increases the skills of those who perform the procedures and thus contributes to public health.

The majority of Bangladeshi people live in rural villages. Most people are poor and cannot afford the cost of treatment if they are hospitalized or advised to purchase essential lifesaving medicines. Although there are government medical centers in some villages from which the villagers can obtain medication for temporary curable diseases, they cannot find any help there for serious diseases. Other villages in the country are too far away from such services. People in remote villages are especially unable to access medical treatment, and they suffer from many kinds of curable and incurable diseases due to a lack of opportunities, knowledge, capacity, and good medical doctors, nurses, and health technicians. To combat these prevailing problems in rural areas of the country in

---

5 It has not been possible to confirm the present status of all of these activities due to the challenges faced by the Islamic Bank in 2018, but such activities have been in their program for years. The current status of some of the activities mentioned in the subsequent chapters is uncertain as well.

terms of health care and medical treatment, Islami Bank hospitals and Islami Bank community hospitals, along with the financial support and cooperation of Islamic Bank Foundation, have introduced some timely and necessary initiatives targeting the health of poor and marginalized people in remote villages. For instance, under the Rural Health Worker Training Project, both Islami Bank hospitals and Islami Bank community hospitals are executing such health-care programs as the establishment of medical centers throughout the country to give free advice to poor patients, to support already established charitable dispensaries, and to provide lump-sum financial support for treatment.

Drinking pure and clean water is among the essential preconditions for good health, and adequate sanitation as well as an overall hygienic environment are key to preventing disease. As a response, both of the aforementioned types of hospitals are providing financial support to poor people in rural areas for tube well and sanitary latrine construction. Thus through such programs and activities under the Rural Health Worker Training Project, these hospitals are trying to improve the health of poor people living in remote villages. This involves providing them with advice and financial support for purchasing medicines and for creating a hygienic environment. As a result, some marginalized and very poor people across the country are able to adhere to the basic rules of public health, maintaining their health and fitness to work.

3. Ibn Sina Trust and Ibn Sina Hospitals

Under the umbrella of the Ibn Sina Trust (Ibn Sina Medical College 2018, "About Ibn Sina Trust"), founded in 1980, a group of people inspired by the values of Islam devoted their lives to serve humanity through providing medical facilities and health-care services. In this spirit, the trust has built hospitals, laboratories, consultation centers, a medical college, and pharmaceutical companies all over the country. From its inception, the trust has served to alleviate suffering and engage in welfare-oriented activities (Ibn Sina Trust 2018). With its social welfare programs, health-care services, and medical facilities, the Ibn Sina Trust has been a pioneer in private medical services. The trust has set itself ambitious goals, toward which it has been working since its establishment in 1980.

The trust runs one medical college, four hospitals, six diagnostic and consultation centers, one pharmaceutical company, one nursing college, and two medical checkup centers—among many other health-care services across the country.[6] The trust has been popular with people due to the health care, medical services, and many other social activities it offers. The trust has three free medical centers in Dhaka. It also gives financial assistance to other free medical centers located in different parts of Bangladesh. The trust has a large budget set aside for such purposes and a separate budget to facilitate free investigation and hospitalization services for those in need. The trust undertakes free operations and treatment for cleft-lipped children. A large budget is kept for the purpose of financial assistance to the disabled, the unemployed, the widowed, and families in distress. Thus while paying special attention to public health, the trust has also been conducting numerous social welfare activities throughout the country to meet some of the basic needs of the poor.

The Ibn Sina Hospital was established in July 1983, keeping pace with the continuous development of medical technologies. The hospital offers services in the field of medicine (internal medicine, neurology, nephrology, gastro-liver, cardiology, oncology, endocrinology, general surgery, gynecology, neurosurgery, spinal surgery, Coloradan surgery, orthopedics surgery, urology, etc.). It provides tertiary medical care in those fields. It also undertakes laparoscopic abdominal and colorectal surgery. For an affordable cost, it offers services to the ever-increasing number of kidney patients through its dialysis unit equipped with modern equipment. Ibn Sina Hospital has an intensive care unit providing twenty-four-hour services with the help of sophisticated equipment supported by skilled, efficient, and dedicated doctors, nurses, and other staff members. The hospital has eight well-equipped operating theaters.

After founding Ibn Sina hospitals across the country, the board of the Ibn Sina Trust felt the need to establish a nursing college to produce nurses with excellent professional and interpersonal skills. As a part of this endeavor, the Ibn Sina Nursing Institute started its journey in 2010 with fifty students. Already, three cohorts of Ibn Sina nurses are in service.

---

6 Please check the updated data on Ibn Sina Trust (2018). There has been turmoil in the organization, especially in its relations to the Islamic Bank, in 2018 (*Dhaka Tribune* 2018).

4. Comparing Faith-Based Hospitals with Public and Private Hospitals: The Quality of Care

As mentioned earlier, the quality of service and the sincerity and commitment to the work in faith-based hospitals such as Islami Bank hospitals and Ibn Sina hospitals have ensured their popularity among the people. Even if their services have not reached the global standards consistently, they have done a lot to serve those who suffer. It is also true that Bangladeshi people are more or less religiously oriented and appreciate the opportunity of being treated in faith-related institutions. Not only in the health sector but also in education, faith-based initiatives are doing well: people's faith in such service providers has endured. Many Christian missionary schools, colleges, and universities are also familiar to people all over the country due to their services to humanity.

These institutions do have their commercial interests—otherwise, they would not be able to maintain their present position. As a matter of fact, no major institution in Bangladesh can really function stably on charity donations alone. Smooth service with a spiritual component has been possible through reasonable service charges as well as reasonable salaries to the people employed by the service. At the same time, religious donations and other sponsorships are also received on the condition that the money is spent on the patients unable to pay the charges. According to Professor Mohammad Yunus (2010, xiv–xxv), this kind of business is called a social business. Such business is not primarily about profit making but about accessible and continuing service provision.

These kinds of social businesses are gaining popularity day by day all over the world. Yet there remains a big difference between the concept of a social business in general and that of faith-based social businesses. Usually in social businesses, the donors get their money back in the form of capital without any interest. But in religiously oriented social businesses, the donation is provided permanently and there is no stipulation about its return to the donor. This difference is possible due to the motivation of faith that can, at least in the best case, reach beyond the social motivation characteristic of social businesses.

In Bangladesh there is no such secular form of social business in the field of health care, although Professor Yunus (2010, 95–109) is planning to launch such health-care servicing centers or hospitals in countries like Bangladesh. If his plans are realized, many people will definitely benefit from those centers. That would be a great initiative and act by Professor

Yunus for the Bangladeshi people—akin to the microcredit system and Grameen Bank, a bank for the poor. Until then, we are to observe how effectively the existing health services provided by business institutions are able to play their role for people seeking health care.

However, the health facilities in the private sector, in Bangladesh, are numerous and of various kinds. According to a report by the Directorate General of Health Services (DGHS 2013), there were 4,020 private hospitals and clinics all over the country, including those in the Dhaka division, 1,505; Rajshahi, 928; Chittagong, 526; Khulna, 661; Barishal, 49; Sylhet, 115; and Rangpur, 236. By 2018, the total number of registered private hospitals and clinics had risen to 5,054 (DGHS 2018, 4). Thus far, few of them have been equipped with highly modern health technologies or have rendered high-quality services to the patients. And despite some positive developments, they have been inaccessible to the common people. While these private hospitals are expensive, their cost is no guarantee against misconduct or irregularities in their activities.

There are a huge number of public health-care services across the country, although their amount is insufficient in relation to the number of people. As of 2018, the total number of government facilities under the DGHS (2018, 4) was 2,258. Most of them were primary-level facilities (2,004, excluding community clinics), however. The total number of secondary and tertiary facilities was no more than 254.[7] These hospitals are fully supported by government money and are deemed to extend the required health and medical services to the common people of the country, but due to rampant corruption and inefficient administration, people are not really getting the expected services there. Visiting patients are often treated with disrespect. Therefore, people have difficulty placing their trust in public hospitals with regard to their treatment, and as a result, they are motivated to go to other health facilities. The affluent have no problem accessing highly expensive private hospitals for their treatment, but this is very different for the poor and middle-income people.

Indeed, midlevel, privately owned hospitals have unofficial brokers and agents to persuade health care-seeking people to have their treatment at the hospitals they work for. Such persistent persuasion means that many people are partly unwillingly convinced to use lower-quality

---

7 DGHS (2018, 4) is pleased with the increased number of health facilities and adds that "teaching and training centre[s] for health care and the seats of these institutions have also been increased."

private health institutions. There, however, doctors may suggest to patients unnecessary tests and other costly services. All this indicates that privately owned hospitals are running the hospitals for mainly business purposes rather than for the noble service of humanity. In their quest for profit, these hospitals are unfortunately often guilty of many kinds of misconduct and unethical practices in terms of health care and medical services.

Faith-based hospitals are pursuing the objective of serving health care–seeking patients in Bangladesh. As they are based on a religious spirit and operate within the guidelines set for them, they are not profit oriented; rather, they are service oriented. The people working for these hospitals are motivated to serve and are therefore better in their approach and behavior. In addition, the rates charged for the services are also very reasonable compared with the privately owned hospitals. Faith-based hospitals like Islami Bank hospitals and Ibn Sina hospitals have therefore become popular among all classes of people across the country. The financial sustainability of this way of operating, however, is not easy to maintain.[8] Their capacity to provide good-quality services at reasonable prices should not be taken for granted in economically turbulent times.

5. Concluding Remarks

Based on the discussion in this chapter, it is quite clear that faith-based hospitals play a significant role in the promotion of health-care services in Bangladesh as an alternative to public- as well as business-based services. In addition, faith-based hospitals like Islami Bank hospitals and Ibn Sina hospitals are also rendering their services for treatment-seeking people in a relatively satisfactory manner.

These hospitals are doing their best to provide better services to patients, and they charge fees that are lower than those of the privately owned hospitals. The patients also have a broadly shared experience that the staff in the faith-based hospitals behave gently—the patients have not often complained about their care. Although the public hospitals take just a nominal fee from patients, the attitude and behavior of their personnel have tended to be unpleasant to a degree that has continually pushed the needy to seek treatment elsewhere.

8 See, for example, the *Daily Star* on the economic challenges of the Islamic Bank Foundation (*Daily Star* 2018).

It is not easy to obtain broad and transparent reports on the functioning of faith-based hospitals in Bangladesh because of government surveillance. The further success of such institutions would not fit the political agenda of the present secularly oriented government of the country. Faith-based hospitals are nevertheless a very functional option in terms of health-care services. If these kinds of hospitals were really recognized by the government as well as by foreign development agencies, other hospitals could even be inspired to accept them as models for health service provision. This chapter thereby urges both national and international authorities to recognize faith-based hospitals as important alternative institutions in the process of improving health services for all in Bangladesh.

References

Aminuzzaman, Salahuddin, and Sumaiya Khair. 2014. "National Integrity Assessment Bangladesh 2014." Transparency International Bangladesh. Accessed August 9, 2018. https://tinyurl.com/yy8rzywh.

Crisp, Nigel. 2010. *Turning the World Upside Down: The Search for Global Health in the 21st Century*. London: Royal Society of Medicine.

Daily Star. 2019. "Islami Bank's Default Loans Double in Three Months." June 30, 2019. Accessed September 16, 2019. https://tinyurl.com/y3nxy526.

Dhaka Tribune. 2018. "Ibn Sina Trust to Sell Off All Islami Bank Shares, Worth Nearly Tk100cr." April 26, 2018. Accessed October 1, 2018. https://tinyurl.com/y5mcetz4.

Directorate General of Health Services (DGHS), Government of the People's Republic of Bangladesh. 2013. "Secondary and Tertiary Level Hospitals All over the Country." Accessed 2014. http://www.hsmdghs-bd.org/Govt_Hospital.htm.

———. 2018. *Health Bulletin 2018*. Dhaka: Management Information System, DGHS. Accessed September 13, 2019. https://tinyurl.com/y3yf4tpr.

Economist. 2017. "The Government Initiates a Coup at Bangladesh's Biggest Bank." April 6, 2017. Accessed August 8, 2018. https://tinyurl.com/y2kvh3dz.

General Economics Division of Bangladesh Planning Commission. 2014. *Millennium Development Goals: Bangladesh Progress Report 2013*. Accessed September 16, 2019. https://tinyurl.com/od9tn8v.

Government of the People's Republic of Bangladesh. 2017. *Eradicating Poverty and Promoting Prosperity in a Changing World: Voluntary National Review (VNR)*. Accessed August 8, 2018. https://tinyurl.com/y4by4xkw.

Ibn Sina Medical College. 2018. "From Ibn Sina Trust to Ibn Sina Medical College." Accessed September 9, 2018. https://ismc.ac.bd/ibn_sina_trust.php.

Ibn Sina Trust. 2018. "Ibn Sina Trust: Pioneer in Health Care." Accessed August 9, 2015. http://www.ibnsinatrust.com.

Islamic Bank Bangladesh Limited (IBBL). 2018. "All about IBBL." Accessed August 2018. https://tinyurl.com/y4vd3e7x.

Islamic Bank Foundation (IBF). "Islamic Bank Foundation." Accessed August 9, 2018. http://www.ibfbd.org.

Nabi, Golzare, Aminul Islam, and Asma Akter. 2015. "Islamic Banking in Bangladesh: Current Status, Challenges and Policy." Researchgate. Accessed August 8, 2018. https://tinyurl.com/y5tc7d5y.

Salahuddin, Yousuf, Ariful Islam, and Rayhan Islam. 2014. "Islamic Banking Scenario of Bangladesh." *Journal of Islamic Banking and Finance* 2 (1): 23–29. Accessed August 8, 2018. https://tinyurl.com/y348wk5x.

Transparency International. 2018. "Corruption Perceptions Index 2017." Accessed August 6, 2018. https://tinyurl.com/y48xvhmn.

United Nations. 2015. *The Millennium Development Goals Report 2015.* Accessed September 16, 2019. https://tinyurl.com/p92xdd3.

——. 2019. "About the Sustainable Development Goals." Accessed September 13, 2019. https://tinyurl.com/y5b6xalg.

United Nations Development Programme (UNDP). 2019. "Human Development Reports, All 2016 HDR Data." Accessed September 13, 2019. http://hdr.undp.org/en/composite/HDI.

World Health Organization (WHO). 2019. "Domestic General Government Health Expenditure (GGHE-D) as a Percentage of Gross Domestic Product (GDP)." Accessed September 13, 2019. https://tinyurl.com/y63byspu.

Yunus, Muhammad. 2010. *Building Social Business.* New York: Public Affairs.

Zaman, Hassan, Dewan Alamgir, Nagavalli Annamalai, Irajen Appasamy, Mirza Hasan, Naomi Hossain, Safi Khan et al. 2007. *Economics and Governance of Nongovernmental Organizations in Bangladesh: World Bank Study.* Dhaka: The University Press Limited.

Zaman, Mohammed Ameeruz. 2011. *In Quest of Fairness.* Dhaka: University Press.

12

―――――

Islamic Health Justice for Women in Saudi Arabia

Hana Al-Bannay

ABSTRACT

Following a recent mandate of gender equality in the Kingdom of Saudi Arabia (KSA), Saudi women have attained new rights that can potentially enable them to enjoy a healthy living. In 2018, the ban on women driving was lifted, and women were permitted to travel outside the country without the consent of a male guardian. These changes correspond with the teachings of a more moderate form of Islam that has been recently introduced in the KSA to replace a conservative one. In light of Islamic principles of social justice and the rights of Muslim women, this chapter proposes reform actions for women's health in the KSA. Improving women's health in the KSA aligns with Saudi Arabia's "Vision 2030."

1. Introduction

Over the past four decades, the sociopolitical systems in the Kingdom of Saudi Arabia (KSA) had strictly limited women's independence. For example, Saudi women were required to obtain consent from a male guardian in order to enroll in a university, be issued a passport, or travel outside the country. Women in the KSA were treated as second-class citizens, as they had to rely on male relatives to lead their lives. According to the "Gender Inequality Index" (United Nations Development Programme

[UNDP] 2017), the KSA is ranked 39 on a list of 189 world countries, with a value of 0.23 (the highest value is 0.649 in Niger and lowest is 0.004 in Norway). Saudi women's participation in the labor market is estimated at 23.37 percent, and a small number of women (30 women of 150 members) hold seats in the Consultative Assembly—called the Shura Council (World Bank 2018). Of the total number of women in the KSA, 69.88 percent are enrolled in universities compared to 66.34 percent of male university students (UNESCO 2019).

With respect to social and public lives in the KSA, religious regulations obligated women to wear a black loose dress called an abaya when they showed in public. Saudi women were prohibited from engaging in public physical activities such as running, jogging, riding a bike, or enrolling in sports competitions. These regulations are broken down with a recent announcement made by the crown prince, Mohammad bin Salman, who stated that women do not need to wear abayas. Although clothing does not necessarily restrict women from physical activities, restricting women to certain kinds of clothing can limit their opportunities to engage in physical activities in public and outdoors. Health reports are alarmed by an increased rate of health conditions among Saudi women as a result of sedentary lifestyle (Mahmood 2018).

In the KSA, childbirth- and pregnancy-related mortality rates have decreased over the decades. According to 2017 statistical reports, of every one hundred thousand live births in the KSA, seventeen women die from pregnancy-related factors. The life expectancy for Saudi women is 76.5 years, and their healthy life expectancy is 66 years (Knoema n.d.). Recently, a legislation of gender equality has abruptly transformed the lives of women in the KSA, and the status of Saudi women has been receiving a great amount of attention by the Saudi sociopolitical systems. Nonetheless, the health needs of Saudi women have not adapted to the transition in the Saudi culture. This chapter discusses the provision of health justice to women in the KSA in reference to Islamic feminism and social justice.

2. The Modern Culture of Saudi Arabia

The KSA has shifted toward a progressive Muslim culture. This transformation collides with a previous conservative form of Islam that had shaped the Saudi culture over the past four decades. Attempting to preserve the pure version of Islam from latter invocations, the religious authority in the KSA had obliged men and women to follow the lifestyles of early Muslims. Conservative religious traditions made the situation of women in the KSA a unique social context (Hamdan 2013).

The Saudi government has recently permitted women to drive. Lifting the ban on driving has increased women's mobility and engagement in social public life. Public life in the KSA is no longer required to be segregated by gender. The authority of the religious police to regulate social public life in the KSA has come to an end. Women in the KSA are now permitted to engage in physical activities such as biking and jogging publicly. Gender segregation in schools and universities has become optional. School curricula are currently under review to remove conservative interpretations of Islam and related teachings on gender roles. Until recently, some academic fields such as electrical and civil engineering and law were not available to female university students. Gender-based regulations in education and the workforce are gradually replaced with new gender-equality regulations.

The Saudi jurisdiction has recently legislated gender equality. Women in the KSA are now permitted to drive and travel outside the country without an official signed permission by an immediate male family member. Saudi women are gradually sharing top decision-making positions with men. In 2013, the Consultative Assembly—called the Shura Council—has elected 30 women members to join 120 men members. Very recently, Princess Reema bint Bandar was appointed as an ambassador to the United States, becoming the first female envoy in Saudi history.

3. Women in Pre-Islamic Arabia

Before the advent of Islam, women in the Arab pagan culture were treated as the property of men. When a father dies, for instance, his sons would share his wives as an inheritance (Women in Islam 2012; Keddie 2007). Women were deprived of their rights of inheritance (Engineer 2011). The birth of a girl was considered a shame, and girls were buried alive to avoid poverty and prevent them from marrying men from other tribes (Women in Islam 2012; Keddie 2007). Moreover, while women were not allowed to choose their husbands or remarry if they became widowed, men had no limit over the number of wives and could give women away to other men (Women in Islam 2012; Keddie 2007). The Qur'an addressed women's status in the Arabian culture before Islam, saying, "When the news of [the birth of] a female is brought to any of them, his face becomes dark, and he is filled with inward grief! He hides himself from the people because of the evil (and shame) of that which he has been informed. Shall he keep her with dishonor, or bury her in the dirt?" (16:58–59). The Qur'an utterly prohibits the act of burying girls alive and considers it a crime. The Qur'an said, "And when the female buried alive shall be questioned. For what sin was she killed?" (81:8–9). It also said, "And kill not your children for fear of poverty. We provide for them and you. Surely, the killing of them is a great sin" (17:31).

The Arab pagan culture was male dominant, undermining women's social capabilities (Women in Islam 2012; Keddie 2007; Sidani 2005; Engineer 2011). Men perceived excessive control over women as a necessity to guarantee the honor and pride of their tribes (Engineer 2011). Women's secondary status to men had contributed to their lacking of basic human rights. They sometimes were prevented from consuming certain types of food at times of food scarcity (Women in Islam 2012; Keddie 2007). To this, the Qur'an said, "And they say: What is in the bellies of such cattle (whether milk or fetus) is for the male alone, and forbidden from our females" (6:139).

After Islam, the situation of women was drastically reformed, and the Qur'an had specified full chapters to describe the rights of Muslim women. One chapter (Surah An-Nisa) discusses the significant roles of women in their families and societies, women's entitlements to inheritance, their rights in marriage, and the boundaries of receiving fair treatment and emotional security (Al-Mannai 2010). Another chapter (Surah Maryam) tells the story of Saint Mary and presents her as a role model to women of all worlds.

4. Women in Islam

Islam has provided women with equal opportunities to men with respect to education and social inclusion (Al-Mannai 2010; Koehler 2011; Syed 2008; Omair 2008; Uthman 2010; Badawi 1995). Prophet Muhammad said, "Seeking knowledge is an obligation for all Muslims including men and women." Muslim women are entitled, but not required, to work and contribute to the household income (Hamdan 2013). In contrast to the Western view that women should be entitled to the same work opportunities as men, Islam avoids burdening women with excessive physical duties. Islam pardoned women from the requirement of contributing to the household income so they wouldn't be burdened with responsibilities outside the home. Men, on the other hand, are obligated to provide financial and emotional securities to women (Badawi 1995). Muslim women are entitled to receive financial support given that they are more likely to become poor (Benn and Hyder 2002).

Islam treats women and men equally in being (their souls). Women in Islam have similar capabilities to men in spirituality and performing good deeds (Hamdan 2013; Al-Mannai 2010; Badawi 1995). Men and women have similar moral and spiritual obligations, and both have the capacity for self-realization in this life and the hereafter. Despite the significant role of Muslim women in building Muslim societies, moral regulations start off with men. The Qur'an said, "Tell the believing men to lower their gaze and be modest. That is purer for them. Lo! Allah is aware of what they do. And tell the believing women to lower their gaze and be modest" (24:30–31). The Qur'an also said,

> Surely the men who submit and the women who submit, and the believing men and the believing women, and the obeying men and the obeying women, and the truthful men and the truthful women, and the patient men and the patient women and the humble men and the humble women, and the almsgiving men and the almsgiving women, and the fasting men and the fasting women, and the men who guard their private parts and the women who guard, and the men who remember Allah much and the women who remember—Allah has prepared for them forgiveness and a mighty reward. (33:35)

Both men and women have responsibilities toward each other (Badawi 1995). The Qur'an said, "And women shall have rights similar to the rights against them, according to what is equitable; but men have a degree (of responsibility) over them" (2:228). On the same grounds, Prophet Muhammad said, "O People, it is true that you have certain rights over your women, but they also have rights over you."

Motherhood is an honorable role in Islam. Mothers in Islam are granted higher status compared to fathers. In relation to this, the Qur'an said, "And We have enjoined (upon) man for his parents—carried him his mother (in) weakness upon weakness, and his weaning (is) in two years that. Be grateful to Me and to your parents" (31:14). Prophet Muhammad also said, "Paradise lies beneath the feet of the mother."

Women in early Islam played significant social and political roles. For instance, Khadija, the first woman in Islam and the wife of the Prophet, was noble and wealthy and was a businesswoman (Ullah, Mahmud, and Yousuf 2013; Koehler 2011; Kabir 2007). She donated her wealth to the cause of Islam. "Islam would not have risen without Khadija's wealth,"

Prophet Muhammad said. Khadija was the first role model for Muslim women (Haylamaz 2007).

Fatima bint Mohammad, like her mother, Khadija, had an active role in her society and was gathering with other women to educate them about Islamic values, of which she had learned from her father (Kashani-Sabet 2005). She, along with other prominent women, such as the Prophet's wives after Khadija, Aisha bint Abu-Baker and Um-Salama, had reported a large number of the hadith—the sayings and behaviors of the Prophet—that are documented in major Islamic sources (el-Aswad 2014). Aisha was the youngest wife of the Prophet and the daughter of the first caliph, Abu-Baker. She was a prominent social and political figure. She opposed the third caliph, Uthman bin Affan, and rode a camel in a battle she led against the fourth caliph, Ali bin Abi Talib (Geissinger 2011; Scott 2009; Gilani 2013). Two centuries later in 859 CE, a pious, devout, and educated Fatima Al-Fihri dedicated her wealth to benefit her society and endowed her property to become the founder of the very first world university, Al-Karaouine University in Morocco (Gray 2013; Das and Das 2013).

Islam recommended men to revere, respect, and be kind to women. Prophet Muhammad said, "The best among you are those who treat their wives well." The Prophet himself was a role model for Muslim men with respect to the treatment of women. He used to stand up and kiss the forehead of his daughter Fatima to greet her respectfully (Ordoni 2014). Fatima was married to Ali bin Abi Talib, a man of great respect to women (Haylamaz 2015; Ordoni 2014). Ali was the Prophet's cousin and the first boy to believe in Islam (Haylamaz 2015). He grew up in the household of Prophet Muhammad and later became an advocate for women's rights (Haylamaz 2015; Ordoni 2014). Ali reportedly said, "Woman is a delicate creature with strong emotions who has been created by the Almighty God to shoulder responsibility for educating society and moving toward perfection. God created woman as a symbol of His own beauty and to give solace to her partner and her family" (Ataya 2015). Ali and Fatima's children, Al-Hassan and Al-Hussain, grew up in a household that was very respectful to women. Al-Hussain, for instance, used to stand up to greet his sister Zainab and would give his seat to her (Askari 2015). In brief, Islam called for women's emancipation and opposed pre-Islamic attitudes and practices that deprived women of their equal rights to men (Hamdan 2013; Das and Das 2013).

Equality, social justice, and human dignity are integral to Islamic teachings and are featured prominently in the Qur'an (Anwar 2013; Crow 2013). Drawing on these principles, Muslim feminists are working to eliminate inequalities against women and enhance their dignity (Hamdan 2013; Das and Das 2013; Shah 2006). Islam treats women and men equally in spirituality and morality. Nonetheless, cultural and traditional norms have infiltrated Islamic teachings of women's rights. Muslim feminists of today continue to struggle with patriarchal attitudes that place women under the control of men (Uthman 2010; Rouse 2004).

In contrast to Western feminists, Muslim feminists seek to attain gender equity and emphasize family as a core social system where women contribute the most to influencing the present society and generating a new one (Uthman 2010; Shah 2006). In line with this, Muslim feminists do not oppose Islamic teachings, with their traditional gender roles and heterosexual relations. They believe that Islam is an ideal social system for emancipating women from oppression (Shah 2006; Rouse 2004). They are calling for an egalitarian interpretation of the Qur'an in relation to Muslim women's roles and rights that fit in the modern world (Uthman 2010; Shah 2006; Rouse 2004). Simply put, Islamic values of feminism, which are taught by the Prophet and his family and companions over fourteen hundred years ago, do correspond with modern human rights.

5. Islam, Human Rights, and Justice

Islamic teachings align with human rights and justice. It prohibited any form of discrimination on the grounds of gender, race, skin color, language, religion, nationality, or social and economic status (Khan 2011; Williams and Zinkin 2009; Syed 2008). Prophet Muhammad reportedly said, "All mankind is from Adam and Eve, an Arab has no superiority over a non-Arab nor a non-Arab has any superiority over an Arab; also a white has no superiority over a black nor a black has any superiority over white except by piety and good deeds." Opposing discrimination is a fundamental concept in Islamic justice. The Qur'an said, "God commands justice and fair dealing" (16:90).

Human rights in Islam imply equal treatment to people based on justice principles and regardless of differences in gender, race, or social status (Naim 2005; Saeed 2007). The Qur'an addressed this, saying, "Stand out firmly for justice, as witnesses to Allah, even if it be against yourselves, your parents, and your relatives, or whether it is against the rich or the poor" (4:135). Islam treats people as born-free humans with equal rights. Hence it recommended Muslims to treat each other humanely with the spirit of brotherhood (Williams and Zinkin 2009). The Qur'an said, "The believers are nothing else than brothers" (49:10). Social justice, on the other hand, considers individual differences as factors to be accounted for when providing fair treatment (Rogers and Kelly 2011).

Social justice can be defined as the fulfillment of individuals' needs and considering individual differences with respect to potentials (Rogers and Kelly 2011; Hofriichter 2005). Social justice promotes equal distributions of power and wealth and mandates charities to the needy through welfare systems (Benn and Hyder 2002). Social justice distributes resources and needs to people equally but relative to individuals' capabilities and potentials (Rogers and Kelly 2011). For instance, social justice in health care implies that health-care resources are distributed equally to people by taking into account individuals' health needs that vary by gender, age, and health status (Rogers and Kelly 2011; Kirby 2011; Bates, Hankivsky, and Springer 2009). These individual differences are addressed in the theory of health capability (Khoo 2013; Marchand, Wikler, and Landesman 2001).

6. Health Capability and Health Justice

The theory of health capability—also called the capability to be healthy—was proposed by Sridhar Venkatapuram in 1993 (Khoo 2013; Abel and Frohlich 2012; Chapman 2015). According to this theory, health is related to social justice, whereas illnesses and premature death are attributed to injustice (Khoo 2013). This theory corresponds with the International Classification of Functioning, Disability and Health (ICF). In the ICF model, restrictions on the functioning and participation of the human body can be due to social and environmental factors in addition to personal ones (WHO 2018). In this respect, social justice in health care implies providing not only adequate biomedical medicine for the treatment of physical bodies but also social and environmental support to enable the functioning and participation of individuals (Khoo 2013; Marchand, Wikler, and Landesman 2001).

In the absence of social justice, people's capabilities to be healthy are reduced (Khoo 2013; Faden and Powers 2011). For example, impoverished people may not have access to healthy food options and leisure activities; therefore, their health and well-being might be below the average. In these situations, providing access to health care without eliminating poverty will not optimize people's health and well-being. Health justice penetrates the roles and responsibilities of governments, societies, communities, and business agencies (Gil 2006; Faden and Powers 2011). Ministries of Health in particular have a pivotal role in social and political reforms to health standards (Day 2010; Kirby 2011). Environmental and sociocultural barriers such as limited transportation, language barriers, and unequal distribution of services affect health behaviors and therefore should be eliminated (Gil 2006; Light 2000; Pham, Vinck, and Weinstein 2010). Social, political, economic, and environmental influences are referred to as social determinants of health (Marmot et al. 2012).

In the spirit of promoting health justice, the World Health Organization has convened a Commission on Social Determinants of Health in 2005 (WHO 2008). The World Health Organization defines health as "a state of complete physical, mental, and social wellbeing and not merely the absence of disease or infirmity" (De Jong and Rutten 1983, 1085). Health in this view is considered a fundamental human right of which individuals are entitled to attain. Enabling access to high-quality health care must be a global goal that can be achieved through a collaborative action between social, economic, and health sectors (1085). Public health therefore should aim to make "needed and effective services available to everyone, regardless of their health conditions, risk, and ability to pay" (Light 2000, 65).

Health justice overlaps with human rights and is bound to both equity and equality (Resnik and Roman 2007; Benn and Hyder 2002; Badawi 1995). Health equality can be defined as allocating equal health needs to people regardless of individual differences (Resnik and Roman 2007). Health equity, on the other hand, is an allocation of health needs while taking into account individual differences (Resnik and Roman 2007; Bates, Hankivsky, and Springer 2009). Individual differences can be related to differences in education, occupation, income, gender, capabilities, inclusion, social factors, social justice, and health development (Fox and Thomson 2013; Marmot et al. 2012). According to the human rights code, these differences are legitimate rights to everyone.

Health and well-being are basic human rights, and people are entitled to the highest standard of health that their state can provide (Benn and Hyder 2002). Health and well-being are contingent on social justice for the attainment of "physical, intellectual, social, emotional, and spiritual potentials" (Littlefield et al. 2002). People's basic needs such as food, shelter, and security have to be met to increase their potential for health (World Health Organization 2017; Littlefield et al. 2002).

7. Reform Actions to the Health of Women in the KSA

In the KSA, the government provides health-care services that are free of charge to Saudi citizens and are regulated by the Ministry of Health at three levels. The primary level provides health care for mothers and newly born children and refers to conditions that require special care to public hospitals at the secondary level (Almalki, Fitzgerald, and Clark 2011). When they receive complex cases, hospitals at the secondary level will refer them to specialized care at the tertiary level (Almalki, Fitzgerald, and Clark 2011). Currently, the Saudi government is preparing to privatize health care in their attempt to improve service standards according to Saudi Arabia's "Vision 2030" (Rahman and Al-Borie 2020).

Reform actions to women's health in the KSA align with the rights of women in Islam and Islamic social justice. Those reform actions can be highlighted through the social-ecological model that views health behaviors as dependent on interactions between people and their environment at various levels, including economy, society, and politics (Glanz, Barbara, and Kasisomayajula 2008). Clearly, adapting the social and economic systems in the KSA to the principles of Islamic feminism and social justice may warrant the provision of women's health needs.

Literature suggests improving the conditions of daily living as an initial step to the provision of health justice (Kirby 2011; Day 2010). No accurate data on poverty in the KSA is available. Some reports claim that the Saudi government does not provide transparent data about the poverty rate in the KSA (United Nations 2017). Saudi society is based on a class system, and the majority of the Saudi population falls in the middle class (Niblock 2015). Power and excessive wealth in the KSA are concentrated in a small upper class, and the gap between the rich and poor is gradually increasing (Niblock 2015). Poverty in the KSA, if not eliminated, will create devastating impacts on women's daily activities.

The absence of public transportation in the KSA makes it difficult for poor and low-income women to afford driving or the expenses of hiring private drivers for their daily errands. The social norms of women's public behaviors in the Saudi culture restrict women from having equal social and leisure activities to men's. For example, it is not appropriate for women in the KSA to get together in a park to run like men do. Isolation and exclusion have devastating outcomes on women's health that include psychosocial conditions, poor health behaviors, illnesses and diseases, and possibly death (Fox and Thomson 2013; Reid, Frisby, and Ponic 2002). Averting patriarchal cultural attitudes that undermine women's capabilities and do not correspond with Islamic values will enable Saudi women to boost their confidence in maintaining control over their lives. Patriarchy, unequal distribution of wealth, and the lack of the strict application to women's entitlement of financial support not only contradict Islamic values but also may impact negatively on the health and well-being of Saudi women.

In alignment with the World Health Organization's suggestions, the technique of tackling problems and providing solutions can be used to implement health justice globally (Pham, Vinck, and Weinstein 2010). In the KSA, women's barriers to adopting health behaviors are cultural, social, and environmental. For instance, the cost of transportation can be a social problem for low-income women in particular. Reform actions to health justice for women in the KSA can benefit men, families, and society overall.

Drawing on the World Health Organization's recommendations, reform actions to the health of Saudi women can include the following: First, providing healthy food options to all people (men, women, and children) and restricting unhealthy food. Second, providing safe and affordable housing to everyone and subsidized housing to the needy. Indeed, the latter is being considered by the Ministry of Housing. Third, increasing employment opportunities for everyone, increasing job securities, and creating more work opportunities for women. Fourth, providing protection for women from work hazards that include both physical injuries and psychological stresses. Fifth, increasing public awareness of work-life balance, legislating for maximum working hours, and allowing the option of early retirement for women. Sixth, promoting social pensions, especially for women. Research shows that social pensions contribute to empowering older women, integrating them into their communities, and promoting gender equality (Fox and Thomson 2013; Duflo 2011). Seventh, reaching out to impoverished women and encouraging them to attend social and religious events in mosques and community centers. Scientific studies show that poor women encounter discrimination and are discouraged from participating in their communities (Fox and Thomson 2013; Grollman 2012). Eighth, involving poor women in health promotion campaigns to make them empowered in voicing their needs (Mohajer and Earnest 2010; Bates, Hankivsky, and Springer 2009). Ninth, planning public transportation everywhere in the country. Tenth, establishing affordable and free-of-charge women-only recreation centers in each neighborhood. Eleventh, involving Saudi families, especially women, in public health projects to address barriers, plan solutions, and evaluate outcomes. Twelfth, increasing the scope of public health programs for prevention. Presently, health promotion in the KSA is focused more on infectious diseases and less on the prevention and management of lifestyle health behaviors (Almalki, Fitzgerald, and Clark 2011; Al-Khaldi and Khan 2000). Thirteenth, applying up-to-date scientific and technical findings in environmental health like accessibility to wheelchairs in urban planning. Fourteenth, increasing awareness about women's rights in Islam and the distinction between Islamic values and patriarchal cultural attitudes toward women (Arnez 2010). Finally, advocating gender equality in schools, mosques, and religious seminars and encouraging men of all ages to promote women's rights.

8. Conclusion

The United Nations proclaimed the importance of gender equality to health development globally (Fox and Thomson 2013; Connell 2012). Women are more likely to become poor, dependent on men, and marginalized and excluded from decision-making (Chant and Sweetman 2012). Patriarchal attitudes that contradict Islamic values of feminism are embedded in the Saudi Arabian culture (Hamdan 2013; Zamberi 2011; Mobaraki and Soderfeldt 2010). Young Saudi women of today, particularly the millennials, have increased awareness of their rights and the devastating social impacts of patriarchy, which entitles men to certain privileges over women. Raising the awareness of the orchestration of gender equality with Islamic feminism and social justice will empower Saudi women. What's good for women is good for society. Healthy women raise healthy children. Considering Islamic principles of feminism and social justice in the promotion of the health and well-being of women in the KSA accords with Saudi Arabia's "Vision 2030" (KSA n.d.) and will potentially benefit men, families, and society overall.

References

Abel, T., and K. L. Frohlich. 2012. "Capitals and Capabilities: Linking Structure and Agency to Reduce Health Inequalities." *Social Science & Medicine* 74 (2): 236–244.

Al-Khaldi, Y., and M. Y. Khan. 2000. "Audit of a Diabetic Health Education Program at a Large Primary Health Care Center in Asir Region." *Saudi Medical Journal* 21 (9): 838–842.

Almalki, M., G. Fitzgerald, and M. Clark. 2011. "Health Care System in Saudi Arabia: An Overview." *Eastern Mediterranean Health Journal* 17 (10): 784–793.

Al-Mannai, S. S. 2010. "The Misinterpretation of Women's Status in the Muslim World." *Digest of Middle East Studies* 19 (1): 82–91.

Anwar, S. M. 2013. "Normative Structure of Human Rights in Islam." *Policy Perspectives* 10 (1): 79–104.

Arnez, M. 2010. "Empowering Women through Islam: Fatayat NU between Tradition and Change." *Journal of Islamic Studies* 21 (1): 59–88.

Askari, S. H. 2015. *Syeda Zainab (SA).* Vol. 5 of Islamic Mobility. Accessed September 13, 2020. https://tinyurl.com/y5debmep.

Ataya, S. 2015. "Islam: Peace & Terrorism, Brief History, Principles and Beliefs." Morrisville, NC: Lulu.

Badawi, J. 1995. *Gender Equity in Islam.* Plainfield, IN: American Trust. Accessed October 10, 2019. https://tinyurl.com/y5cmjmqu.

Bates, L. M., O. Hankivsky, and K. W. Springer. 2009. "Gender and Health Inequities: A Comment on the Final Report of the WHO Commission on the Social Determinants of Health." *Social Science & Medicine* 69 (7): 1002–1004.

Benn, C., and A. A. Hyder. 2002. "Equity and Resource Allocation in Health Care: Dialogue between Islam and Christianity." *Medicine, Health Care and Philosophy* 5 (2): 181–189.

Chant, S., and C. Sweetman. 2012. "Fixing Women or Fixing the World? 'Smart Economics,' Efficiency Approaches, and Gender Equality in Development." *Gender & Development* 20 (3): 517–529.

Chapman, A. 2015. "The Foundations of a Human Right to Health: Human Rights and Bioethics in Dialogue." *Health & Human Rights: An International Journal* 17 (1).

Connell, R. 2012. "Gender, Health and Theory: Conceptualizing the Issue, in Local and World Perspective." *Social Science & Medicine* 74 (11): 1675–1683.

Crow, K. D. 2013. "Closed-Door Roundtable Discussion on Human Rights and Islam (Kuala Lumpur, 20 November 2012)." *Islam and Civilisational Renewal (ICR)* 4 (2).

Das, K., and M. Das. 2013. "A Glimpse of Muslim Women in Assam." *Asian Journal of Multidisciplinary Studies* 1 (5).

Day, L. 2010. "Health Care Reform, Health, and Social Justice." *American Journal of Critical Care* 19 (5): 459–461.

De Jong, G. A., and F. F. H. Rutten. 1983. "Justice and Health for All." *Social Sciences Medicine* 17 (16): 1085–1095.

Duflo, E. 2012. "Women Empowerment and Economic Development." *Journal of Economic literature* 50 (4): 1051–1079.

el-Aswad, E. S. 2014. "Muhammad." In *Encyclopedia of Psychology and Religion*, edited by D. A. Leeming, 1148–1151. Boston: Springer. Accessed September 13, 2020. https://doi.org/10.1007/978-1-4614-6086-2_9333.

Engineer, A. A. 2011. "Rights of Women and Muslim Societies." *Socio-legal Review* 7:44.

Faden, R., and M. Powers. 2011. "A Social Justice Framework for Health and Science Policy." *Cambridge Quarterly of Healthcare Ethics* 20 (4): 569–604.

Fox, M., and M. Thomson. 2013. "Realising Social Justice in Public Health Law." *Medical Law* 21 (2): 278–309.

Geissinger, A. 2011. "A'isha bint Abi Bakr and Her Contributions to the Formation of the Islamic Tradition." *Religion Compass* 5 (1): 37–49.

Gil, D. G. 2006. "Reflections on Health and Social Justice." *Contemporary Justice Review* 9 (1): 39–46.

Gilani, S. S. 2013. "Aiesha Bint Abu Bakr." *Defence Journal* 16 (7): 50.

Glanz, K., K. Barbara, and V. Kasisomayajula, eds. 2008. *Health Behavior and Health Education Theory, Research, and Practice*. San Francisco: Jossey-Bass.

Gray, D. H. 2013. "Political Women in Morocco–Then and Now." *Journal of North African Studies* 18 (4): 617–618.

Grollman, E. A. 2012. "Multiple Forms of Perceived Discrimination and Health among Adolescents and Young Adults." *Journal of Health and Social Behavior* 53 (2): 199–214.

Hamdan, A. 2013. "Arab Women's Education and Gender Perceptions: An Insider Analysis." *Journal of International Women's Studies* 8 (1): 52–64.

Haylamaz, R. 2007. *Khadija: The First Muslim and the Wife of the Prophet Muhammad*. Somerset, NJ: Tughra Books.

———. 2011. *Ali ibn Abi Talib: The Hero of Chivalry (Leading Companions of the Prophet)*. Clifton, NJ: Tughra Books.

Hofriichter, R. 2005. "Review of the Book Health and Social Justice: Politics, Ideology, and Inequity in the Distribution of Disease." *American Journal of Epidemiology* 16 (4): 399–400.

Jones, T. C. 2011. "Saudi Arabia versus the Arab Spring." *Raritan* 31 (2): 43.

Kabir, K. S. 2007. "Towards an Islamic Framework of Women Empowerment." *Tafhim: IKIM Journal of Islam and the Contemporary World* 2 (2).

Kashani-Sabet, F. 2005. "Who Is Fatima? Gender, Culture, and Representation in Islam." *Journal of Middle East Women's Studies* 1 (2): 1–24.

Keddie, N. R. 2007. *Women in the Middle East: Past and Present*. Princeton, NJ: Princeton University Press.

Khan, T. S. 2011. *Human Rights and Islam*. New Delhi: Murari Lal & Sons.

Khoo, S. 2013. "Health Justice and Capabilities: A Turning Point for Global Health." *International Sociology* 28 (2): 155–167.

Kingdom of Saudi Arabia. n.d. "Vision 2030." Accessed September 13, 2020. https://www.vision2030.gov.sa/en/programs.

Kirby, M. 2011. "Health Care and Global Justice." *International Journal of Law in Context* 7 (3): 273–284.

Knoema. n.d. "World Atlas Data." Accessed October 10, 2019. https://tinyurl .com/yyzyulan.

Koehler, B. 2011. "Female Entrepreneurship in Early Islam." *Economic Affairs* 31 (2): 93–95.

Light, D. W. 2000. "Fostering a Justice-Based Health Care System." *Contemporary Sociology* 29 (1): 62–74.

Littlefield, D., C. C. Robison, L. Engelbrecht, B. González, and H. Hutcheson. 2002. "Mobilizing Women for Minority Health and Social Justice in California." *American Journal of Public Health* 92 (4): 576–579.

Mahmood, F. M. 2018. "Prevalence and Prevention of Lifestyle-Related Diseases in Saudi Arabia." *International Journal of Health Sciences* 12 (5): 1–2.

Marchand, S., D. Wikler, and B. Landesman. 2001. "Class, Health, and Justice." *Milbank Quarterly* 76 (3): 449–467.

Marmot, M., J. Allen, R. Bell, E. Bloomer, and P. Goldblatt. 2012. "WHO European Review of Social Determinants of Health and the Health Divide." *Lancet* 380 (9846): 1011–1029.

Mobaraki, A. E., and B. Söderfeldt. 2010. "Gender Inequity in Saudi Arabia and Its Role in Public Health." *Eastern Mediterranean Health Journal* 16 (1): 113–118.

Mohajer, N., and J. Earnest. 2010. "Widening the Aim of Health Promotion to Include the Most Disadvantaged: Vulnerable Adolescents and the Social Determinants of Health." *Health Education Research* 25 (3): 387–394.

Naim, A. A. A. 2005. "The Interdependence of Religion, Secularism, and Human Rights: Prospects for Islamic Societies." *Common Knowledge* 11 (1): 56–80.

Niblock, T., ed. 2015. *State, Society and Economy in Saudi Arabia (RLE Saudi Arabia).* London: Routledge.

Ordoni, A. M. 2014. *Fatima the Gracious.* Morrisville, NC: Lulu.

Pham, P. N., P. Vinck, and H. M. Weinstein. 2010. "Human Rights, Transitional Justice, Public Health and Social Reconstruction." *Social Science & Medicine* 70:98–105.

Rahman, R., and H. M. Al-Borie. 2020. "Strengthening the Saudi Arabian Healthcare System: Role of Vision 2030." *International Journal of Healthcare Management*, 1–9. https://doi.org/10.1080/20479700.2020.1788334.

Reid, C., W. Frisby, and P. Ponic. 2002. "Confronting Two-Tie Community Recreation and Poor Women's Exclusion: Promoting Inclusion, Health, and Social Justice." *Women Studies* 21 (3): 88–94.

Resnik, D. B., and G. Roman. 2007. "Health, Justice, and the Environment." *Bioethics* 21 (4): 230–241.

Rogers, J., and U. A. Kelly. 2011. "Feminist Intersectionality: Bring Social Justice to Health Disparities Research." *Nursing Ethics* 18 (3): 397–407.

Rouse, C. M. 2004. *Engaged Surrender: African American Women and Islam.* Oakland: University of California Press.

Saeed, A. 2007. "Trends in Contemporary Islam: A Preliminary Attempt at a Classification." *Muslim World* 97 (3): 395–404.

Scott, R. M. 2009. "A Contextual Approach to Women's Rights in the Qur'ān: Readings of 4:34." *Muslim World* 99 (1): 60–85.

Shah, N. A. 2006. "Women's Human Rights in the Koran: An Interpretive Approach." *Human Rights Quarterly* 28 (4): 868–903.

Sidani, Y. 2005. "Women, Work, and Islam in Arab Societies." *Women in Management Review* 20 (7): 498–512.

Syed, K. T. 2008. "Misconceptions about Human Rights and Women's Rights in Islam." *Interchange* 39 (2): 245–257.

Ullah, M. M., T. B. Mahmud, and F. Yousuf. 2013. "Women Entrepreneurship: Islamic Perspective." *European Journal of Business and Management* 5 (11): 44–52.

UNESCO Institute of Statistics. 2019. "Data for Sustainable Development Goals." Accessed October 10, 2019. http://uis.unesco.org/en/country/sa.

United Nations. 2017. *Report of the Special Rapporteur on Extreme Poverty and Human Rights on His Mission to Saudi Arabia.* United Nations Human Rights Council. Accessed September 12, 2020. https://digitallibrary.un.org/record/1298754?ln=en.

United Nations Development Programme (UNDP). 2017. "Gender Inequality Index." In *Human Development Reports.* Accessed October 10, 2019. http://hdr.undp.org/en/composite/GII.

Uthman, I. O. 2010. "A Triadic Re-reading of Zaynab al-Ghazali and the Feminist Movement in Islam." *Islamic Studies* 49 (1): 65–79.

Williams, G., and J. Zinkin. 2010. "Islam and CSR: A Study of the Compatibility between the Tenets of Islam and the UN Global Compact." *Journal of Business Ethics* 91 (4): 519–533.

Women in Islam. 2018. "Women in the Pre-Islamic Societies and Civilization." Accessed October 10, 2019. https://tinyurl.com/y5drkbl7.

World Bank. 2018. "Saudi Arabia's Economic Outlook—April 2018." Accessed October 10, 2019. https://tinyurl.com/yy8p3r26.

World Health Organization (WHO). 2008. *Closing the Gap in a Generation: Health Equity through Action on the Social Determinants of Health.* Accessed October 10, 2019. https://tinyurl.com/nmaqfkd.

———. 2017. "Human Rights and Health." Accessed October 10, 2019. https://tinyurl.com/yymwk7uo.

———. 2018. "International Classification of Functioning, Disability and Health (ICF)." Accessed October 10, 2019. http://www.who.int/classifications/icf/en.

Zamberi, A. S. 2011. "Evidence of the Characteristics of Women Entrepreneurs in the Kingdom of Saudi Arabia: An Empirical Investigation." *International Journal of Gender and Entrepreneurship* 3 (2): 123–143.

13

Ethics of HIV/AIDS and Religion in Africa

A SYSTEMATIC LITERATURE REVIEW

Sahaya G. Selvam

ABSTRACT

The role of religion in the prevalence and the prevention of HIV and in the care of people living with HIV/AIDS and children orphaned by HIV is well researched. The objective of the present systematic literature review is to examine the ethical issues underpinning the relationship between HIV/AIDS and religion in Africa. Carrying out a literature search in Academic Search Premier, a digital database of academic journals, twenty-two articles were selected based on some specific inclusion and exclusion criteria. The selected articles were analyzed in order to identify patterns in the emerging themes related to the objective of the review. Three major themes were picked up. These include (1) the ethics of the influence of religion on behavior related to HIV prevalence and treatment; (2) the impact of religion on social stigma and discrimination related to HIV/AIDS; and (3) the experience of internalized conflict yet feeling supported by religion. The themes are explained and supported by evidence from literature. The implication of these themes for the interaction between religion and health justice is also discussed.

1. Introduction

There is an undeniable interaction between HIV/AIDS and religion in Africa. The underlying reason for this dynamic relationship is that "religion plays an important role in the life of many Africans" (Ntetmen-Mbetbo 2013, 76). Not only in indigenous societies in Africa but also in contemporary urban societies, the causes of illness are often related to supernatural sources. Hence the association between religion and HIV/AIDS does not have to be forced. As a consequence, religion is also an important determinant in the spread of HIV in sub-Saharan Africa (Manzou, Schumacher, and Gregson 2014). In short, the role of religion in the prevalence, diagnosis, and prevention of HIV and in the care of people living with HIV and children orphaned by HIV is well researched empirically.

Often the association between religion and HIV seems very ambiguous, with mixed outcomes. For instance, a study that reviewed literature on the influence of religion on psychologically coping with HIV/AIDS suggested that, on the one hand, belief in a higher power, prayer, and collaboration between themselves and the higher power might facilitate healthy coping and, on the other hand, some beliefs and practices in religion (such as the belief in miracles) may amount to unhealthy forms of coping "that may make them feel good initially but ultimately leave them feeling empty" (Pargament et al. 2004, 1204). There is also the issue of people living with HIV/AIDS being discriminated against and at the same time embraced by religion.

Such situations raise many ethical questions: Does religion serve for good in its fight against HIV/AIDS in Africa? Or in order to overcome HIV/AIDS, is it better to keep religion out of the frontline? While caring for people living with HIV/AIDS, does religion also create guilt in the hearts of the beneficiaries while giving the impression of being compassionate to them? The objective of the present chapter, therefore, is to examine the ethical issues underpinning the relationship between HIV/AIDS and religion in Africa through a meta-analysis of academic literature.

The general research question that guided the present literature review was, How does academic literature deal with justice issues related to HIV/AIDS and religion? More specifically, What themes relevant to ethics emerge in the sampled HIV/AIDS and religion literature?

2. Methodology

Systematic literature reviews are common in medical sciences and psychology. In these fields of human knowledge, the procedure of meta-analysis, as it is also referred to, attempts to statistically analyze quantitative data to identify, appraise, and synthesize available evidence and, on that basis, propose some conceptual or hypothetical conclusions. Often a systematic literature review is a quantitative procedure. However, qualitative systematic literature reviews are also increasingly being employed in social sciences (Selvam 2014, 2015). While quantitative systematic reviews help in evaluating the strength of available evidence in terms of numbers, the qualitative reviews are beneficial in systematically schematizing the emerging themes within the selected studies in relation to the research question of the review. Three steps are followed in a systematic literature review: (1) searching and selecting the available literature, (2) analyzing the sources, and (3) reporting the emerging themes. The following sections of the present chapter report these three steps in the examination of the underpinning ethical issues in academic literature that discuss the relationship between religion and HIV/AIDS in Africa.

2.1. Literature Search and Selection

In June 2015, a search was run on Academic Search Premier, a digital database of literature and a component of the EBSCOHost Services. Academic Search Premier is a multidisciplinary database that provides full text for nearly thirty-nine hundred peer-reviewed journals. Studies were considered eligible for inclusion in the present review if they were published in peer-reviewed scholarly journals and in English and if full texts were freely available. A search of "HIV Africa religion" yielded a list of nine entries. This was considered insufficient for a review. When the search term was expanded to "HIV religion," the result was a list of eighty-four entries. This list was further filtered for scholarly peer-reviewed journals, and this resulted in a list of seventy-seven entries; when it was again filtered for full texts, the list was narrowed to forty-one entries.

A cursory reading of the abstracts of these forty-one peer-reviewed articles revealed that twelve of them were not directly related to Africa or Africans; in fact, five of the twelve studies involved people of African descent living in the United States, the United Kingdom, or the Caribbean; none of these studies were included for analysis. A further seven entries were rejected because they did not directly discuss either ethical or religious issues. Finally, twenty-two full texts were downloaded in pdf format for analysis. The years of publication of the selected literature ranged from 2004 to 2011. Table 13.1 provides some detail on the selected literature. The sources represent data drawn from a good spread of countries across sub-Saharan Africa.

2.2. Literature Analysis: Qualitative Thematic Analysis

The selected articles were read in detail to cull out patterns of themes. This process followed the method of thematic analysis that Sahaya G. Selvam and Joanna Collicutt (2013) have explained and employed in a study elsewhere. "Thematic analysis is a method of identifying, analysing and reporting patterns (themes) within data" (Braun and Clark 2006, 79). Often this approach goes beyond identifying and analyzing to interpreting various aspects of the data on the basis of the research topic (Boyatzis 1998). In simple words, thematic analysis consists of coding the data systematically and finally reporting patterns that emerge from the data. In the present study, the selected articles were treated as the data for thematic analysis. The following section reports the emerging themes from this analysis. The discussion section will point out the implication of the findings in the context of the theme of the present book.

3. Findings

In all, three themes were identified as emerging from the selected literature. The present section lists the themes and provides substantial evidence from the sampled literature. In this section, an attempt is made to strengthen an argument furnished by one literature source with evidence from another source from among the twenty-two academic articles selected for the analysis.

3.1. Theme 1: Ethics of the Influence of Religion on Behavior Related to HIV Prevalence and Treatment

Two important points emerge under this theme in the literature. First, the more proscriptive a religious tradition is about sexual behavior, the more likely that there is a lower prevalence of HIV among the adherents of that religion or sect. Second, the attitude toward prayer and miracle healing has a mixed outcome on HIV testing and seeking treatment. These two points are elaborated later.

Table 13.1. Description of selected literature

Series number	In-text reference	Source of sample	Source journal	Type and focus of study
1	Afolabi et al. 2011	Nigeria	*Educational Research Quarterly*	Empirical (n = 215 university students); to study the influence of neuroticism, agreeableness, extraversion, and HIV awareness on risky sexual behavior
2	Agardh et al. 2011	Uganda	*PLoS ONE*	Empirical (n = 980 university students); to investigate the relationship between sociodemographic and religious factors and their impact on sexual behavior
3	Aguwa 2010	Nigeria	*Crosscurrents*	Conceptual; to examine how religious teachings and policies affect the implementation of HIV preventive programs
4	Allain et al. 2004	Ghana	*Vox Sanguinis*	Empirical (n = 39 blood donors); to investigate the role of religion and religious practice in containing HIV
5	Awoyemi 2008	African continent	*Conservation Biology*	Editorial; the role of religion in HIV/AIDS intervention in Africa: a possible model for conservation biology

(*continued*)

Table 13.1. Description of selected literature (*continued*)

Series number	In-text reference	Source of sample	Source journal	Type and focus of study
6	Dilger 2007	Tanzania	*Journal of Religion in Africa*	Empirical—qualitative; role of practices of healing and community building in neo-Pentecostal churches in the context of globalization, modernity, and HIV/AIDS
7	Fakoya et al. 2012	United Kingdom	*HIV Medicine*	Empirical (n = 246 Africans in London); to describe the association of religion with HIV outcomes in newly diagnosed Africans living in London
8	Hallfors et al. 2013	Zimbabwe	*Ethnicity & Health*	Empirical (n = 328 orphan girls); to examine the influence of religion on attitudes, behaviors, and HIV infection among rural adolescent women
9	Manzou, Schumacher, and Gregson 2014	Zimbabwe	*PLoS ONE*	Empirical (4,418 and 6,609 men aged 17–54 years and on 5,424 and 9,893 women aged 15–44 years in the baseline survey [1998–2000] and the follow-up survey [2003–5]); to compare changes in HIV prevalence between major religious groups in eastern Zimbabwe

Series number	In-text reference	Source of sample	Source journal	Type and focus of study
10	Ntetmen-Mbetbo 2013	Cameroun	*Culture, Health & Sexuality*	Empirical—qualitative (n = 45 gay men aged between 18 and 40 years); to the explore the extent to which African gay men feel free to express and enjoy their faith while simultaneously acknowledging their sexual orientation
11	Olusanya, Afe, and Onyia 2009	Nigeria	*Acta Pædiatrica*	Empirical (n = 266 newborns and 1330 controls); to establish the characteristics of infants with HIV-infected mothers enrolled under a two-stage universal newborn hearing screening program
12	Opio et al. 2013	Uganda	*PLoS ONE*	Empirical (n = 911 participants from 46 fishing communities); to determine the prevalence and risk factors of HIV infection among fishing communities
13	Pargament et al. 2004	General	*Southern Medical Journal*	Literature review; to review the literature on religious coping among individuals with HIV

(*continued*)

Table 13.1. Description of selected literature (*continued*)

Series number	In-text reference	Source of sample	Source journal	Type and focus of study
14	Platter and Meiring 2006.	Namibia	*AIDS Care*	Empirical—qualitative (n = 10 interviews); to explore how people infected with HIV cope psychologically with this life-threatening virus
15	Rankin et al. 2004	Malawi	*Health Care for Women International*	Empirical—qualitative (n = 39 women in 3 focus groups); to explore the familial, cultural, and religious influences on women that contribute to HIV/AIDS
16	Regnerus, and Salinas 2007	Six sub-Saharan African Countries	*Review of Religious Research*	Data from Demographic and Health Surveys of Ethiopia, Kenya, Malawi, Namibia, Zambia, Zimbabwe; to evaluate the effect of religious affiliation on different forms of AIDS-based discrimination, paying close attention to possible confounding effects

Series number	In-text reference	Source of sample	Source journal	Type and focus of study
17	Smith 2004	Nigeria	*Culture, Health & Sexuality*	Empirical—mixed method (survey among 863 and interview with 20 Igbo-speaking young migrants); to examine the intersection of HIV/AIDS and Christianity, focusing on understanding the social processes whereby HIV risk is equated with religious immorality
18	Stockemer and LaMontagne 2007	Forty-three African countries	*Contemporary Politics*	Meta-analysis—data from 43 African countries; to uncover the social, economic, and political contexts in which HIV/AIDS survives or perishes and to explain why certain countries have higher rates than others
19	Trinitapoli 2006	Malawi	*Review of Religious Research*	Empirical—qualitative data from 85 Christian and Muslim congregations in 59 villages; to explore the role religion plays in HIV transmission, focusing on the place of religious organizations in shaping HIV risk behavior

(continued)

Table 13.1. Description of selected literature (*continued*)

Series number	In-text reference	Source of sample	Source journal	Type and focus of study
20	Trinitapoli and Regnerus 2006	Sub-Saharan Africa	*Journal for the Scientific Study of Religion*	Empirical (n = 960); to examine whether AIDS risk behavior and perceived risk are associated with religious affiliation or with religious involvement
21	Watt et al. 2009	Tanzania	*AIDS Patient Care & STDs*	Empirical— qualitative data from interviews with 36 clients receiving antiretroviral drugs (ARVs); to identify opportunities for religious organizations to support the psychological well-being of people living with HIV/AIDS
22	Zou et al. 2009	Tanzania	*BMC Public Health*	Empirical (n = 438); to probe associations between religious beliefs and HIV stigma, disclosure, and attitudes toward ARV treatment

Religion emerges as an important determinant of sexual behavior among adherents. This has been supported by several studies. In a study carried out among Ugandan university students by Anette Agardh and colleagues (2011), with those who rated religion as less important in their family, the probability of early sexual activity and having a high number of lifetime partners increased by a statistically significant amount (odds ratio [OR] = 1.7; 95 percent confidence interval [CI]: 1.2–2.4 and OR = 1.6; 95 percent CI: 1.1–2.3, respectively). However, the role of religion seemed to have no impact on condom use.

Focusing on particular religious traditions, emerging from a survey among a fishing community in Uganda, Alex Opio and colleagues (2013) report that Muslims had lower HIV prevalence (14.4 percent) as compared to Christians (25.2 percent). A similar finding was also reported in a study carried out in Nigeria (Olusanya, Afe, and Onyia 2009, 1292): "There was more than 50% increased risk of HIV among Christian mothers compared to their Muslim counterparts (OR: 1.59; 95% CI: 1.13–2.24)." In a meta-analysis of literature, Daniel Stockemer and Bernadette LaMontagne (2007, 369) have confirmed that "the higher the percentage of Muslims in a country, the lower the HIV prevalence rate." Although the Islamic religion's allowance of polygyny and discouragement of condom use could run counter to a reduction in HIV prevalence, many scholars have found that affiliation with Islam is negatively associated with HIV prevalence.

The study reported by Jenny Trinitapoli and Mark D. Regnerus (2006) is more nuanced. Their analysis of data from the Malawi Diffusion and Ideational Change Project reveals substantial variation according to religious affiliation and religious involvement. Men belonging to Pentecostal churches consistently report lower levels of HIV risk behavior as compared to men belonging to other Christian denominations and people from the Muslim tradition. In general, regular attendance at religious services is associated both with reduced odds of reporting extramarital partners and with lower levels of perceived risk of infection.

What is at the heart of these effects? Taken together, the influence of religion on the sexual behavior of its adherents could be attributed to the proscriptive role of religion. Vehement preaching and the fear of stigma might prevent risky sexual behavior. It could also promote a sense of moral responsibility or even guilt toward sexual behavior that is considered immoral by religions, which is also termed as risky behavior in the context of HIV. Such an argument is furnished by J.-P. Allain and colleagues (2004) with the data from Ghana. In this study, irrespective of their HIV status or religion, 95 percent of the respondents believed that extramarital sex was a sin, and 79 percent of those tempted to have an extramarital affair considered that their religious beliefs helped them abstain.

In a second related subtheme, much of the selected literature (Aguwa 2010; Hallfors et al. 2013; Smith 2004; Zou et al. 2009) examined the association between people's faith in prayer and healing and their attitude toward testing and treatment for HIV. The literature shows very mixed findings. A study carried out in Zimbabwe (Hallfors et al. 2013) suggests that young women belonging to a church known as Apostolic Church are at increased risk of HIV infection due to early marriage. Moreover, most Apostolic sects discourage medical testing and treatment in favor of faith healing. This again can increase the risk of undiagnosed HIV infection for young married women and their infants in high-prevalence areas (see also Smith 2004). On the other hand, the participants in an exploratory study carried out in Tanzania (Zou et al. 2009) had a more balanced view of prayer and seeking treatment. Although the majority of respondents (80.8 percent) believed that prayer could cure HIV, almost all (93.7 percent) said that they would begin antiretroviral (ARV) treatment if they became infected with HIV. The study further established that the participants' willingness to begin ARV treatment was not significantly associated with the belief that prayer could cure HIV or with other religious factors. On the contrary, the refusal of ARV treatment was related to the lack of formal education and the lack of knowledge about ARVs themselves.

3.2. Theme 2: Impact of Religion on Social Stigma and Discrimination Related to HIV/AIDS

Stigma is an expression of social injustice. It might begin with branding and naming and end with social discrimination and seclusion. The association between social stigma and public health in general and HIV/AIDS in particular has been very well discussed in literature for a long time (i.e., Guttman and Salmon 2004). For the purposes of the present review, the contributing role of religion in social stigma and discrimination was considered.

Literature related to faith healing and HIV has already been reviewed in the previous section. One negative implication of the practice of faith healing is to attribute one's health status to one's state of sin and moral flaw, present or past, which has attracted the anger of the supernatural powers. Often the possibility of a cure is promised only when the individual takes the blame. Among the selected literature, several studies have alluded to this connection between religion and stigma. The evidence for the argument ranged from Nigeria (Aguwa 2010) to Tanzania (Zou et al. 2009; see also Watt et al. 2009). In this context, women are more likely to suffer seclusion than men.

However, there are also very subtle distinctions made about the role of religion and social stigma. For instance, the study carried out by James

Zou and colleagues (2009) in Tanzania revealed that most participants (over 84 percent) also acknowledged that they would disclose their HIV status to their pastor or congregation if they became infected. This indicated that the participants did not fear being stigmatized by the leaders or their congregation. This could also imply that the origin of the stigma is probably associated with perceived religious beliefs rather than the believing community itself.

Similarly, Mark D. Regnerus and Viviana Salinas (2007) present some telling insights into the relationship between religion and AIDS-based discrimination. Based on data from the annual Demographic and Health Surveys of six sub-Saharan African countries, the authors point out possible confounding effects. According to them, ethnicity is a far more consistent predictor of discrimination than religion. There are also other confounding variables such as age, education, work status, and rural/urban distinctions. For instance, people from rural areas may be more discriminatory than those from urban setups in their attitude toward those who are open about their HIV status. Where religion does play a role, Islam is reported to exhibit more discriminatory tendencies than Catholicism and Protestantism. Another study from Malawi, which only used a sample of female participants, points out that given that women are often kept out of the leadership role of organized and indigenous religions, women living with HIV might feel more discriminated against than their male counterparts (Rankin et al. 2005). Given these variations, Regnerus and Salinas's (2007) conclusion seems meaningful: that organized religion as such cannot be completely blamed for generating discriminatory sentiments. Social stigma and discrimination have various antecedents.

3.3. Theme 3: Experiencing Internalized Conflict Yet Feeling Supported by Religion

Some reviewed studies have moved deeper into examining the internal processes within religious adherents in the context of HIV/AIDS. As regards these psycho-religious processes, on the one hand, there are negative affective states such as guilt, internal moral conflict experienced by individuals who take religion seriously (Ntetmen-Mbetbo 2013), while on the other hand, there are also positive perceptions that include meaning-making support provided by religion when diagnosed with HIV (Plattner and Meiring 2006) and a sense of hope sustained by prayer and religious faith that could facilitate improved effects of ARV treatment (Watt et al. 2009).

After exploring the experiences and perceptions of forty-five gay men in Cameroun between the ages of eighteen and forty years, Ntetmen-Mbetbo (2013) points out that most of the participants claimed that their faith and their sexual orientation were two important dimensions of their identity, and therefore, they found it difficult to choose between the two. In this context, religion could be a source of stress. At the same time, the participants also claimed that organized religion's attitude toward homosexuality did not seem to make religious life less important for these gay men in Africa.

In another qualitative study (Plattner and Meiring 2006) that involved ten participants in Namibia who had been diagnosed with HIV, the participants, while accepting that the virus was a test or punishment from God, did not blame God for their situation. On the contrary, eight out of the ten participants stated that their HIV infection had brought them closer to God. In that study, almost all participants also reported that having been diagnosed with HIV, religion became very important to them. Religious beliefs provided hope for a good outcome and made their status more meaningful and purposeful. Almost as if in a replicated study (Watt et al. 2009), thirty-six participants in a qualitative study in Tanzania claimed that their personal faith positively influenced their experience of living with HIV and that religious organizations had neutral or negative influences. On the positive side, prayer gave hope to those living with HIV, and still others claimed that prayer supported their adherence to medications.

4. Discussion and Conclusion

The present review began with the following research question: How does academic literature deal with justice issues related to HIV/AIDS and religion? Stated more specifically, What themes relevant to ethics do emerge in the sampled HIV/AIDS and religion literature related to Africa? In answer to these questions, three themes have been presented: (1) the influence of religion on behavior related to HIV prevalence and treatment; (2) the impact of religion on social stigma and discrimination related to HIV/AIDS; and (3) the experience of internalized conflict among adherents while still feeling supported by religion.

It emerges that apparently there is an ambiguous association between HIV/AIDS and religion. Probably the negative dimension of the association emerges from religious beliefs that attempt to present universal principles of morality, and the positive association can be attributed to compassion that religious people are expected to extend to the rest of humanity. In other words, while religious belief and organizational structures might generate a negative stigmatization or guilt, the believing community itself extends its support and understanding to people living with HIV (Ntetmen-Mbetbo 2013; Zou et al. 2009).

How could this paradoxical association between religion and HIV/AIDS exist? Seen from within religious circles, most religious adherents might look up to religion as providing a moral compass. This moral directive is often achieved, as Émile Durkheim (1951) and Max Weber (1963) have previously argued, by means of social cohesion, social control, and emotional support. All agents of socialization—including family, schools, governments, and media—may use these strategies; however, the combination could be stronger in religion, especially in traditional societies as in sub-Saharan Africa. Religion, by offering emotional support, helps people endure suffering and deprivation while also providing answers to the ultimate questions of life, death, and suffering. Religion conditions individuals by strengthening their bonds with the group. In this way, religion not only provides a sense of belonging to its adherents but also steers them toward acceptable social behavior. It is perhaps these dynamics that participants in the reviewed studies are expressing in the context of HIV/AIDS. Religion might create a sense of guilt in them for the apparent breakup of moral order, but at the same time, it also compassionately embraces them. What this interaction could imply is that religion tends to elicit moral behavior through compassion.

On a pragmatic level, it could also be true that, as Stephen M. Awoyemi (2008) argues, "Christian churches [and by extension, religions] are beginning to understand that their basic assumption that preaching and moralizing about HIV/AIDS would solve the problem of behaviour change is not fool proof" (811). In the early decades of the emergence of HIV, religions might have tended to be more discriminatory and judgmental toward people diagnosed with HIV; however, having realized that the power of institutional control exerted by religions has its limitations, religions themselves have changed their strategies in the control of the spread of HIV. They provide training and counseling in prevention work among the uninfected people and compassion and treatment in the care of those already infected.

In conclusion, what Hansjörg Dilger (2007) claims to be the role of neo-Pentecostalism in Tanzania could be extended to the role of religion in Africa:

Religion in the context of AIDS is more than just a source of ambiguity in the ways in which societies in [Africa] deal with the disease. Christianity's role has often been described by policy-makers and social scientists either with regard to the stigmatising attitudes of churches or with reference to the charitable acts that are associated with Christian organisations in the context of the epidemic. . . . The "negative" and the "positive" or "constructive" dimensions of religion with regard to HIV/AIDS cannot be understood as separate or decontextualised aspects of the ways in which [institutionalized religion has] established itself in [Africa]. (78)

What we have observed in the context of AIDS is only a symptomatic outcome of the role that religions play in the larger social context of Africa. Institutionalized religions are playing a vital role in accompanying the African peoples in their negotiation with accelerated social change that has been brought about by social processes such as westernization, urbanization, and globalization. Religions meet many of the conflicting needs and desires of its members in the larger social context. Religions provide social identity to new migrants who are otherwise facelessly anonymous in the fast mushrooming urban contexts. They mobilize the rural masses for collective development. Religions, for the African peoples, act as the moral guardians in order to provide continuity, stability, and hope in the context of uncertainty, ambiguity, and ruptures caused by conflicting messages of the media, governments, and their own traditions. What the present literature review has demonstrated is that in this complicated social context, the role of religions in their relationship with HIV/AIDS is also likely to remain complex and at times ambiguous—and defying any oversimplified conclusions.

References

Afolabi, Olukayode Ayooluwa, and Ayobami Adekunle Adesina. 2011. "Transformations in HIV Awareness in Nigeria: An Empirical Investigation of Personality and Risky Sexual Behaviour Among Undergraduates." *Educational Research Quarterly* 35 (2): 23–42.

Agardh, Anette, Gilbert Tumwine, and Per-Olof Östergren. 2011. "The Impact of Socio-Demographic and Religious Factors upon Sexual Behavior among Ugandan University Students." *PLoS ONE* 6 (8): 1–12.

Aguwa, Jude. 2010. "Religion and HIV/AIDS Prevention in Nigeria." *Cross Currents* 60 (2): 208–223.

Allain, J.-P., M. Anokwa, A. Casbard, S. Owusu-Ofori, and J. Dennis-Antwi. 2004. "Sociology and Behaviour of West African Blood Donors: The Impact of Religion on Human Immunodeficiency Virus Infection." *Vox Sanguinis* 87 (4): 233–240.

Awoyemi, Stephen M. 2008. "The Role of Religion in the HIV/AIDS Intervention in Africa: A Possible Model for Conservation Biology." *Conservation Biology* 22:811–813.

Boyatzis, Richard E. 1998. *Transforming Qualitative Information: Thematic Analysis and Code Development*. London: Sage.

Braun, Virginia, and Victoria Clarke. 2006. "Using Thematic Analysis in Psychology." *Qualitative Research in Psychology* 3 (2): 77–101.

Dilger, Hansjörg. 2007. "Healing the Wounds of Modernity: Salvation, Community and Care in a Neo-Pentecostal Church in Dar Es Salaam, Tanzania." *Journal of Religion in Africa* 37 (1): 59–83.

Durkheim, Émile. 1951. *Suicide: A Study in Sociology*. New York: Free Press.

Fakoya, I., A. Johnson, K. Fenton, J. Anderson, N. Nwokolo, A. Sullivan, P. Munday, and F. Burns. 2012. "Religion and HIV Diagnosis among Africans Living in London." *HIV Medicine* 13 (10): 617–622.

Guttman, Nurit, and Charles T. Salmon. 2004. "Guilt, Fear, Stigma and Knowledge Gaps: Ethical Issues in Public Health Communication Interventions." *Bioethics* 18 (6): 531–552.

Hallfors, Denise D., Hyunsan Cho, Bonita J. Iritani, John Mapfumo, Elias Mpofu, Winnie K. Luseno, and James January. 2013. "Preventing HIV by Providing Support for Orphan Girls to Stay in School: Does Religion Matter?" *Ethnicity & Health* 18 (1): 53–65.

Manzou, Rumbidzai, Christina Schumacher, and Simon Gregson. 2014. "Temporal Dynamics of Religion as a Determinant of HIV Infection in East Zimbabwe: A Serial Cross-Sectional Analysis." *PLoS ONE* 9 (1): 1–11.

Moore, J. F. 2003. "The Prospect of a Global Ethic on HIV/AIDS: The Religions and the Science-and-Religion Dialogue." *Zygon: Journal of Religion & Science* 38 (1): 121–124.

Ntetmen-Mbetbo, Joachim. 2013. "Internalised Conflicts in the Practice of Religion among Kwandengue Living with HIV in Douala, Cameroun." *Culture, Health & Sexuality* 15:76–87.

Olusanya, Bolajoko O., Abayomi J. Afe, and Ngozi O. Onyia. 2009. "Infants with HIV-Infected Mothers in a Universal Newborn Hearing Screening Programme in Lagos, Nigeria." *Acta Paediatrica* 98 (8): 1288–1293.

Opio, Alex, Michael Muyonga, and Noordin Mulumba. 2013. "HIV Infection in Fishing Communities of Lake Victoria Basin of Uganda—a Cross-Sectional Sero-Behavioral Survey." *PLoS ONE* 8 (8): 1–10.

Pargament, Kenneth I., Shauna McCarthy, Purvi Shah, Gene Ano, Nalini Tarakesh-war, Amy Wachholtz, Joan Duggan, et al. 2004. "Religion and HIV: A Review of the Literature and Clinical Implications." *Southern Medical Journal* 97 (12): 1201–1209.

Plattner, I. E., and N. Meiring. 2006. "Living with HIV: The Psychological Relevance of Meaning Making." *AIDS Care* 18 (3): 241–245.

Rankin, Sally, Teri Lindgren, William Rankin, and Joyce Ng'oma. 2005. "Donkey Work: Women, Religion, and HIV/AIDS in Malawi." *Health Care for Women International* 26 (1): 4–16.

Regnerus, Mark D., and Viviana Salinas. 2007. "Religious Affiliation and AIDS-Based Discrimination in Sub-Saharan Africa." *Review of Religious Research* 48 (4): 385–400.

Selvam, Sahaya G. 2014. "Influence of Family on Youth's Relationship with God: A Systematic Review of Psychology Literature." In *Youth and Family in Today's India*, edited by Sahayadoss Fernando and Jesu Pudumai Doss, 65–80. Chennai: Don Bosco Publications.

———. 2015. "Positive Psychology's Character Strengths in Addiction-Spirituality Research: A Qualitative Systematic Literature Review." *The Qualitative Report* 20:376–405.

Selvam, Sahaya G., and Joanna Collicutt. 2013. "The Ubiquity of the Character Strengths in African Traditional Religion: A Thematic Analysis." In *Well-Being and Cultures: A Positive Psychology Perspective*, edited by Hans Knoop and Antonella Delle Fave, 83–102. Heidelberg: Springer.

Smith, Daniel Jordan. 2004. "Youth, Sin and Sex in Nigeria: Christianity and HIV/AIDS-Related Beliefs and Behaviour among Rural-Urban Migrants." *Culture, Health & Sexuality* 6 (5): 425–437.

Stockemer, Daniel, and Bernadette LaMontagne. 2007. "HIV/AIDS in Africa: Explaining the Differences in HIV Prevalence Rates." *Contemporary Politics* 13 (4): 365–378.

Trinitapoli, Jenny. 2006. "Religious Responses to AIDS in Sub–Saharan Africa: An Examination of Religious Congregations in Rural Malawi." *Review of Religious Research* 47 (3): 253–270.

Trinitapoli, Jenny, and Mark D. Regnerus. 2006. "Religion and HIV Risk Behaviors among Married Men: Initial Results from a Study in Rural Sub-Saharan Africa." *Journal for the Scientific Study of Religion* 45 (4): 505–528.

Watt, Melissa H., Suzanne Maman, Mark Jacobson, John Laiser, and Muze John. 2009. "Missed Opportunities for Religious Organizations to Support People Living with HIV/AIDS: Findings from Tanzania." *AIDS Patient Care & STDs* 23 (5): 389–394.

Weber, Max. 1963. *The Sociology of Religion*. Boston: Beacon Press.

Zou, James, Yvonne Yamanaka, Muze John, Melissa Watt, Jan Ostermann, and Nathan Thielman. 2009. "Religion and HIV in Tanzania: Influence of Religious Beliefs on HIV Stigma, Disclosure, and Treatment Attitudes." *BMC Public Health* 9:1–12.

14

Traditional, Christian, and Modern Approaches to Masculinity

HEALTH-CARE VOLUNTEERS IN TANZANIA

Auli Vähäkangas

ABSTRACT

This chapter analyzes the construction of masculinity among the male volunteers of a Christian palliative care program in Tanzania. Various researchers have identified three different cultural categories working hand-in-hand in contemporary Tanzania (Hasu 1999; see also Comaroff and Comaroff 1991). These categories, which Tanzanians also use in their everyday language, can be classified as *kienyeji* (traditional), *kikristo* (Christian), and *kisasa* (modern). These cultural categories make identity construction demanding, and for that reason, there is a special need to analyze how these various categories influence the construction of masculinities in the HIV/AIDS context. The Selian Hospice and Palliative Care Program volunteers act as a good example of transforming masculinities in the HIV/AIDS era. These types of practical examples, which indicate that the construction of masculine identity needs flexibility between various cultural categories, are clearly needed on the African continent in order that the more theoretical discourse on construction of masculinities will continue on both local and intercontinental levels.

1. Three Cultural Categories in Encountering HIV/AIDS

The recent AIDS research in Africa has noted that an important part of the whole problem on the continent is unclear identifications of masculinity. Masculinity in Africa can be grouped into three types: (1) hegemonic masculinity, (2) soft patriarchy, and (3) liberation theological masculinity (Chitando 2012; Chitando and Chirongoma 2012; Colvin, Robins, and Leavens 2010; Van Klinken 2013; Wyrod 2008). The focus of these previous studies is transforming the masculinities of individuals, not as members of their communities. Another problem is that the previous studies do not take notice of the changing situation where the masculinities are constructed. Adrian Van Klinken (2013) determines that significant social transformations take place in and through religious discourse in Africa; the religious setting is, however, many times lacking in the previous research on masculinity in Africa.

The present study analyzes the construction of masculinity among the male volunteers of a Christian palliative care program in Tanzania. Various researchers have identified three different cultural categories working hand-in-hand in contemporary Tanzania (Hasu 1999; see also Comaroff and Comaroff 1991). These categories, which Tanzanians also use in their everyday language, can be classified as *kienyeji* (traditional), *kikristo* (Christian), and *kisasa* (modern). Tanzanian men construct their personal and social identities based on the cultural categories discussed earlier. Usually, an individual creates his personal identity from at least two of these categories. The same individual can change his approach during the course of his life; older people tend to rely more on *kienyeji*, while younger, urban people rely more on *kisasa*. The situation, however, is much more complicated than just age or rural-urban differences. The label "modern" in connection with masculinity construction is not always a positive description. It seems to carry an idea of something coming from the outside and being too Western to fit into Tanzanian society, but at the same time, it also seems to be attractive to many younger, urban people. The previously discussed cultural categories make identity construction demanding, and for that reason, there is a special need to analyze how these various categories influence the construction of masculinities in contemporary Tanzania.

This study analyzes the role of volunteers as an aspect of African communality in serving the poor in the Selian Hospice and Palliative Care Program in Arusha, Tanzania. This program launched the "Tanzanian model" and is renowned for its success and multidisciplinary approach in caring for dying patients. The number of patients had increased rapidly, and in April 2012, this program was serving approximately five thousand patients, the largest group being those with AIDS but also those with tuberculosis (TB) and those with cancer The Selian program uses trained volunteers who make regular home visits and who help provide day-care service while the multidisciplinary team visits the sick in the villages.

Previous research on volunteers that provide care and support for people living with HIV/AIDS indicates that most volunteers in Africa are women (Kasimbazi and Sliep 2011, 95–110). However, one interesting aspect among the Selian volunteers is that almost half of them are men. Furthermore, previous research on volunteering has emphasized that the pattern of volunteering may be rather different between men and women (Edgardh 2011; Taniguchi 2006). The aim of this chapter is to find out the following:

- How do the traditional, Christian, and modern cultural categories contribute to the construction of masculinities in Tanzania?

- How does the role of male health-care volunteers contribute to the discussion of masculinities in the HIV/AIDS context?

2. Volunteer Interviews in the Selian Hospice and Palliative Care Program

The data of this study was collected in April 2012. I had done fieldwork on the Selian Hospice and Palliative Care Program previously in 2009 and thus had all the necessary contacts already for this second fieldwork period. In addition to that, I had lived ten years in Tanzania and spoke fluent Swahili. During 2012, I attended day care in two rural villages, one a mining community and one a plantation community, as well as in a semiurban village outside the town of Arusha. In addition, I visited the sick in the Arusha Lutheran Medical Centre, which is a hospital in the town of Arusha, and attended meetings of the professional team and of the volunteers in one of the districts.

The total number of interviewed volunteers was forty, out of whom twenty-two were females and eighteen were males. The interviews were conducted using a semistructured interview scheme in which the first theme dealt with motives for volunteering, the second theme with the rewarding aspects of volunteering, and the concluding theme with the hardships of volunteering. Interviews were conducted while the volunteers were on service, which made them quite brief. Interviews with volunteers lasted from fifteen to thirty minutes. The participants' ages ranged from twenty-three to sixty-five years old, and they came from varying ethnic and religious backgrounds. Five of those interviewed—three women and two men—were Muslims. The rest of the interviewed volunteers were members of different Christian denominations, the majority belonging to the Lutheran Church.

In addition to the volunteers' interviews, I interviewed five team members on the role of volunteers. These team members included the leader of the program, a nurse, a social worker, an evangelist, and a pastor. The interviews were supplemented by participant observations as well as countless informal conversations with team members, volunteers, and patients concerning the role of volunteers in the Selian Hospice and Palliative Care Program. All interviewees gave their informed consent prior to their inclusion in the study. All details that could identify a volunteer have been omitted.

Interviews were tape-recorded and selectively transcribed. As the interviews were conducted in Swahili, I had to translate the direct quotations used in this chapter into English. All data were analyzed using qualitative content analysis in which coding categories are derived directly from the text data (Hsied and Shannon 2005). In the content analyses, three major categories of results were identified: (1) motivation to volunteer, (2) rewarding aspects in volunteering, and (3) obstacles to volunteering. In all these major categories, special attention was given to gender.

3. Male Identity in a Changing Tanzanian Society

In many ways, the traditional situation no longer exists in Tanzania because urbanization has changed its society. It is no longer a question of a small community where everyone knows one another and in which it is possible to offer or receive social support (Dilger 2006, 111–12). Indeed, this social change has affected the generational and gender hierarchies in Tanzania, but these hierarchies seem to influence gender roles in volunteering in modern society as well. Some aspects of the traditional village-setting communality nonetheless have survived in the newly established community organizations. The lack of communal support creates a strong need for organized support from groups such as the Selian Palliative Care Program and from church communities.

In traditional Tanzanian societies, male identity was constructed not only at home but in terms of the larger community as well. The attributes that have long been central to this male identity have been fighting skills and leadership within the age group together with the clan system (von Bülow 1995, 7). This is because in a collective culture, identity is not a question of a single individual, as the community is also involved in the process of identity construction. In an African context, identity is continuously constructed and transformed within a discursive process that involves discourses that are ethnic and religious (von Bülow 1995, 3). While female behavior has traditionally been seen as being home centered, male behavior is oriented out toward the larger community. Today, contemporary society does not value fighting skills as highly, but the qualities these skills represent, bravery and success, continue to command respect. Another important contributor to the high status of males is wealth (Howard and Millard 1997). Additional contributors to high status are proper occupation, in the traditional sense, and good moral behavior. Philip Setel, who has studied the male population in the Kilimanjaro area in northern Tanzania, reported that some occupations are more valued than others. For example, farming is viewed as being honest and tiring work. Other occupations are not as highly valued, such as being a businessman or a petty trader (Setel 1995, 41).

The Swahili term *heshima* explains gender roles in Tanzania also in relation to the gender roles in volunteering. *Heshima* is a broader concept than the English word *honor; heshima* can also mean respect and dignity. This means that a woman's *heshima* is connected to correct moral behavior and is mainly related to female sexual behavior. In contrast, honor is much more than an individual's estimation of self-worth. Instead, a woman is judged by the society in terms of her honor (Silberschmidt 1999, 166). While *heshima* is interpreted as an important aspect of female sexual behavior, it is not very frequently connected to male sexual behavior. In fact, male sexual behavior does not necessarily have to adhere to the Christian sexual moral code, because social status is more important for male *heshima.* Thus with regard to female behavior, *heshima* seems to refer more to personal dignity, whereas for male behavior, *heshima* is a mark of community respect. Traditional and Christian moral behavior and its influence on the construction of masculinities in the Arusha region are discussed more later on in this chapter.

4. Gender Differences in Volunteering

Male and female volunteers were both very motivated in their volunteering. Their reasons for motivation, however, differed quite a lot. A major motivation to continue volunteering seemed to be the community-related benefits. This was especially the case for the male volunteers, as they emphasized many times how important volunteering was for their status in the community. One of the female volunteers expressed this as follows: "I like to serve the community." One male volunteer explained a similar idea differently: "Many come to ask my advice. They see that I can guide and counsel them." The female focus was on the service and on the community members, while the men seemed to be contented with their own role and additional status in the community. Another male volunteer explained, "They like me and give good feedback on my service." Two additional women focused again on the community in their comments on how they enjoy seeing how the neighborhood also responds to help the patients and how this interaction reduces the stigma in the community.

Many of the volunteers expressed that their service entailed spiritual benefits. This resembled the prosperity gospel concept of giving. These male and female volunteers stated that they devote their time to the service of others and that in return, God will give back to them. One explained that she visits the sick one week, and the next, God blesses her business. Another female volunteer explained how her volunteering meant that her whole family was blessed. Another male volunteer explained how God had protected him from being infected with HIV when he helped a patient bathe and the gloves broke. With this story of the poor protection of gloves, this volunteer wants to stress the fear of being infected himself. He himself had to be tested twice for HIV. The caregiver tested negative for HIV, which he saw as a miracle from God.

Leadership and counseling roles were clearly evident among the Lutheran evangelists, all of them men, participating in the program. This was especially apparent during the day care organized in church surroundings and was also apparent during the volunteers' monthly meetings, which opened with a prayer by one of the evangelists. During the interviews, some volunteers emphasized the importance of peer support when faced with difficult psychological or social challenges, but no one stated explicitly that some peer support was actually the support from those volunteers who had trained as evangelists and who had experience in counseling.

Previous research has reported that volunteering is also considered to be a responsibility, or including various challenges (Jack et al. 2011; Taniguchi 2006, 84). This responsibility aspect was evident throughout the various challenges—practical, psychological, and social challenges—encountered in the present study. The volunteers who were interviewed listed various practical challenges that they faced while serving the sick in their community. The men mentioned more often than the women the challenges of transportation and recounted how the bicycles that they had been assigned earlier were either stolen or broken. Many women commented that they could walk or use their transportation money to travel by bus if a sick person lived farther away. Both men and women stated that the major practical problem that they faced was the lack of medicine or other medical supplies. Medicines were available in Tanzania during the field research period; the problem was distribution. Many interviewees complained about how the local nurses who should distribute these medicines did not do their work properly.

Only men explained how difficult it was to wake up during the night when they had to travel to visit a sick person, and they did not even have a flashlight. I did not ask the women volunteers if they needed to visit the sick during the night or if they merely coped with the darkness of the night. Both men and women explained the practical challenges of the rainy season during the interviews. For example, they mentioned the obstacles they encountered reaching patients' homes through mud and floods.

Both men and women considered their own financial situation as being a challenge for volunteering. If they did not have anything to bring when visiting a patient, they would be asked why they came empty-handed. Additionally, many of the patients seemed to harbor the misunderstanding that the volunteers were compensated for their services, or at least they were given some food to be distributed to the patients. I also discussed this issue of food distribution with the team, and they told me that this aspect of the program warrants further patient education. Food is distributed only during day care and given directly to the patient. In those few cases when the patient is too ill, someone from the team ensures that the food reaches the patient's home. Financial challenges and unrealistic expectations of the patients were also reported in a study of the palliative care volunteers in Uganda (Jack et al. 2011, 713).

5. Transforming Masculinities
through Care Role in Community

The gender differences in volunteering that were previously discussed reveal that the Selian program has succeeded in inviting both male and female volunteers to assume the palliative care role in their communities. This further raises the question of how and whether the male volunteers transform their masculine identities during the process of their service. Recruitment of volunteers from both genders at the same time is an explicit decision of the program to promote gender equality and to try to reduce stigma in the community. Another explicit action to reduce stigma is the decision to serve patients suffering from illnesses other than AIDS in the program. According to interviews, this has reduced stigma, especially in the beginning, when medication was not available and an HIV-positive test result meant the rapid death of a patient. AIDS patients have even better chances to live than, for example, most of the cancer patients.

The male volunteers seem to construct their masculine identities primarily from a traditional male identity, and the central feature is their leadership and the role of counseling in the community. However, at the same time, men adopt a modern masculine identity when accepting their roles as caregivers in their community. Accepting a caregiving role in an African setting is extraordinary (Chindomu and Matizamhuka 2012; Fynn 2011). Moreover, previous research in European contexts has discovered that, for example, men in Greece would not consider joining care programs as volunteers (Edgardh 2011, 86).

Selian masculinities could be interpreted as following what is called "soft patriarchy," which is a concept that was coined by van Klinken (2010) in his analyses of the approaches of masculinities in Africa. The transformation of masculinity in Selian's case occurs within a patriarchal framework that does not support the feminist theological vision of masculinity transforming beyond patriarchy. Van Klinken's case study of a Pentecostal church in Zimbabwe illustrates a similar approach to the transformation of masculinity within the patriarchal framework. This is referred to as the "soft patriarchy" model, and it does not seem to be officially planned but rather is a result of being open to both respecting traditions as well as wanting to face new challenges in volunteer work in Tanzania. Furthermore, previous research in the South African context has revealed that the new masculinity in Africa looks to history as a model and is traditionalist (Morrell, Jewkes, and Lindegger 2012, 25). In contrast, the Selian masculinities are not based on history or tradition, even though they respect the local African traditions and offer men the opportunity to build strong social capital through volunteer work in their community.

This soft patriarchy could further be evaluated by adopting Ninna Edgardh's (2011, 83–88) analysis of the ideal and existing gender roles in church-related social work. Yet what is the ideal in the Selian case is not openly explained. In other words, evidence suggests that the ideal is that both women and men are to be selected from their local communities, and through this selection process, the program promotes gender equality in volunteer work. This equality does not require that men lose their masculinity. The departure point of the Selian case seems to be the idea that there is a need to transform slightly the existing gender roles but not to transform them into unrealistic ideals that would deter men from joining as care volunteers.

6. Healing—Restored to Wholeness

The transformation of masculinities among the studied health-care volunteers seems to reflect the search for wholeness, in which the goal is not only a physical cure but to reach a balance in life. In many Tanzanian ethnic societies, an adult is described as *mtu mzima* (a whole person; Mbiti 1973, 11; Pobee 1986, 17). This wholeness (*uzima*) refers to more than an individual's age; *uzima* is a broader concept than the English word *wholeness*. It can be translated as vitality, adulthood, completeness, energy, existence, maturity, and perfection. An important part of male wholeness is the reproduction of a son (Vähäkangas 2009). A pathway leading to successful coping in the African context is the concept of healing. Healing has been and remains an important part of life. Healing is not limited to health, and one of its central elements is the restoration to wholeness (Harjula 1989, 131). While searching for healing, the African people need not only medical healing but also the liberation and restoration of their entire life.

Steve de Gruchy has called attention to healing and its great importance to all Christians in Africa, but according to de Gruchy, social justice is not considered to have much theological importance. This fundamental relationship of health and social justice demands attention in the time of AIDS (de Gruchy 2007, 63–65). Reconciliation in one's own community and with one's own past is an important part of wholeness and should also be considered while dealing with the construction of masculinities.

Social relations are essential to one's well-being. An old African saying defines the essence of social identity as one's personal identity: "I am because we are; and since we are, therefore I am" (Mbiti 1969, 108–9). This saying stresses the African worldview of community. The image and personality of an individual become important within the context of a community. Musa Dube refers to this old saying and raises concern for a more communal approach in HIV and AIDS prevention projects. Dube's further analysis shows that the communal approach—in her example, Adinkra, which is a space of justice, solidarity, and liberation—is an ideal, and much work must be done to bring it about (Dube 2006, 139–41). A more communal approach would also be needed for the construction of male identity in contemporary Tanzania.

Some writers promote the African community spirit—for example, *ujamaa* in Tanzania or *ubuntu* in South Africa—as a solution to almost all problems on the continent (see Bujo 1998). Frans Wijsen points out that these theologies take the need to justify African traditions too far. Wijsen (2005) further concludes that there has to be a balance of commitment and criticism—in other words, it is a question of both continuity and discontinuity between gospel and culture (141). In the cultural categories used in this chapter, the good values of *kienyeji* have to be used in supporting the construction of male identities. The use of African traditions, the roots of the people, has been widely discussed in the African theologies, especially among the female theologians. Only quite recently, this discussion has, however, started to focus on masculinities and their African roots.

7. Conclusion

This chapter had two aims. The first aim was to analyze how the cultural categories contribute to the construction of masculinities in Tanzania. The findings of this study indicate that the male volunteers seem to construct their masculine identities primarily from a traditional male identity, and the central feature is their leadership and the role of counseling in the community. However, at the same time, men adopt a modern masculine identity when accepting their roles as caregivers in their community. This indicates a strong use of modern behavior among the studied palliative care volunteers. Christian masculine behavior was not explicitly explained during the interviews. This does not, however, mean that the Christian churches would not have any influence on the discussion of masculinities in present-day Tanzania. This was just not clearly addressed during the interviews and would need further study to find out the importance of churches to the construction of masculinities.

The second aim evaluated the role of male health-care volunteers in the discussion of masculinities in the HIV/AIDS context. Already the decision of the Selian program to recruit both genders is a strong contribution toward gender equality in the local communities. This example shows the communities that men are also capable and needed in health-care work among AIDS patients. In addition, it seems that this is also a way to reduce stigma in the studied communities. Male volunteers themselves were very motivated in their role of giving social, psychological, spiritual, and even physical support to the dying and their near relatives. Modern values seem to be expressed in that context in terms of care and compassion rather than those of social justice.

The Selian health-care volunteers act as a good example of transforming masculinities in the HIV/AIDS era. These types of practical examples that indicate that the construction of masculine identity needs flexibility between various cultural categories are clearly needed on the African continent so that the more theoretical discourse on construction of masculinities will continue on both the local and the intercontinental levels.

Acknowledgments

I am grateful to the Selian Hospice and Palliative Care Program team in Arusha, Tanzania.

References

Bujo, Benezet. 1998. *The Ethical Dimension of Community: The African Model and the Dialogue between North and South.* Nairobi: Paulines Publications Africa.

Bülow, Dorthe von. 1995. "Power, Prestige and Respectability: Women's Groups in Kilimanjaro, Tanzania." CDR Working Paper 95.11. Copenhagen: Centre for Development Research.

Chindomu, Charles, and Eunica E. Matizamhuka. 2012. "Challenging African Men to Be 'Man Enough to Care' in the HIV Era: Special Focus on the Anglican Diocese of Manicaland, Zimbabwe." In *Redemptive Masculinities: Men, HIV, and Religion*, edited by Erza Chitando and Sophie Chirongoma, 423–446. Geneva, Switzerland: World Council of Churches.

Chitando, Ezra. 2012. "Even When There Is No Rooster, the Morning Will Start: Men, HIV and African Theologies." *Journal of Feminist Studies in Religion* 28 (2): 141–145.

Chitando, Ezra, and Sophie Chirongoma. 2012. "Introduction: On the Title." In *Redemptive Masculinities: Men, HIV, and Religion*, edited by Erza Chitando and Sophie Chirongoma, 1–30. Geneva, Switzerland: World Council of Churches.

Colvin, Christopher J., Steven Robins, and Joan Leavens. 2010. "Grounding 'Responsibilisation Talk': Masculinities, Citizenship and HIV in Cape Town, South Africa." *Journal of Development Studies* 46 (7): 1179–1195.

Comaroff, Jean, and John Comaroff. 1991. *Of Revelation and Revolution: Christianity, Colonialism, and Consciousness in South Africa*. Vol. 1. Chicago: University of Chicago Press.

de Gruchy, Steve. 2007. "Re-learning Our Mother Tongue? Theology in Dialogue with Public Health." *Religion & Theology* 14:47–67.

Dilger, Hansjörg. 2006. "The Power of AIDS: Kinship, Mobility and the Valuing of Social and Ritual Relationships in Tanzania." *African Journal of AIDS Research* 5 (2): 109–121.

Dube, Musa. 2006. "Adinkra! Four Hearts Joined Together: On Becoming Healing-Teachers of African Indigenous Religion/s in HIV/AIDS Prevention." In *African Women, Religion, and Health: Essays in Honor of Mercy Amba Ewudziwa Oduyoye*, edited by I. A. Phiri and S. Nadar, 131–156. Maryknoll, NY: Orbis.

Edgardh, Ninna. 2011. "A Gendered Perspective on Welfare and Religion in Europe." In *Welfare and Religion in 21st Century Europe*. Vol. 2 of *Gendered, Religious and Social Change*, edited by Anders Bäckström et al., 61–106. Surrey: Ashgate.

Fynn, Sharl. 2011. "Experiences of Social Support among Volunteer Caregivers of People Living with HIV/AIDS." In *Response-Ability in the Era of AIDS: Building Social Capital in Community Care and Support*, edited by Wenche Dageid, Yvonne Sliep, Olagoke Akintola, and Fanny Duckert, 111–128. Bloemfontein, South Africa: Sun Media.

Harjula, Raimo. 1989. "Curse as a Manifestation of Broken Human Relationships among the Meru of Tanzania." In *Culture, Experience and Pluralism, Essays on African Ideas of Illness and Healing*, edited by Anita Jacobson-Widding and David Westerlund, 125–137. Uppsala Studies in Cultural Anthropology 13. Uppsala, Sweden: University of Uppsala.

Hasu, Päivi 1999. "Desire and Death: History through Ritual Practice in Kilimanjaro." *Transactions of the Finnish Anthropological Society* 42. PhD diss., Finnish Anthropological Society, Helsinki, Finland.

Howard, Mary Theresa, and Ann V. Millard. 1997. *Hunger and Shame: Child Malnutrition and Poverty on Mount Kilimanjaro.* New York: Routledge.

Hsied, H.-F., and S. E. Shannon. 2005. "Three Approaches to Qualitative Content Analysis." *Qualitative Health Research* 15 (9): 1277–1288.

Jack, Barbara A., et al. 2011. "A Bridge to the Hospice: The Impact of Community Volunteer Programme in Uganda." *Palliative Medicine* 25 (7): 706–715.

Kasimbazi, Anette Kezaabu, and Yvonne Sliep. 2011. "Unpaid Volunteers and Perceived Obstacles in Ensuring Care and Support of People Living with HIV/AIDS." In *Response-Ability in the Era of AIDS: Building Social Capital in Community Care and Support,* edited by Wenche Dageid, Yvonne Sliep, Olagoke Akintola, and Fanny Duckert, 95–110. Bloemfontein, South Africa: Sun Media.

Mbiti, John S. 1969. *African Religions and Philosophy.* Nairobi: Heinemann Kenya.

———. 1973. *Love and Marriage in Africa.* London: Longman.

Morrell, Robert, Rachel Jewkes, and Graham Lindegger. 2012. "Hegemonic Masculinity/Masculinities in South Africa: Culture, Power, and Gender Politics." *Men and Masculinities* 15 (1): 11–30.

Pobee, John S. 1986. "Life and Peace: An African Perspective." In *Variations in Christian Theology in Africa,* edited by Carl Hallencreutz and John Pobee, 14–31. Nairobi, Kenya: Uzima.

Setel, Philip. 1995. "The Social Context of AIDS Education among Young Men in Northern Kilimanjaro." In *Young People at Risk: Fighting AIDS in Northern Tanzania,* edited by Knut-Inge Kepp, Paul M. Biswalo, and Aud Talle, 49–68. Oslo, Norway: Scandinavian University Press.

Silberschmidt, Margrethe. 1999. *"Women Forget That Men Are the Masters": Gender Antagonism and Socio-economic Change in Kisii District, Kenya.* Uppsala, Sweden: Nordiska Afrikainstitutet.

Taniguchi, Hiromi. 2006. "Men's and Women's Volunteering: Gender Differences in the Effects of Employment and Family Characteristics." *Nonprofit and Voluntary Sector Quarterly* 35:83–101.

Vähäkangas, Auli. 2009. *Christian Couples Coping with Childlessness: Narratives from Machame, Kilimanjaro.* American Society of Missiology 4. Eugene, OR: Pickwick.

van Klinken, Adriaan S. 2010. "Theology, Gender Ideology and Masculinity Politics: A Discussion on the Transformation of Masculinities as Envisioned by African Theologians and a Local Pentecostal Church." *Journal of Theology for Southern Africa* 138:2–18.

———. 2013. *Transforming Masculinities in African Christianity: Gender Controversies in Times of AIDS.* Farnham, UK: Ashgate.

Wijsen, Frans. 2005. "The Practical-Theological Spiral." In *The Pastoral Circle Revisited: A Critical Quest for Truth and Transformation,* edited by Frans Wijsen,

Peter Henriot, and Rodrigo Mejia, 129–147. Nairobi, Kenya: Paulines Publications Africa.

Wyrod, Robert. 2008. "Between Women's Rights and Men's Authority: Masculinity and Shifting Discourses of Gender Difference in Urban Uganda." *Gender & Society* 22:799–823.

15

Theological and Ethical
Reflections on HIV/AIDS

PERSPECTIVES FROM INDIA

George Zachariah

ABSTRACT

Theological and ethical reflections on HIV and AIDS should begin with
a critical review of the way we problematize the pandemic and the
politics of our interventions and ministries of care. The dominant notion
that HIV infection is caused by sexual immorality continues to legitimize
the demonization of the infected and to reduce Christian engagement
in this soul-saving business. This chapter proposes an alternative methodological standpoint by privileging the perspectives of the infected bodies.
Such a perspective invites us to develop an intersectional approach in
the very understanding of the problem. It calls us to interrogate patriarchy, heteronormativity, Victorian sexual morality, and globalization.
When infected bodies read Scripture and tradition, informed by their
experiences of stigma, discrimination, and representation, alternative
theological reflections happen that disrupt the status-quo theology and
give birth to transformative and therapeutic theological reflections that
can bring about healing, wholeness, and restoration in the lives of the
infected. It also transforms the ecclesia into a community that celebrates
the wholeness of all.

1. Introduction

The chair of the Health Commission of the Catholic Bishops' Conference of India said the following:

> All the Catholic Healthcare Institutions, as we are serving the Lord, will admit and care for the people living with HIV. As Blessed Teresa of Calcutta used to say, "A person affected by HIV and AIDS is Jesus among us. How can we say no to Him?" These statements do not make any sense to me personally. I approached the Director of Health Commission of the Catholic Bishops Conference of India and explained to him about my status. He said, "You sinned and therefore you must be ready to face all the consequences. You should not go about from one NGO to another revealing your status and if you do so, you will have a tough time with the church." I was asked to keep silent about my HIV status. (GBI 2013, 14–15)

This is the voice of a fifty-year-old HIV-positive Roman Catholic priest from India exposing the contradiction of a faith community that is at the forefront of serving people living with HIV and AIDS. When our ministries of compassion and care are informed by the dominant theological and biblical perspectives, the church fails to become a therapeutic presence in the lives of the infected and affected communities. This chapter is therefore an attempt to initiate alternative theological and ethical reflections on HIV and AIDS, affirming the epistemological privilege of the infected bodies.

Familiarity with and excessive reliance on the dominant versions of the pandemic of HIV and AIDS tend to lead us to a taken-for-granted attitude that prevents us from problematizing it by analyzing critically the dominant diagnosis and the solutions prescribed. Underscoring the importance of restudying the problem, Amartya Sen (2008) opines that "it not only requires informed and determined action, but demands, first of all, a broader and more foundational cognizance of the nature of the affliction that attacks us from its safe haven of dense fog" (1). Said differently, a politically committed ethical discernment of the HIV and AIDS experience involves a new discernment of its epistemology that affirms the infected bodies as the site of knowledge that can provide healing, wholeness, and restoration and create community.

2. Theological and Ethical Reflections
on HIV and AIDS: A Critical Review

A theological and ethical reflection on HIV and AIDS is as old as the disease itself. The churches and other faith-based organizations have been at the forefront of responding to the pandemic through ministries of care, compassion, and support. However, it is important for us to critically evaluate the ways in which our dominant theological and ethical discourses continue to problematize HIV and AIDS.

Often, we tend to understand HIV infection as contracted through the irresponsible behavior of the infected persons. It is a common belief that an HIV infection could have been avoided if the person had led a highly moral life. Such an approach reduces responsibility to the personal behavior of the infected and demonizes them as sinners. This is the reason for perceiving HIV and AIDS as an issue of immorality and sexual promiscuity in our dominant theological discourses. Reverend Jerry Falwell has articulated it better than anybody else: "AIDS is a lethal judgment of God on the sin of homosexuality and it is also the judgment of God on America for endorsing this vulgar, perverted, and reprobate lifestyle. . . . God destroyed Sodom and Gomorrah primarily because of the sin of homosexuality. Today He [sic] is again bringing judgment against this wicked practice through AIDS" (Gill 2007, 11). The perception of HIV and AIDS as "wages of sin" and divine judgment is the logical conclusion of problematizing the disease as an issue of sexual immorality. The liberal Christian attempt to reach out to infected people based on the slogan "Love the sinner but hate the sin" is also problematic. The famous ABC (Catholic Bishops' Conference of India [CBCI] 2005, 17) approach to address the issue of HIV and AIDS (A is for abstinence, B is for "be faithful," and C is for condoms) too emerges from a moralistic diagnosis of the problem. The emphasis in the church documents on the need for marital fidelity, abstinence from premarital sex, and self-discipline also reinforces the same moralistic position. What we find here is the assumption that behavior is always a matter of free choice. Such a problematization underscores the view that the pandemic can be confronted only through strictly following the standardized Christian (Victorian) sexual morality.

Since the Bible is considered the authoritative source to inform us in our theological and ethical reflections, it is important to explore how the dominant Christian discourses use the Bible as the source. In our efforts to redeem our communities from the pandemic, we often present the Bible as a "two-thousand-year-old vaccine" that can guide the lost to the words that will heal them. Churches and Christian organizations, in their campaign to create awareness about the pandemic, use biblical texts that give scriptural validity to abstinence and being faithful. These texts either condemn sexual immorality and unrighteousness (1 Cor 6:18–20; Eph 5:1–3) or lift up the courage to abstain from sexual immorality (Gen 39). "Guilt, repentance, and forgiveness" is another motif that we find in the biblical reflections on HIV and AIDS. "If we confess our sins, he is faithful and just and will forgive us our sins and *purify* us from all *unrighteousness*" (1 John 1:9 NIV; italics mine) is a text that is used in the liturgy of the mainline Protestant churches. This prayer also reinforces a moralistic understanding of sin and guilt.

As Gerald West (2011) rightly observes, in the early stages of the epidemic, informed by theologies of retribution, HIV was interpreted biblically as "a manifestation of human sinfulness, . . . fulfilling the curses cited in Deuteronomy 28:27. . . . The failure to develop a vaccine to cure HIV has been taken by some as confirming God's punishment of a stubborn and sinful generation" (136). Liberal engagements with the Bible are centered on Jesus and his healing ministry. There you find a strong message to engage in ministries of prevention, awareness, and care. However, these interpretations fail to understand the transformative politics of Jesus's healing ministry. The Bible is also being used in the dominant Christian discourses to help the dying endure the pain and suffering, invoking Jesus's suffering and death. The fundamental problem with this hermeneutical method is that the Bible is being perceived as a book of ready-made answers to all our contemporary questions of moral ambiguity.

In our approach to HIV and AIDS, informed by the perspective of the "perfect" and "able-bodied" people, we tend to consider people living with HIV (PLHIV) as an empirical category, who are in need of our mercy, charity, and care. The PLHIV are being constructed as the "other" of us, the "pure" and the "able bodied" in our theological and ethical discourses on HIV and AIDS, to be saved by our interventions. They are at the receiving end of our projects and programs that we design and execute for them. We still call our ministry the ministry *to* the PLHIV. In such a ministry, they can never be the agents of their lives; rather, they can be the beneficiaries of our goodwill and philanthropy. Problematizing PLHIV as an empirical category to be acted upon through our interventions of charity and care is the hallmark of our dominant theological and ethical approach to HIV and AIDS. Our attempt to reflect upon ethical discernment and praxis in the context of HIV and AIDS experience invites us to look for alternative ways of problematizing the pandemic for transformative praxis.

3. Methodological Transgressions: Moral Agency of the Infected Bodies

Our critical discernment about the dominant theological discourses on HIV and AIDS invites us to engage in methodological transgressions informed by the everyday living experiences of the infected bodies. Said differently, the infected bodies of the PLHIV have to become the locus of our theological and ethical reflections on HIV and AIDS. These are the bodies that endure pain, stigma, exclusion, assault, poverty, and representation. The infected bodies ostracize them and make them dependent on the welfare programs of the state and the church. At the same time, those infected bodies do enable them to organize themselves as fellowships of PLHIV to resist all inhumane interventions of exclusion, stigma, assault, and apathy. This is the scandal of the infected bodies of the PLHIV. The very symbol of their exclusion becomes the source for a new affirmation of life with dignity. Any attempt to theologically engage with the HIV and AIDS pandemic hence should consider the infected bodies of the PLHIV as authentic texts that can inform us in our theological deliberations and ethical discernment and praxis. Enabling the moral agency of the infected bodies is therefore the primary act of healing and restoration. Such a methodological transgression provides us the epistemological key to engage in alternative theological and ethical reflections and praxis. When we problematize HIV and AIDS from the standpoint of the PLHIV, we create a radical discontinuity with our dominant rhetoric on HIV and AIDS, because infected bodies see reality differently.

4. Interrogating Patriarchy and Heteronormativity

In our discernment that socioeconomic factors and patriarchy contribute to the spread of HIV and AIDS, we need to go beyond the dominant diagnosis that identifies sexual immorality as the cause for HIV infection. In fact, in India, the sacred institution of marriage has become one of the major causes of the spread of HIV infection. So the church's prescription of ABC as the panacea for HIV and AIDS does not really address the problem in countries like India. When the dominant approach proposes abstinence as the safest method against the spread of the pandemic, women who face sexual abuse and rape both within the family and in the public space do not have the luxury to choose abstinence. It is important to note here that the union minister of state for home affairs in India made a statement in the Parliament that "marital rape cannot be criminalized in India as marriages are sacred in the country" (Venkat 2015).

"Be faithful to your partner" is yet another moralistic prescription that has failed miserably in addressing the issue. According to a United Nations Development Programme (UNDP) and Joint United Nations Programme on HIV/AIDS (UNAIDS) document (2001), 80 percent of women in long-term stable relationships who are HIV positive were infected by their partners (22). Safe sex through using condoms is also not an option for most of the women in India, as they do not have control over their bodies and sexuality. As Aruna Gnanadason (2016) rightly observes, in India, "good women are expected to be ignorant about sex and passive during sexual intercourse, which makes it difficult for them to be informed about risk reduction or, even when informed, makes it difficult for them to be proactive in negotiating safe sex" (157). Married women, in general, lack power over their own sexual lives. In the context of the pandemic, it is not safe for women in patriarchal societies to get married. Compared to housewives, sex workers are more empowered to protect themselves from HIV infection because they can insist on safer sexual practices. All these narratives categorically underscore the naked reality that the major factor for the spread of the pandemic is the powerlessness of women. As long as they lack control over their bodies and sexuality and are unable to make decisions about their life because of economic dependency and patriarchal values and norms, the pandemic cannot be controlled. The seedbed for the tragic infection is hence the families, the churches, and all other civil society institutions that perpetuate inequality among men and women.

It is also important to see the impact of religious doctrines on the life of the people. The documentary *Can Condoms Kill?* portrays the story of Harriet Nakabugo, a Ugandan woman married to an infected man. She refused to use condoms because, as Catholics, "we are not allowed to use them. I would miss all of God's blessings, and my reward would definitely be hell." When reporters asked Cardinal Emmanuel Wamala whether it would be better to die than to use condoms, he replied, "If that's one's belief, yes, it's better. Christ's teaching has never been easy" (Gill 2007, 112). All this underscores the very fact that "with the HIV and

AIDS epidemic, heterosexual marriages have turned out to be one of the deadliest institutions due to its patriarchal distribution of power" (Dube 2004, 9). Religion functions as a sacred canopy that sanctions and legitimizes this gendered genocide by invoking the suffering of Christ and exhorting women to imitate him so that they can find meaning in their tragic suffering and death. So a perspective from the infected bodies of the PLHIV challenges us to resist all attempts to moralize the issue and rather to look for insights from the infected bodies. HIV is nothing but a virus, neither a moral condition nor a moral issue.

The classification of certain communities as "high-risk groups" is yet another misconception perpetrated by a moralistic approach. Commercial sex workers, men having sex with men, and injecting drug users (IDUs) belong to this category. In the public discourses, they are portrayed as vessels of immorality, vectors of disease, and objects of pity. They are being criminalized by our law and order system and demonized by our dominant moral codes. Section 377 of the Indian Penal Code imposed by the British in 1860 states that "whoever voluntarily has carnal intercourse against the order of nature with any man, woman, animal shall be punished with imprisonment for life, or with imprisonment of either description for a term which may extend to 10 years, and shall be liable to fine." When heterosexuality is canonized as normative, any deviant sexual behavior, even between consensual adults, can be demonized as immoral and illegitimate, subject to rigorous punishment under the law.

Researches on HIV infection and sex workers help us demystify the myth that sex workers and sexual minorities are the major carriers of the pandemic. According to statistics from India, female sex workers constitute less than 1 percent of the infected female population in India. HIV prevalence among female sex workers in the Indian state of Maharashtra has dropped from over 54 percent to 23 percent. There is also a decrease nationally among IDUs, from 13.3 percent in 2003 to 10.16 percent in 2005. As "high-risk groups," they are the target of several HIV-related interventions, which will alienate them instead of empowering them to combat HIV and AIDS. The story of the women sex workers associated with Sampada Grameen Mahila Sanstha (SANGRAM) in Maharashtra proved that when sex workers were able to take control of their lives, they could help each other and prevent the spread of the pandemic. Realizing the risky behavior involved in their profession, they focus on their responsibilities in sexual relations and help other sex workers protect themselves from HIV and AIDS. An alternative approach to HIV and AIDS, therefore, challenges us to stop criminalizing and demonizing the sex workers and, instead, network with them as partners in ministry to combat the spread of HIV and AIDS.

5. Infected and Affected Children:
Toward an Ethic of Care and Compassionate Justice

India has the largest number of AIDS orphans in the world. The number is increasing day by day. Parent-to-child transmission is the most common form of spread of HIV and AIDS in Asia. As of 2007, according to UNICEF statistics, only sixty-four thousand Asian children who are living with HIV and AIDS received antiretroviral treatment (ART). On average, only one in five children receive ART, and even in countries where the provision for treatment is 100 percent, many children living and affected by HIV and AIDS are deprived of treatment because of the stigma and discrimination attached to the disease.

Most of the children contract the virus from their mothers at birth. A single dose of nevirapine given to the mother in labor and the baby at birth and a caesarian delivery and formula feeding can bring down the risk of contracting the virus to less than 2 percent. Since it is so simple, only less than three hundred children were born with HIV in all rich countries combined in 2005. But thousands of children are born with the infection every year in the Southern Hemisphere. When it comes to the treatment of the infected children, the pharmaceutical companies are not interested in developing pediatric medications because there are fewer children infected in the developed nations.

The stigma and discrimination attached to the disease are more cruel and painful than the disease itself. The civil society considers orphaned children with HIV/AIDS or children who have parents dying from HIV/AIDS as untouchables. Even our sacred spaces and sanctuaries are not inclusive enough to welcome them. Novelist Jaspreet Singh (2008) narrates his conversation with the principal of an elite school in south Delhi: "A child with AIDS is a child with special needs," the principal says. "In our classrooms we have children with dyslexia, Down's syndrome and even leukemia." Singh asks, "But would you admit an HIV positive kid?" He pauses to think. "It's a hard question," he says. "I have no problems, but I don't know how my teachers might respond." Singh then asks, "But would you be bold enough to admit someone from an HIV positive care home?" He responds, "The thing is . . . I don't want to treat the child like a guinea pig" (136). He is right. The founding principle of all elite schools is discrimination between the rich and the poor. The children infected with HIV and AIDS are denied their constitutional right to free and compulsory education due to stigma and discrimination.

In the Indian context, there is a disturbing link between casteism, patriarchy, children, religion, and HIV and AIDS. The Devadasi system (the age-old practice of temple prostitution) is the best example to look at children and HIV and AIDS at the interface of religion, caste, and patriarchy. The Devadasis are girls and young women from *dalit* communities dedicated as courtesans in the Brahmanical temples. Through casteist manipulations, dalit parents are forced to dedicate their female children to religiously sanctioned temple prostitution. These young girls finally end up in the red-light areas in the big cities. What we find in the Devadasi system is a religiously sanctioned casteist and patriarchal practice that increases the vulnerability of subaltern girls to HIV and AIDS.

Theological and ethical discernment and praxis informed by the experiences of the orphaned children with HIV demand from us an ethic of care and compassionate justice. It inspires us to challenge our worldview, which stigmatizes and discriminates against the children at risk. It calls for an ethic of care where we welcome them into our communities, our sanctuaries, and our homes. The theological and ethical imperative before us is to become angels that brighten the lives of the orphaned children with HIV.

6. Interrogating Globalization: Toward an Ethic of Justice and Equality

A perspective from the infected bodies affirms the right of the PLHIV to health care. Article 47 of the Indian Constitution envisions public health as one of the primary responsibilities of the government. But the reality is different. Hospitals are the worst places for people living with HIV in India. If they disclose their HIV status, treatment for even common diseases is denied to them. When it comes to treatment for HIV and AIDS, it is not accessible to common people in India. In spite of the fact that the drugs can prolong the life of an infected person, people are not in a position to access it. The drugs need to be taken with a high-protein, high-fat meal, which an average individual cannot afford daily. HIV and AIDS require lifelong treatment, and people should have access to newer drugs to give them alternatives when they experience side effects or when they develop a resistance to the drug. A second-line treatment procedure is required when they develop a resistance to the first-line treatment.

There are a variety of ways through which the right to health care of the common people is taken away from them. The pharmaceutical companies are not interested in investing in research and development of new drugs for diseases such as malaria and TB, which affect millions of people in developing countries. In fact, about one-third of the world's population does not have access to essential medicines. Eighty percent of the world's population lives in developing countries but consumes less than 20 percent of all medicines (Martin 2007). Even treatments can affect a family in diverse ways, particularly in the context of prevailing health-care disparities and deprivation of basic health needs based on demographics and income inequality. Lack of confidentiality in the treatment protocols can lead to social ostracization of the patients. Without a governmental commitment to universal health care, survival has become the luxury of those who can afford to pay.

Globalization has a direct impact on the availability and accessibility of treatment to infected people. Amartya Sen (2008) talks about the "bitter irony" of PLHIV in India struggling to get access to medications while Indian companies produce drugs at a cheaper price. "No country has done more than India in cheapening the production cost of known antiretroviral drugs, and yet most HIV affected people in India cannot afford to get and use these drugs" (9). Intellectual property rights through patents set the price of essential drugs for HIV/AIDS at a level that is far beyond PLHIV's reach. Lifesaving drugs thus became a commodity for accumulating profit.

The major health problems that we face in India are directly related to the way we organize our social relations. Access to nutritious and sufficient food, mosquito control, proper sanitation facilities, and availability of clean drinking water can prevent the major epidemics that kill hundreds of thousands of people every year. In our vertical approach, we try to tackle each disease without recognizing the wider social factors that contribute to its prevalence and spread. HIV and AIDS are also approached in a vertical fashion.

It is observed that diseases such as malaria and TB are linked with HIV and AIDS. That means a campaign against HIV and AIDS has to address the issues of public health and universal health care. With the withdrawal of the state from the public health sector and the monopolization of the HIV and AIDS sector by nongovernmental organizations (NGOs) and corporate houses, the emphasis on public health and universal health care is almost lost. So an ethical discernment and praxis need to address the importance of public health and universal health care and insist that the government be committed to providing the basic amenities for all people to lead a healthy life. At the same time, we need to be conscious of the problems with our "medicalized view of healing." *Restoring Hope*, a publication of the World Health Organization, identifies this problem in the following words: "Unfortunately, the history of public health and medicine is replete with examples of what happens when medicine is reduced to a technology, and when the dimension of care, of decent care, is forgotten or abandoned" (Matic 2008, vii). This is a concern that we need to address immediately in our engagement with the PLHIV.

The demise of the welfare state and the privatization and corporatization of health care are to be understood as the consequence of the current wave of globalization. Globalization has been instrumental in making subsistent communities vulnerable to epidemics through forceful displacement, the withdrawal of subsidies, and the closing down of ration shops. Most of the nations with an alarming rate of HIV prevalence are the ones who spend more on debt servicing than on health care and welfare programs. Every third person infected with HIV and AIDS belongs to a debt-driven country. So an ethic of justice and equality should have the boldness to reject the idolatry of globalization and to join the worldwide movement for jubilee and debt cancellation.

From a conventional understanding, the care, healing, and restoration of the PLHIV are confined to medication and pastoral care. But a perspective from the infected bodies of the PLHIV would enable us to see the need for a multisectoral approach in dealing with the everyday living experiences of the PLHIV. Pastoral care to the HIV/AIDS-infected people, in general, is focused to help them get out of the guilt and to face death with hope. Once a person is infected, death is the only hope in life. A theology of pastoral care informed by the infected bodies is a theology of life—a theology that inspires us to sojourn with the PLHIV in their struggle to live and to live with meaning, joy, and hope. A pastoral care of life and hope does not mean that we should deny the tragic implications of the pandemic. Rather, we should enable the PLHIV to be positive as they battle with destiny every moment of their life. They should be enabled to get out of the haunting stigma and shame associated with the disease. From the shackles of their wounded psyche, they should be led to the sunlight of self-respect and self-love. This desire to be "positive" is therapeutic. The PLHIV, through our ministries of care and compassionate justice, should be enabled to become agents of their lives, rejecting the culture of self-hate and silence. The hope that we find here is not an unrealistic hope that does not recognize the possibility of death. Rather the hope is the ability of the infected bodies to become moral agents.

7. Hermeneutics of Healing from Infected Bodies

Theological and ethical discernment and praxis in the context of HIV and AIDS do not consider the Bible as a timeless and universal moral codebook that can be applied in the context of moral ambiguities. Rather, the Bible has the potential to become a resource in the journey of the infected ones as they try to make sense of their lives in their struggle and search for wholeness. The attempt at the School of Theology at the University of Natal, South Africa, to read the Bible along with the PLHIV is worth mentioning here. "I died when I was diagnosed as HIV positive" was the profound outburst of a PLHIV that inspired the School of Theology to explore along with the PLHIV whether there is life and dignity after the death of someone diagnosed as HIV positive. "Can the Bible be a resource for dignity, life and wholeness when the church is clearly not (yet)?" was the question that they explored together. In their journey together, one PLHIV opined, "I would rather come to the bible study than go to church" (West 2003).

Redemptive readings of sacred texts require a hermeneutical commitment to read the texts from the vantage point of the infected bodies. For Jim Mitulski (2000), the ingredients of an HIV hermeneutic include an understanding of exile and estrangement from family and society and an understanding of blame and shame. But their understandings also include "the innate desire of the soul and the body to overcome adversity and to survive. . . . These insights culled from the social location of living with HIV can make the pages of the Bible come alive. They help us to see and tell our own story as part of divine revelation" (153–54). Ken Stone's (1999) attempt to reread certain lament psalms as texts of resistance is important here. Lament psalms, for Stone, "do not generally acquiesce to suffering. . . . Rather, they complain about it; and this complaint offers readers a subject-position from which an end to suffering and distress can be actively pursued." Differently said, "many of the laments respond to suffering with *resistance*" (20–21). Redemptive readings of sacred texts, therefore, initiate a new hermeneutic from the infected bodies to challenge the dominant theology of retribution and instead, through its deeper engagement with unjustifiable suffering, construct a theology of lament and protest.

A hermeneutic from the infected bodies does not consider the Bible as a book of answers. It is a hermeneutic that reads together the stories of ancient faith communities and the stories of the infected bodies. The stories of the ancient communities speak differently when they are reread by the infected bodies. Such a reengagement with the Bible provides them new insights about the agency of the vulnerable body. They are more than victims; they are the protagonists of a transformative praxis that can arrest the spread of all viruses—viruses of the pandemic, stigma, apathy, economic inequality, patriarchy, and heteronormativity. This sense of moral agency resignifies their life and enables them to believe that it is possible to live with dignity even after the "death of being diagnosed as HIV positive." "Guided by the compassion and justice rather than fidelity to religious orthodoxy, an HIV hermeneutic wrestles with sacred text in diverse ways in order to grasp its redemptive detail and potential," observes West (2011, 156). A hermeneutic from the infected bodies further inspires them to transgress the cultural veils of shame and privacy and to make their infected bodies the site for public policy discourses. Engagement with the biblical narratives leads them to new solidarity networks with communities who also undergo similar experiences (Kanyoro 2004, viii–ix).

8. Living Positively: From Victims to Agents of Change

The metamorphosis of the PLHIV from the state of victimhood to a people with moral agency is not a natural process. Here the narratives of the early faith communities recorded in the pages of the Scripture and the narratives inscribed on the infected bodies have the power to inspire them in their struggles to initiate and sustain this process of transformation. The biblical narratives tell us stories of victims becoming agents of change. We read in the book of Exodus the story of Shiphrah and Puah, two slave women who showed the courage to disobey the orders of the king to midwife the liberation of the people from the fetters of slavery. Similarly, the narratives of the infected bodies also empower us to dream of the possibility of a life beyond the present. Today they realize that "HIV is something you can live with, not something you have to die from." The body of Christ is called to enable HIV-positive people to live positively.

9. Celebrating Infectious Memories

The ethical reflection from the vantage point of the infected bodies of the PLHIV is an ethic of risk that rejects the prevailing dominant ethic of control. "In living out this ethos, we can neither undo the past nor control the future. But we can learn from the past, and we can live creatively, responsibly, and compassionately in the present" (Welch 2000, 37). This ethical responsibility to live creatively in the present is not with the guarantee of the realization of our hope. But it is a hope against hope. It is an ethic of risk because if we do not resist the forces of death and decay, we will lose the ability to dream, care, and mend.

Such an ethic of risk is nourished by the celebration of infectious memories. Infectious memories are the memories of the infected bodies, suffering and struggling with hope to convince the world that life prevails over all infections and stigma and pandemics. Sunday after Sunday, we celebrate the infectious memory of the One who was crucified for dreaming a different world: different from the morality and the law and order of the prevailing regimes. Infectious memories are contagious. We, as the church, are called to subject ourselves to be infected by these memories of lives dedicated to affirm life and negate all manifestations of death. Theological reflections and ethical discernment and praxis in the context of HIV and AIDS should therefore reflect our commitment as the body of Christ to be infected by the memories so that we can be a presence of life and infect our surroundings with the beauty of life. We see the affirmation of this vision in the *Policy on HIV and AIDS* of the National Council of Churches in India: "The Church as an *ecclesia* is called out to live in *koinonia* (fellowship)—seeking not the holiness of a few, but the wholeness of all—thereby catalyzing the realization of *basileia* (kingdom of God) on earth" (2009, 6).

References

Catholic Bishops' Conference of India (CBCI). 2005. *Commitment to Compassion and Care: HIV/AIDS Policy of the Catholic Church in India.* New Delhi: Commission for Health Care.

Dube, Musa W. 2004. "Grant Me Justice: Towards Gender-Sensitive Multi-sectoral HIV/AIDS Readings of the Bible." In *Grant Me Justice: HIV/AIDS & Gender Readings of the Bible*, edited by Musa W. Dube and Musimbi Kanyoro, 3–23. New York: Orbis.

GBI. 2013. "Stand Upright before God, but Unwanted and Sinful before Men." In *Living, Not Just Existing: Stories of Brothers/Sisters Living with HIV*, edited by Alphinus R. Kambodji and Susan Jacob, 2–9. Hong Kong: CCA.

Gill, Peter. 2007. *The Politics of AIDS: How They Turned a Disease into a Disaster*. New Delhi: Viva.

Gnanadason, Aruna. 2016. "Celebrating Sexuality in an Age of HIV and AIDS: A Feminist View." In *Disruptive Faith, Inclusive Communities: Church and Homophobia*, edited by George Zachariah and Vincent Rajkumar. Delhi: ISPCK/CISRS.

Kanyoro, Musimbi R. A. 2004. "Preface: 'Reading the Bible' in the Face of HIV and AIDS." In *Grant Me Justice: HIV/AIDS & Gender Readings of the Bible*, edited by Musa W. Dube and Musimbi Kanyoro. New York: Orbis.

Martin, Greg, Corinna Sorenson, and Thomas Faunce. 2012. *Balancing Intellectual Monopoly Privileges and the Need for Essential Medicines*. BMC. Accessed August 17, 2012. https://tinyurl.com/y3mlp4bz.

Matic, Srdan. 2008. Preface to *Restoring Hope: Decent Care in the Midst of HIV and AIDS*, by Ted Karpf. Geneva, Switzerland: WHO.

Mitulski, James. 2000. "Ezekiel Understands AIDS, AIDS Understands Ezekiel: Or Reading the Bible with HIV." In *Take Back the Word: A Queer Reading of the Bible*, edited by Robert E. Gross and Mona West. Cleveland: Pilgrim.

National Council of Churches in India (NCCI). 2009. *Policy on HIV and AIDS: A Guide to Churches in India*. Nagpur, India: NCCI.

Sen, Amartya. 2008. "Understanding the Challenge of AIDS." In *AIDS Sutra: Untold Stories from India*, edited by Negar Akhavi. New Delhi: Random House India.

Singh, Jaspreet. 2008. "Bhoot Ki Kahaanian (Ghost Stories)." In *AIDS Sutra*, edited by Negar Akhavi. New Delhi: Random House India.

Stone, Kenneth. 1999. "Safer Text: Reading Biblical Laments in the Age of AIDS." *Theology and Sexuality* 10:16–27.

United Nations Development Programme (UNDP) and United Nations Programme on HIV/AIDS (UNAIDS). 2001. *Fact Sheets: United Nations Special Session on HIV/AIDS*. New York: UNDP and UNAIDS.

Venkat, Vidya. 2015. "Anger over Minister's Marital Rape Comment." *Hindu*, April 30, 2015. Accessed September 18, 2015. https://tinyurl.com/y5x4bnm7.

Welch, Sharon D. 2000. *A Feminist Ethic of Risk*. Minneapolis: Fortress.

West, Gerald. 2003. "Reading the Bible in the Light of HIV/AIDS in South Africa." *Ecumenical Review* 55 (4): 335–344.

——. 2011. "Sacred Texts, Particularly the Bible and the Qur'an, and HIV and AIDS: Charting the Textual Territory." In *Religion and HIV and AIDS: Charting the Terrain*, edited by Beverly Haddad. Pietermaritzburg, South Africa: University of KwaZulu-Natal Press.

PART 4

Mental Health

THEME INTRODUCTION

Mari Stenlund

1. Prevalence of Mental Health Disorders

In some countries, mental disorders are being defined as new national diseases, while they appear to be less common in other parts of the world. Mental health or substance use disorders seem to be more common, for example, in New Zealand, Australia, Iran, and the United States, while rates are much lower, for example, in Colombia, Mexico, Vietnam, China, Nigeria, and Russia. However, according to WHO's survey, the majority of those with severe mental disorders receive treatment in the United States and New Zealand, but only a minority in China and Nigeria (Kessler et al. 2007, table 2; Ritchie and Roser 2018). Although it is anything but clear how these results should be interpreted, it seems that culture and the standard of living influence at least the recognized or estimated prevalence of mental health and substance use disorders and the possibility of receiving treatment. However, it is far from simple to say who should learn what and from whom.

2. The Right to Mental Health

When the human right to health is discussed in general, health is usually considered in terms of wholeness, and mental health issues are not focused on.[1] Even though the human rights of persons with mental disorders are a topic, what the right to mental health actually means is not particularly clear in those discussions (WHO 2005). The reason might be that "mental health faded from view as a global health issue until recently," as Jonathan Wolff (2012, 131) puts it. There has also been disagreement about whether mental health is more of an aspirational or rhetorical right than an identifiable, meaningful, operational, and enforceable one. Lawrence Gostin (2001, 271) also notes how an overly broad definition of mental health (the WHO's definition, for example) may lead to the right having ambiguous content, which would reduce its meaningfulness in practice.

The *International Covenant on Economic, Social and Cultural Rights* (ICESCR; United Nations Human Rights 1966, art. 12) recognizes the right of everyone to the highest attainable standard of mental health. Since the right to mental health is in this way listed as a human right, it is not simply a moral claim but rather something that imposes binding obligations on states (Gostin 2001, 271). However, when it comes to the right to mental health, international covenants differ from each other. For example, in the *European Social Charter* (1996, art. 11), the right to mental health is not mentioned separately, but the right to the protection of health in general is.

3. Conditions Necessary for the Mental Health of Individuals and Populations

It seems unclear what the right to mental health means and how this right obligates states, other people, and also religious communities. Lawrence O. Gostin (2001, 271) suggests that the right to mental health might mean the following: "The duty of the state, within the limits of its available resources, to ensure the conditions necessary for the mental health of individuals and populations."

"Conditions necessary for the mental health of individuals and populations" include, first, a sufficiently diverse range of mental health services and other social services that promote people's well-being (Gostin 2001, 272). For example, Wolff (2012, 131) recognizes the challenges of offering mental health treatment, particularly in poor countries.

Second, as Natalie Drew et al. (2005, 81) put it, "Certain sociopolitical and economic conditions need to exist in order to promote the mental

---

1 See, for example, Asher (2010) and Tobin (2012). Compare also with the formulations of the ICESC (1966, article 12).

well-being of the population." Gostin notes that human rights viola-tions such as discrimination, marginalization, and extreme violence also impair mental health. These violations may induce lifelong mental suffering, which is a problem for not only individuals but the whole community and may even pass from generation to generation (Gostin 2001, 265–66).[2] Moreover, poverty, lack of education, unemployment, and restrictions on civil liberties may affect mental health. Conversely, "people's mental health is dependent upon their ability to enjoy and exercise a range of human rights" (Drew et al. 2005, 81). Gostin (2001, 266) expresses it this way: "Some measure of mental health is indispensable for human rights because only those who possess some reasonable level of functioning can engage in political and social life. Similarly, human rights are indispensable for mental health because they provide security from harm or restraint and the freedom to form, and express, beliefs that are essential to mental well-being."

However, as we saw in the data earlier, people in countries with a rela-tively high standard of living and human rights do not seem to have fewer mental health disorders than countries with lower standards of living. If the data are to be taken as such, the opposite would seem to be the case. Moreover, many states have very limited means to ensure the mental health of their citizens. Thus even though the right to mental health imposes a clear obligation on states, the entire mental health issue has often been much more a matter of civil society and communities than one of the state.

4. When Mental Health Meets Religion: Diverse Challenges

Seen globally, a good number of diverse challenges arise when mental health meets religion. In some parts of the world, religion has often been considered difficult to deal with in mental health work. Some people treated in mental health facilities have been afraid to speak about their religious convictions, fearing that their views and experiences would be seen as not sane. Although the ethical principles guiding psychiatry, for example, emphasize that the freedom of religion of persons with mental disorders should be respected,[3] this fear is not completely unfounded. In practice, so-called supernatural experiences can indeed be seen as signs of a mental disorder (and sometimes they are). Moreover, the existential

---

2 See also Wolff (2012, 130–31) and Ahmed and Dein in this volume.
3 See, for example, United Nations (1991, principle 1:5).

considerations of persons with mental disorders may be ignored; they may also be viewed as symptomatic or a result of incorrect medication, for example (Wagner and King 2005, 141). Among neoatheists, it has been suggested that atheism correlates with good mental health and that the belief in God is delusional (see, e.g., Dawkins 2007). Sigmund Freud saw God as a projection of infantile wishes and religion as a cultural pathology. Despite this, psychoanalysis has still had an influence on the pastoral education movement in many countries (Thielman 1998, 16–17).

On the other hand, religious actors also play a significant role in supporting persons with mental disorders. In Finland, for example, mental health challenges are recognized in Lutheran pastoral care and diaconal work. Lutheran hospital pastors work also in psychiatric hospitals, which is one way to support patients but on the other hand raises the question of how equally people from different religious backgrounds receive spiritual help. More generally, religions serve as communities where persons with mental disorders can belong, like anyone else. In practice, however, stigmatization exists within these communities as well, and the social roles of those with mental disorders may be quite limited (Stenlund 2014, 279–81; on addictions, see Nikkinen in this volume).

While in parts of the world, the phenomenon of religion can even be "tabu" in mental health work, in many developing countries, help for mental health problems is often sought primarily from religious actors or traditional healers. Due to relatively poor psychiatric resources, mental health problems are frequently treated by persons other than mental health professionals. As Saeed Farooq and Fareeda A. Minhas (2001) point out, "It can be argued that in the majority of developing countries mental health care is being provided by the community in the true sense of community care" (226–27). When expressed this way, the picture of the right to mental health is far from hopeless in many developing countries.

Numerous studies suggest that being religious often promotes mental health.[4] However, even when mental health workers have a positive attitude toward religion, they often have limited skills to discuss religion with patients and recognize if psychiatric help is needed for problems that someone may manifest through religious language. A patient's problems might at times be better understood by religious actors who may have more suitable instruments to assist the person. With the world becoming more multicultural, understanding people's diverse religiosity is more important and more challenging than ever.

---

4 See, for example, Koenig and Larson (2001). Compare with Stenlund in this volume.

When it comes to mental health justice, a challenging issue is how mental health problems, addictions included, are understood. According to the medical model, disorders must be diagnosed according to official medical standards (*DSM-5* or *ICD-11*) and treated medically. This is accepted by most communities of faith, but there are also specifically religious ways to understand and treat these problems. Moreover, from some religious viewpoints, problems that might suggest mental health disorders (spirit or jinn possessions, for example) are seen as "spiritual illnesses" to be treated spiritually (see Ahmad and Ahmed and Dein in this volume). The question arises on how the individual's right to mental health should be understood in such situations. When does spiritual help for spiritually understood problems respect the right to mental health, and when does it violate it?

5. Toward Mental Health Justice

The chapters in this part of the volume consider, from various viewpoints, the diverse challenges that emerge when mental health justice in particular encounters faith or religion.

Within the multicultural context of South Africa, Ayesha Ahmad observes a traditional mode of healing known as *sangoma*. Ahmad discusses the phenomena of somatization, empathy, and sharedness in sangoma as they relate to Western psychiatry.

Khaldoon Ahmed and Simon Dein look at how Bangladeshi immigrants in Britain have experienced mental illness and present such patients' views concerning jinn, in addition to other spiritual explanations of mental disorders.

The perspective then turns to human rights discourse and cases where people's religious beliefs and activity might negatively affect their mental health. I (Mari Stenlund) present various ways of understanding the freedom of religion and discuss how the right to mental health relates to these different views.

This part concludes with Janne Nikkinen's discussion of addictions and religion in the context of the complicated role that Christian faith-based organizations play in addiction treatment.

References

Asher, Judith. 2010. *The Right to Health: A Resource Manual for NGOs.* The Raoul Wallenberg Institute Professional Guides to Human Rights, edited by Leif Holström. Vol. 6. Leiden: Martinus Nijhoff.

Dawkins, Richard. 2007. *The God Delusion*. London: Black Swan.

Drew, Natalie, Michelle Funk, Soumitra Pathare, and Leslie Swartz. 2005. "Mental Health and Human Rights." In *Promoting Mental Health*, 81–88. Geneva, Switzerland: World Health Organization.

European Social Charter (Revised). 1996. Accessed September 12, 2019. https://tinyurl.com/y4bcdybk.

Farooq, Saeed, and Fareeda A. Minhas. 2001. "Community Psychiatry in Developing Countries—a Misnomer?" *Psychiatric Bulletin* 25:226–227.

Gostin, Lawrence O. 2001. "Beyond Moral Claims: A Human Rights Approach to Mental Health." *Cambridge Quarterly of Healthcare Ethics* 10 (3): 264–274.

Kessler, Ronald C., et al. 2007. "Lifetime Prevalence and Age-of-Onset Distributions of Mental Disorders in the World Health Organization's World Mental Health Survey Initiative." *World Psychiatry* 6 (3): 168–176.

Koenig, Harold G., and David B. Larson. 2001. "Religion and Mental Health: Evidence for an Association." *Internal Review of Psychiatry* 13 (2): 67–78.

Ritchie, Hannah, and Max Roser. 2018. "Mental Health." Our World in Data. Accessed September 26, 2019. https://ourworldindata.org/mental-health.

Stenlund, Mari. 2014. "Freedom of Delusion—Interdisciplinary Views Concerning Freedom of Belief and Opinion Meet the Individual with Psychosis." Doctoral thesis, University of Helsinki. Accessed September 12, 2019. http://urn.fi/URN:ISBN:978-952-10-9747-8.

Thielman, Samuel B. 1998. "Reflections on the Role of Religion in the History of Psychiatry." In *Handbook of Religion and Mental Health*, edited by Harold G. Koenig, 3–20. San Diego: Academic.

Tobin, John. 2012. *The Right to Health in International Law*. Oxford: Oxford University Press.

United Nations. 1991. *Principles for the Protection of Persons with Mental Illness and the Improvement of Mental Health Care*. Accessed September 12, 2019. https://tinyurl.com/y24p86bg.

United Nations Human Rights. 1966. *International Covenant on Economic, Social and Cultural Rights*. Accessed September 12, 2019. https://tinyurl.com/qxqfpj5.

Wagner, Luciane C., and Michael King. 2005. "Existential Needs of People with Psychotic Disorders in Pôrto Alegre, Brazil." *British Journal of Psychiatry* 186:141–145.

Wolff, Jonathan. 2012. *The Human Right to Health*. New York: W. W. Norton.

World Health Organization (WHO). 2005. *WHO Resource Book on Mental Health, Human Rights and Legislation*. Geneva, Switzerland: WHO.

16

Sangomas, Somatization, and Sharedness

Ayesha Ahmad

ABSTRACT

Religious interpretations and meanings around illness, suffering, and healing have gained traction within health system development around the world, with a greater integration of religious-based frameworks in clinical settings. However, the critical analysis and nuances of religious or faith values do continue to lack robustness. In this chapter, I look at the concept of somatization, which is typically perceived through a biomedical paradigm as a negative symptom or presenting a clinical phenomenon in the diagnostic process. However, in the traditional South African sangoma consultation, somatization is a form of sharedness that enables the pain and suffering of the person to be conveyed to the healer. This chapter argues that such a shared narrative enhances empathy and can aid positive religious or faith-based coping strategies. In turn, a greater mode of healing has the potential for a pathway to a more fulfilled health justice.

1. Introduction

Contemporary global contexts are often challenging for health-care practitioners. In the advent of globalization, migration, humanitarian crises, conflict, and increased mobility, modern-day societies are increasingly multicultural. South Africa is a nation of eleven official languages, a colonial history, a relatively recent traumatic apartheid period, and complex oral traditions surrounding morality and medicine. Quite simply, we all carry forth a cultural background and are "cultural bodies." Culture is a phenomenon that is universally present and embodies a "full range of human values, behavior, and social structure indigenous to specific groups around the world that are passed on from one generation to the next" (Boehnlein, Schaefer, and Bloom 2005, 335). However, our contemporary era is characterized in many parts of the world as globalized—this means that within a country's population, people reflect a hybrid of a number of cultural influences rather than statically embody particular traits, beliefs, and practices. Thus a culture is increasingly difficult to define. Moreover, cultural dialogue in a pluralistic belief system about health is challenging for concepts of health justice.

Sangomas are a traditional mode of healing in South Africa even in contemporary times. In this chapter, the sangoma consultation is set up and viewed through a narrative lens. Somatization and sharedness are important elements of the sangoma-patient relationship as well as in the understanding of health and illness. Exploring these concepts against the Western dialects of cause and symptomology, as well as the pathological take on somatization, will highlight an interesting discourse of empathy. Somatization, for a sangoma, is essential for contributing a working empathy to the consultation and promotes a sense of sharedness. The patient is received, therefore, from the embodiment of their narrative. This chapter concludes by suggesting such insights to human relations are beneficial to health-care systems that currently and typically attempt to reduce persons to diseases. Furthermore, it brings the value of the human exchange in healing and medicine into the concept of health justice.

This chapter introduces the working practice of a sangoma to explore the phenomenon of somatization. Moreover, the discussion will flesh out the principle of empathy in therapeutic practice—in both traditional and clinical settings—with the view to illustrating ways that the recognition of somatization as a mode of sharedness can promote health justice. Overall, the chapter challenges current dialogues between Western and non-Western cultural practices of empathy, especially from a psychiatric point of view.

2. Sangomas in South Africa

Sangomas are the backbone of indigenous communities such as the Bantu in South Africa (Cumes 2013, 58). Sangomas are practitioners of a philosophy based on a belief in ancestral spirits called *ngoma*. Ancestors form an integral part of all aspects of being a sangoma. Sangomas, for example, receive a calling to become healers by their ancestors, and their role is to guide and protect the living. Ancestors also are the initiators of morality, and illness is often seen as a form of moral lesson and an opportunity for an individual to reflect on their behavior.

A sangoma is part of an oral tradition and is based on experience. In other words, a sangoma's healing is not derived from scientific knowledge and method. Sangomas are traditional medical practitioners. Traditional medicine is defined by the World Health Organization General Guidelines for Methodologies on Research and Evaluation of Traditional Medicine as "the sum total of the knowledge, skills, and practices based on the theories, beliefs, and experiences indigenous to different cultures, whether explicable or not, used in the maintenance of health as well as in the prevention, diagnosis, improvement or treatment of physical and mental illness." There are an estimated two hundred thousand sangomas in South Africa—compared to twenty-five thousand Western-trained medical doctors (Truter 2007, 56). Decisions regarding the mode of medicine to seek may thus be influenced by availability and accessibility to different forms of treatment.

3. Sangomas: Healers or Clinicians?

In a recent lecture on cultural perspectives of psychiatry, a trainee psychiatrist reflected on a photograph taken of a sangoma in South Africa. The sangoma was robed in traditional clothing, which consisted of a long white cloak. The young psychiatrist, in the midst of his own training, looked at the sangoma, and from his view, he saw a traditional healer who strangely looked like a Western clinician. I found this to be interesting on various levels. Significantly, the interplay of symbolisms found that a comparison was strange. The strangeness originated because of a fundamental distinction—namely, between the healer, the sangoma, and the clinician, the Western doctor. By virtue of the differentiation, there should be no commonality and certainly no resemblance or empathy between these different systems and conceptualizations of the human body.

As a way perhaps to compensate for this uncomfortable comparison and deconstruction of identity, the trainee psychiatrist reasoned that it was in fact the sangoma who looked like the Western doctor, as opposed to the Western doctor being akin to the sangoma. Western medical knowledge is the dominant and prioritized medical structure in our global world. This prioritization raises ethical notions for the normativity of ideas and empathy toward pluralism in treating and viewing the sick and suffering body and mind. Thus a focus for this forthcoming chapter discussion is to bring to light the relationship between the healer/clinician and a patient. Crucial to the notion of healing is the therapeutic alliance resulting from empathy. The aim is to explore empathy in the context of sangomas because somatization becomes a key component in generating empathy, whereas from more Western traditions, somatization is vulnerable to pathologization from contemporary psychiatric frameworks. It is an important function of this chapter to relate empathy to health justice and the ethical nature of the healing relationship in conditions that are associated with both the body and the mind.

4. Healers and Clinicians

The divide between traditional African healers and biomedical practitioners is a visible fracture, even in a society where over 60 percent of the population has consulted with a sangoma (van Wyk, van Oudtshoorn, and Gericke 1999, 10). Sangoma practice involves the transferring of knowledge that has been received experientially rather than derived by empirical method. Thus there is a fundamental divide between traditional healing and scientific medicine. Moreover, the work of the sangoma relies on narrative and is an oral tradition.

Narrative also takes the form of dreams communicated between a sangoma and their ancestor as well as illness being a form of script as an expression to the patient from their ancestor. The meanings invoked in these narratives are subject to the empathy in which they are received. The backbone, then, for the purpose and task of healing by a sangoma is from the sharedness of experience and suffering between ancestors, sangomas, and their patients. In comparison, the doctor-patient relationship with a biomedical clinician has been founded on empirical knowledge that has been scripted and supported by the processes of verification and falsification. The doctor-patient relationship invokes shifts of power between knowledge of suffering and the experience of suffering.

5. Religious and Cultural Issues in Contemporary Clinical Medicine: Defining the Body

The conceptualization of the human body is an integral part of contemporary debates in the philosophy of medicine and biomedical ethics. The human body is the locus, the reference point, and a system for the ethical theory that follows. Thus information about the human body soon surpasses the boundaries of the clinical setting—it becomes, in turn, about the human condition and then the subject matter and an object of concern for philosophical, clinical, religious, and cultural perspectives alike.

The way we structure our (cultural) concept of the body has implications for the ways that the human body is treated within healing practices—such as biomedicine and by sangomas—and these implications originate from even the most fundamental (conceptual and theoretical) of levels. For example, medical ethicist Edmund Pellegrino (2008, 309) pointed out that "man's most daring creations promise to annihilate him as a person unless he can decide who he is and what his existence is for and where it should head." Pellegrino argues that the current context of biomedicine—one whereby the boundaries between life and death are no longer fixed points (Lizza 2009, 1)—requires us to reexamine our understanding of the body. Pellegrino is critical of the biomedical viewpoint of the body, or at least the lens it is viewed through, fearing that the impact of a description about the body that is considered neutral and value-free will forgo a conscientious and responsible analysis of society.

The implicit reference in Pellegrino's observations is that without a conscientious and evaluative analysis of the way that medicine uses the body for its action, both our bodies and our societies may suffer. Furthermore, it implies that how we treat the body reflects our society, a premise from which Michel Foucault (1973) established his conception of ethics. The human condition is not merely experienced; it is enacted. A "good" society, body, ethic, or medicine is not "discoverable" but is "practiced" (Foucault 1973), or alternatively, our understanding of the human condition is formed through practice discourses.

In contemporary clinical practices, the body is considered an inactive, timeless, ageless object. Such a body, as an object, is enacted through medical practices (Mol 2002). In contrast, it is through the embodied person that the effects of medicine are received and experienced—Pellegrino (2008) reminds us that the body has a relation to the human condition and its societal situation and not just its counterpart, the individual person. How we conceptualize the body as a reflection of our own existence, then, has further implications for a pluralistic medical discourse of healing and treating the body in society.

What may we derive from such representations of the body? Is the body in biomedicine the "same" body that is a part of our relation to the world in our human condition, or is the ill, failed, afflicted body a separate body, a "medical" body? The concept of the "body" has become increasingly significant in recent years, where who we are has been succeeded by the normative inquiry of who we should become. New biomedical technologies are resulting in a changing ontology of medical practice, where medicine is no longer confined to the "ill," the "unwell," the "diseased," or the "unhealthy." As Leon Kass (1972, 18) states, the "boundaries" of our "individual" lives are "already subject to considerable manipulation," questioning the notion of a "natural" body privileged through the practices of scientific medicine.

6. The Body in Society

Foucault (1973) argued against the notion that there can be one underlying structure of our existence—we are instead elements of a complex and diverse field. Knowledge, or the organization of our knowledge, has led to different "bodies" throughout history. In *The Birth of the Clinic*, Foucault (1973) traces this development of knowledge within modern medical culture and describes a transition in the objective of medicine—namely, from saving souls to saving bodies. The new modes of scientific knowledge have created a particular phenomenon, the "medical" gaze, which is a central categorization of Foucault's work and is a product of reductionist medicine. The "medical" gaze is that which can deduce objects of symptoms, illness, and disease. The body could be "read" in order to discover its hidden truths, which are revealed so as to manipulate and change the body according to medical norms—a contemporary form of the good-versus-evil metaphysics from pre-nineteenth-century models of our human existence.

The body, then, is constantly in flux. It is not a timeless, ageless object because it is subject to powers and norms external to the clinical environment. The body is not only a "scientific" body; it is also a social body. The body, then, is subject to multiple ontologies, produced rather than given. The space of the body in the clinical gaze is significant for structuring health and socially appropriate understandings of well-being. Understanding the body in society is challenging for clinical practitioners to understand their patients and provide health justice. The body in society highlights the reciprocal nature of healing between the clinician and the patient. The case of sharedness in the next section between the healer and patient in South African contexts will serve as an important example of engaging with nonphysical understandings of the human body, health, and illness.

7. Sharedness of and in Sickness: South African Sangomas

The transformation of medicine from healing to scientific practice—or as described by J. Wreford (2005), to a commitment to radical materialist thinking (Scheper-Hughes 1987, 8)—has fundamentally altered the landscape for sangomas. The ontology of such traditional African healing is redundant compared to dominant medical systems as described earlier in this chapter. Its entire phenomenology is bracketed aside from the physicalist definition of the material body. The sharedness, then, of health and healing within the discourse of sangomas is increasingly a private and exclusive space. The sharedness forms through the concepts of understanding the spiritual constitution of knowledge, relationships, and presence of sickness.

D. Chidester (2012), in tracing the sacred in South Africa, asks,

> But what, exactly, are we tracking? What is the sacred? In the study of religion, the sacred has been defined as both supremely transcendental and essentially social, as an otherness transcending the ordinary world—Rudolph Otto's 'holy,' Gerardus van der Leeuw's 'power,' or Mircea Eliade's 'real'—or as an otherness making the social world. Following Émile Durkheim's understanding of the sacred as that which is set apart from the ordinary, everyday rhythms of life, but set apart in such a way that it stands at the center of community formation (5).

Furthermore, healing relationships in African religion and sacredness have an important element of kinship; the position of a sangoma invokes a calling by paternal or maternal ancestors (Chidester 2012, 201). The nature of healing relationships is thus multiple and crosses over different dimensions of the human condition.

The sacred dynamics of a society, for Chidester, constitute a "wild ambiguity" (2012, 15). In part, this describes the inevitableness of the belief system surrounding sickness in sangoma tradition to fall into the category of a religious familiarity rather than a practice akin to scientific medicine. The phenomenology is of course present in South African society of sangoma healing; however, its role in contributing to health and treatment receives a different recognition than it would if considered to be a form of medicine, thus affecting notions of justice in health. Is the right to health fulfilled through access to sangoma healing? To explore this question and the factors that influence the nature of how it may be answered, it is necessary to delve deeper into the conceptual understandings of sickness in South African society. The premise for this is that the reciprocal nature of healing means that the patient is dependent on the healer/clinician's understanding of their illness experience. What are the requirements to ensure that this aspect of health justice is fulfilled?

8. Spiritual Illness

A preexisting belief system centered on the presence of spirits in the etiology of illness is challenging for biomedicine. Roland Littlewood's (1991) "The New Cross-Cultural Psychiatry" highlights the need for understanding local narratives of illness as well as moral values. However, these remain as additional descriptions to conform to a structure of consulting a patient by diagnosis and treatment. These categories of defining illness are at risk of reducing a person's experience of a disease or form of suffering. Littlewood thus refers to B. J. Good and M. J. D. Good's (1982) emphasis that the "significance of a system of classification emerges only when we take into account not only all the meanings the illness terms connote and relate to, but also the actual context and identities of the people involved" (Littlewood 1990, 314).

Spiritual illness is sometimes associated with spirit possession. Spirit possession manifests through gaining hold of a human being (Boddy 1994, 407). Spirits are typically understood to possess the ability to exert a greater force than the individual who becomes possessed can counteract. Sometimes spirits are invited for the purpose that the person will become possessed. However, this is only undertaken during ceremonies or rituals and under strict regulation. Other forms of spirit possession may align with more malicious and sinister causations such as a curse.

Anthropologist Mary Keller has specialized in possessed bodies, producing the seminal book on the topic, *The Hammer and the Flute*, a culturally and historically comparative study that proposes that a possessed body has "instrumental agency" and is no longer an autonomous agent.

"Instrumental agency" is a concept that Keller develops to explain a possessed person's paradoxical authority—namely, that they obtain their identity, or differentiated power, from their community's view that they are no longer autonomous agents. This shows the communal nature of the status of an individual's ontology. Keller (2003) says, "Possessed bodies are extremely different from the Western model of proper subjectivity" (viii). Thus the possessed body, or at least the body containing or responding to influences from spirits such as ancestral spirits, appears to be very different from the body viewed from an anatomical lens in biomedical contexts by clinicians as well as the role of the body in different relations in society.

The need to recognize the role of spiritual illness in a society where there is a pluralism of health-care systems and a dominant biomedical framework is essential. As Wreford (2005) describes in her thesis on sangoma presence in South African society, "to treat the sick in isolation from 'invisible beings'" (Appiah 1992, 11)—the spiritual community of the ancestors (or indeed, of the living community)—"is almost inconceivable" (Iwu 1986; Ngubane 1977; Yoder 1982). However, in parallel, it is the case that "spirituality rarely finds a place in the practice of biomedicine. Western medicine has increasingly inclined towards the separation of mind and spirit from the body" (4). For an individual whose core understanding of their illness is from a spiritual perspective, there is an ethical dimension to legitimizing suffering with different understandings and reflections than standardized notions of disease and illness. It is thus crucial to lend voice to the traditional South African experience.

9. Somatization

Somatization describes a phenomenon typically within illness contexts about the expression of physical symptoms that do not have an identifiable physical cause or origin. Somatization is an integral feature of a sangoma and patient interaction, but I will suggest that it also offers a way to mediate between the conflicting and coexisting medical systems described so far during this chapter.

Patients who present with somatic symptoms in biomedical settings bring uncertainty and ambiguity and are thus challenging. Requests for investigations and relief from suffering are difficult to manage from patients with somatoform disorders. Consequentially, a biomedical perspective recommends that when a patient reports symptoms that cannot be explained by an underlying organic problem, the primary care provider should consider psychiatric disorders, such as major depression, anxiety disorders, and alcohol and drug abuse, in the differential diagnosis. Cross-culturally, the divide in ways that somatization is understood is interesting. For example, traditional Chinese medicine has no concept of "medically unexplained symptoms," and treatment may be less complicated in Asian patients than in white patients because Asian patients recognize an interconnection between mind and body (Yeung and Deguang 2002, 253). Somatization may be understood, then, as a term relative to particular concepts embodied by members of a particular community.

From the point of entering the field of psychiatry as the mode of treatment interaction with a patient experiencing somatic symptomology, the discourse alters further for the South African patient who is from an indigenous background in the clinical consultation. Perceptions of mental illness among the South African community are related to social taboos, and mental illness is heavily stigmatized. Consequences of a mental health diagnosis have ethical implications subject to the context that the person receiving the diagnosis is situated in. Depending on the connotation that forms the stigma, there is potential for further harm to a vulnerable individual. In addition, the experiencing of symptomology in a dualistic sense makes it difficult to engage in the typically dualistic language of psychiatry. Suffering in a South African context may not necessarily be identified as either physical or mental but rather as being present in the person's lived experience. Understanding narrative, then, is an important aspect of the clinical encounter where a sharedness of experience may be absent.

The need for health-care professionals to understand religious and cultural taxonomies of illness and the use of traditional healing as a mode of treatment is required as well as a greater understanding of the nature of mental illness stigmatization (Mohamed-Kaloo and Laher 2014, 1). Misunderstanding expressions of suffering affects diagnosis, and mental distress may be mirrored in somatic symptoms leading to the diagnosis of medical conditions such as hypertension or backache. In relation to the previous discussion of spiritual illness, spirit possession may be considered a cause of mental illness.

10. Mental Illness and Culture

Culture is an essential consideration of the clinical interview, case formulation, and treatment of an individual. It is correct, therefore, to allow for a space in the clinical encounter for an individual to bring forth nonclinical explanations. This invariably means that nonclinical discourses are subject to the clinician's understanding and judgment for how the individual's subjectivity is bearing on their symptom presentation. When we use the term *psychiatry*, we are referring to the medical treatment of the mind to heal. Yet for a sangoma, the presence of pain and suffering is not described as pathology. Pathology is a normative value of a description of a person's suffering and an organizing principle for narrating pain.

Psychiatry places the origins of pain in a dichotomous position—namely, the traditionally dualistic concepts of physical and mental. Pain is a physical sensation invoking suffering. Psychosomatic pain is classified as an expression of psychosocial stress or as displaying medically unexplained symptoms. These are symptoms that are inconsistent with an identifiable medical diagnosis.

The causal model of medicine requires a physical origin of pain. Pain that is defined as psychopathological pain is considered to be a mood state. In somatization, it is imperative that the meaning and experience of pain is expressed and understood. Narration of people's experiences of pain can reveal the organization and structure in which their symptoms manifest, enabling the "witnessing and helping to order the experience to be of therapeutic value" (Kleinman 1989).

A pain that has a psychic origin emphasizes the importance of constructing the narrative of a person's experience of pain. In narratives, the meaning of pain is dispersed away from its origin, therefore annihilating the necessity for classifying pain as physical or mental. Instead, narratives need to be examined as if they are the body of the mind, the revealer, and the locus of the relationship between the person and their pain.

An example of such healing is *isibongo* poetry by sangomas in South Africa. A poem is, after all, in the words of Jonathan Culler (2005), "not simply a series of sentences; it is spoken by a persona, who expresses an attitude to be defined." Such poetry permits incompatibilities between different types of pain—physical or psychosomatic—to be irrelevant, and consequently the sharing and recognition of pain are dispersed through the communication of verse. Psychosomatic pain transcends the boundaries of the individual through the development of poetry, offering a role in medicine to discuss medically unexplained symptoms independently of the categories of physical or psychosomatic pain.

Concepts of cures search for a terminus, a process whereby there is a telos of removing a possession or a ghost or resetting the actions of certain molecules or chemical levels in traditional African healing and biomedicine, respectively. However, the conference talks yielded insights into the intricacies of the mind's voice. Thus the meaning of stories can aid health-care professionals in societies such as South Africa that are often underresourced and deal with patients who are living in impoverished conditions.

11. Acts of Healing

Between a doctor and a patient, there is a very special and unique relationship contained in an exclusive realm. The connection is formed from the presenting of an illness, and the sick are drawn to the healing. The healer in turn aspires to release the sick from their symptoms and pain. On a wider spectrum, acts of healing signify and reflect the experiential aspects of the human condition—namely, connection and relation to other individuals and empathy and compassion toward suffering. The following scenario describes the intensity of the sangoma and patient encounter:

A woman sits opposite a white-robed sangoma in an exclusive space contained within a rural village. The woman, an elder, is experiencing acute chest pain. She can locate the pain to her heart, but the pain is all-encompassing. It conducts through the whole of her body and smashes through one cell to another, carrying destruction to reach all of her being. The energy from the pain—its heat and the awareness of the body's aliveness—transpires into a particular state. In this state, the sangoma focuses on expelling the pain that she believes is a curse. The pain's momentum is experienced as the speed of a spirit that has possessed her body. The body and the spirit are two separate entities that on this occasion have become entangled in her life force. The sangoma is not powerful enough to kill the curse. He can only direct it toward the woman, sitting opposite him. The pain, or curse, is propelled from the body, and it is invited to be absorbed into the body of the healer. The healer becomes possessed by the curse, and the elder woman is born back into life. The healer labors through the curse. The curse has entered his body, but his powers of healing prevent it from identifying with his physicality. In a heightened trance, the curse is combated. Slowly the healer begins to relax, and the curse is dissipated.

Culture is a natural entity of which individuals are part. The medicinal world that the woman elder and the healer belong to is as real and ingrained in experience as our hospital setting is in our experience. Yet the narratives of each show a common illumination of our human discrepancy. While biomedicine prescribes a third party into our medical relationships—namely, that of chemical (pills), or physical (radiotherapy/ imaging), or biological (transplants)—to embody the pain that illness causes, the presence that there has been an invasion of the human body is a commonality between biomedicine and African views of illness in South Africa (Helman 2007). It is through the presence of pain that both the sangoma and the clinician develop the skills to reach and help another person. How that experience is conveyed, whether through ritual or narrative or diagnostic charting, is only ever a symptom of what belies the curse of illness—namely, the gift of the relationship between the sick and the healing.

12. Conclusion

Traditional African healing such as the practice provided by sangomas in South Africa as well as scientific biomedical services forms a constellation of beliefs, theories, treatments, understandings of disease, and the experience of suffering. The need has been highlighted throughout this chapter for a systematic dialogue between health practitioners in providing health justice.

Somatization and sharedness are significant parts of the conceptual and practice models of treatment for both traditional healers and clinicians. Narrative in the form of expression of symptoms, distress, and suffering and the sharedness of a relationship between a healer/clinician and a patient are fundamental aspects of health justice. Patients need to be understood and received in a way that relates to their narrative and their worldview in order to provide respect, dignity, and compassion. In this sense, sangomas enrich the medicalized discourse of health, and providing adequate and appropriate platforms for traditional medicine and healers in society will help medical practitioners work within both cultural and clinical encounters while attempting to provide the right to health to all members of a society.

References

Appiah, K. A. 1992. *In My Father's House: Africa in the Philosophy of Culture.* London: Methuen.

Boddy, J. 1994. "Spirit Possession Revisited: Beyond Instrumentality." *Annual Review of Anthropology* 23:407–434.

Boehnlein, J. K., M. N. Schaefer, and J. D. Bloom. 2005. "Cultural Considerations in the Criminal Law: The Sentencing Process." *Journal of the American Academy of Psychiatry and the Law Online* 33 (3): 335–341.

Chidester, D. 2012. *Wild Religion: Tracking the Sacred in South Africa.* Berkely: University of California Press.

Cook, C. T. 2009. "Sangomas: Problem or Solution for South Africa's Health Care System." *Journal of the National Medical Association* 101 (3): 261–265.

Cumes, D. 2013. "South African Indigenous Healing: How It Works." *EXPLORE: The Journal of Science and Healing* 9 (1): 58–65.

Fabrega, H., 1982. "A Commentary on African Systems of Medicine." In *African Health and Healing Systems: Proceedings of a Symposium,* edited by P. S. Yoder, 237-252. Los Angeles: Crossroads.

Foucault, M. 1973. *The Birth of the Clinic.* London: Tavistock.

Good, B. J., and M. J. D. Good. 1982. "Toward a Meaning-Centered Analysis of Popular Illness Categories: 'Fright Illness' and 'Heart Distress' in Iran." In *Cultural Conceptions of Mental Health and Therapy,* 141–166. Dordrecht: Springer Netherlands.

Helman, C. G. 2007. *Culture, Health and Illness.* Cleveland: CRC.

Iwu, M. 1986. *African Ethnomedicine.* Nigeria: UPS.

Kass, L. 1972. "Making Babies: The New Biology and the 'Old' Morality." *Public Interest* 26:1346–1350.

Keller, M. 2003. *The Hammer and the Flute: Women, Power, and Spirit Possession.* Baltimore: Johns Hopkins University Press.

Kleinman, A. 1988. *The Illness Narratives: Suffering, Healing, and the Human Condition.* New York: Basic Books.

Littlewood, R. 1990. "From Categories to Contexts: A Decade of the 'New Cross-Cultural Psychiatry.'" *British Journal of Psychiatry* 156 (3): 308–327.

Lizza, J. P., ed. 2009. *Defining the Beginning and End of Life: Readings on Personal Identity and Bioethics.* Baltimore: Johns Hopkins University Press.

Mohamed-Kaloo, Z., and S. Laher. 2014. "Perceptions of Mental Illness among Muslim General Practitioners in South Africa." *SAMJ: South African Medical Journal* 104 (5): 350–352.

Mol, A. 2002. *The Body Multiple: Ontologies in Medical Practice.* Durham, NC: Duke University Press.

Ngubane, H. 1977. "Body and Mind in Zulu Medicine: An Ethnography of Health and Disease." In *Nyuswa-Zulu Thought and Practice*. London: Academic.

Pellegrino, E. D. 2008. *The Philosophy of Medicine Reborn: A Pellegrino Reader*. Bloomington, IN: University of Notre Dame Press.

Scheper-Hughes, N. 1987. "The Mindful Body: A Prolegomenon to Future Work in Medical Anthropology." *Medical Anthropology Quarterly* 1 (1): 6–31.

Truter, I. 2007. "African Traditional Healers: Cultural and Religious Beliefs Intertwined in a Holistic Way." *SA Pharmaceutical Journal* 74 (8): 56–60.

van Wyk, Ben-Erik, Bosch van Oudtshoorn, and Nigel Gericke. 1999. *Medicinal Plants of South Africa*. Pretoria, South Africa: Briza.

Wreford, J. 2005. *Negotiating Relationships between Biomedicine and Sangoma: Fundamental Misunderstandings, Avoidable Mistakes*. South Africa: Centre for Social Science Research, University of Cape Town.

Yeung, A., and H. Deguang. 2002. "Somatoform Disorders." *Western Journal of Medicine* 176 (4): 253–256.

Yoder, P. 1982. "Commentary on African Systems of Medicine." In *African Health and Healing Systems: Proceedings of a Symposium*. UCLA, African Studies Center, African Studies Assoc., Office of International Health. https://tinyurl.com/y5qwa84j.

17

The British Bangladeshi
Experience of Mental Illness

Khaldoon Ahmed and Simon Dein

ABSTRACT

Bangladeshis are a large South Asian Muslim migrant group in the United Kingdom with distinctive health needs due to relative social exclusion and high rates of psychosis. Islam and religious identity are important, and ethnographic research shows that prayer, traditional healing, and belief in jinn (spirits) are common in those who experience mental illness. This chapter reviews existing research on the British Bangladeshi experience of mental illness and presents new research by Dr. Khaldoon Ahmed on the experience of psychosis in the community. There is evidence that in the younger bilingual group, traditional Islamic/Bengali idioms of distress and help seeking occur in parallel with psychiatric health services or are replaced or transformed in contact with them.

1. Introduction

1.1. Bangladeshis in the United Kingdom

Bangladeshis are one of the largest ethnic minorities in the United Kingdom, numbering almost half a million in the 2011 Census (Office for National Statistics [ONS] 2011). To understand the distinct patterns of illness beliefs and behaviors requires looking at religious practices, adaptation to life in the UK, and the unique relationship this diaspora group has to its country of origin. This is a relatively young population of whom around half were born in Bangladesh. They predominantly identify as practicing Muslims and are clustered in often deprived inner-city parts of London.

The site of Professor Simon Dein's research is Tower Hamlets, a borough situated just to the east of London. Dr. Khaldoon Ahmed's research takes place in Camden and Islington, two small inner-city boroughs just north of the center. People of Bangladeshi origin in Tower Hamlets number 81,377, forming 32 percent of the population. In Camden and Islington, the populations are 12,500 (5.7 percent) and 4,662 (2.3 percent), respectively (ONS 2011).

Large-scale migration to the United Kingdom from Bangladesh began in the 1970s, the vast majority originating from Sylhet, a hilly region of almost three million people in the northeast of Bangladesh. The migrants to the United Kingdom settled mostly in London but also in Oldham and Birmingham in northern England (Peach 2006). The first, second, and third generations of this community have a generally impoverished economic and educational profile as compared to the white British population but also when compared with the other South Asian migrant populations of Indians and Pakistanis (Peach 2006). This is despite a growing cohort of financially successful families and individuals who move to suburbs, often following advanced educational attainment (Yasmin 2015). The important demographic feature to note in the young profile of the population is that 37 percent of people of Bangladeshi origin were under fifteen in the 2001 Census in Camden (London Borough of Camden [LBC] 2007).

A striking feature of the community is the constant travel between the United Kingdom and Bangladesh. Visits for family events like weddings and virtual communication in the form of phone calls and sending money give rise to a unique translocal globalized identity, with religious and cultural influences traveling in both directions (Eade and Garbin 2006). There are religious trends unique to British Bangladeshis and some that overlap with the wider Muslim population in the United Kingdom. There has been a rise in a religiosity and observance that in its interpretation is stricter and self-consciously "purer" than the traditional Sufi/mystic and Hindu-influenced Bengali Islam as practiced by the first generation. There is a tension between new British Islamic practices influenced by puritanical Sunni Salafism and the older South Asian culture (Dein et al. 2008).

1.2. Mental Illness and British Bangladeshis

A number of epidemiological psychiatric studies have outlined patterns of biomedically defined mental illness in British Bangladeshis. The ethnic minority psychiatric illness in the community (EMPIRIC) study is a large recent investigation that looked at common mental disorders (CMD), anxiety, and depression. It found no statistical difference in rates of illness between white groups and Bangladeshi men (Weich et al. 2004). The study interestingly found lower rates in Bangladeshi women. This is in contrast to middle-aged Indian and Pakistani men and older Indian and Pakistani women, who had significantly higher rates of CMD than their white counterparts. Turning from CMD to psychosis, however, a different picture emerges. The incidences of psychoses faced by all Black and minority ethnic (BME) groups appear significantly elevated (Fearon et al. 2006). When adjusted for age and gender, the first-episode psychosis elevated risk in Bangladeshis was 2.1 (incidence rate ratios [IRR] 1.4–3.1; Kirkbride 2008). This study had particular power as it included large numbers of Bangladeshis in inner-city London, including Tower Hamlets, and distinguished between different migrant South Asian groups. This high risk is clearly a public health concern that requires a response from researchers and mental health services.

1.3. Explanations of Illness and Help Seeking

Ethnographic research in Bangladesh and the United Kingdom has looked at cultural understandings and responses to mental illness. British psychiatrist and anthropologist Alyson Callan conducted a study in Sylhet (2003). *Fagolami* is the general term used for madness. It can be caused by *zadutona* (sorcery) or *nozor* (the evil eye). Jinn (spirit) possession was thought to be a common reason for madness. Callan found that those afflicted by *fagolami* were taken to both the *kabiraj* (traditional healer) and the *daktar* (biomedically trained doctor). There were very few psychiatrists in Sylhet. Other healers consulted were the *fir* (living saint), *mullah* (priest), *guinine* (exorcist), homeopathic practitioner, and *hakim* (Unani or Greek/Islamic medicine practitioner). Treatments would involve recitation of verses of the Qur'an; the blowing over the patient, known as *foo*; and the use of *tabiz* (amulets).

How these beliefs and practices are re-created and transformed in a diasporic setting in London was investigated by Dein, Alexander, and Napier (2008). In this study, forty people of Bangladeshi origin in East

London were interviewed. It was found that physical and psychological problems as well as misfortunes in life were strongly associated with jinn. This was regardless of age, although younger informants did see these beliefs as "superstitious." Muslims of Bangladeshi origin generally believe in Islamic ideas of jinn as entities separate from humans that include demons, satanic beings, and angels. They can take multiple forms and can potentially possess people. The informants of the study attributed various behavior and experiences to jinn influence or possession. For example, low mood, withdrawal, "speaking rubbish," and change in behavior were thought to be caused by possession.

Informants in Dein's study consulted different types of healers at the same time. This included biomedical doctors, *hakims*, *kabiraj*, and *mullahs*. Folk healers used amulets, blew over the patient, and recited Qur'anic verses. Imams in the community often gave mixed recommendations—advising people to see a Western medical doctor or sometimes to see an exorcist. These were spiritual healers from Africa and South Asia who advertised in the local Bangla-language press and often charged extortionate rates for healing.

Belief in jinn as a cause for illness appears to be common across Muslim populations in Britain, as shown by N. Khalifa et al. (2011). In this study, 111 individuals of South Asian, Middle Eastern, and North African background answered a questionnaire on beliefs in jinn, black magic, and the evil eye. The majority of respondents believed these phenomena existed and could cause "schizophrenia, depression, anxiety, behavioral changes, personality changes, epilepsy, blood pressure problems, fever and bruises."

While Dein's ethnographic research focused on a single ethnic group, a qualitative comparison of the experience of six ethnic groups in the United Kingdom was published by W. O'Connor and J. Nazroo (2002). This was part of the study of EMPIRIC commissioned by the Department of Health (UK). The six groups were Bangladeshi, Caribbean, Indian, Irish, Pakistani, and white. In-depth interviews were held to elicit narratives of cause, idioms of mental distress, coping mechanisms, and use of services. The authors were surprised by similarities in ideas of illness causation. In most groups, social causes were thought to result in mental illness, like family, racism, employment, finances, and poor physical health. Specific South Asian idioms of distress were found with descriptions of "stress," "worry," "nervousness," "pressure," and "illness in the head." This study reinforces the premise that regardless of ethnic group, causation of mental illness is important for an unwell individual, and this does not usually fit into an encapsulated, culture-specific "explanatory model."

2. The New Research Study in Camden and Islington

2.1. Aim and Hypothesis

Dr. Ahmed's study looks at the experience of psychosis of Bangladeshis in London using semistructured ethnographic methods to investigate how psychosis is described, named, and thought to be caused and where healing is sought. Past ethnographic research has focused on the religious and cultural explanations. This study begins with the hypothesis that in an overwhelmingly young British Bangladeshi population with a growing second and third generation, there will be increasing adoption of biomedical explanations and help seeking for mental illness.

This population has a risk of more than double for psychosis than in white British groups (Kirkbride 2008), yet there is little qualitative research that looks specifically at the unique experience of British Bangladeshis. Existing research shows a resort to often exploitative traditional healers (Dein et al. 2008). Research is needed to establish patterns of help seeking for health services to meet the needs of this community with its higher rates of illness.

The study therefore provides a much-needed snapshot of the interaction between culture, illness, and psychiatric health care in British Bangladeshis today.

2.2. Methods

From the range of methodologies and tools available to look at these questions, the Short Explanatory Model Interview (SEMI) was chosen. This is a semistructured interview derived from ethnographic approaches and developed by Lloyd et al. (1998). It includes the following:

- personal and cultural background
- nature of the problem
- help the subject is seeking
- interaction with physician/healer
- beliefs related to mental illness

This tool was chosen as it is brief and tested and validated in a number of cultural settings. R. McCabe and S. Priebe (2004b) used it to investigate explanatory models (EMs) in four UK ethnic groups—white, African-Caribbean, Bangladeshi, and West African. It was found that Bangladeshis were more likely to have a social or supernatural EM. Whites were more likely to have a biological EM, and this was related to greater treatment satisfaction and therapeutic relationships.

The highly influential concept of "explanatory models" was proposed by A. Kleinman (1980). EMs are the "notion about an episode of sickness and its treatment that are employed by all those engaged in the clinical process." This concept has driven a great deal of research in culture and illness in the past three decades.

The clinical relevance of the concept has been highlighted by research that shows that when clinicians understand the patients' EMs, outcomes are better (Callan and Littlewood 1998). A number of research methods, including the SEMI, have been developed to look at EMs, such as the EMIC (Explanatory Model Interview Catalogue; Weiss 1997), the MINI (McGill Illness Narrative Interview; Groleau et al. 2006), and most recently, the BEMI (Barts Explanatory Model Inventory; Rudell, Bhui, and Priebe 2009).

These semistructured approaches, however, have some limitations and can be contrasted with longitudinal ethnography—an example of which is James Wilce's work (2004). He uses a linguistic-anthropological analysis of videotape recordings of a woman with schizophrenia in Matlab in Bangladesh.

There is not an expectation in Dr. Ahmed's study to use it to find a discrete and bounded EM for Bangladeshis in the United Kingdom who experience psychosis.

Research in EMs is vulnerable to bias and has failed to provide convincing evidence of a stable set of beliefs around the experience of mental illness. McCabe and Priebe (2004b) found that the concept and cause of illness were inconsistent when eight participants from four ethnic groups were interviewed at a one-year interval. In a study from the Netherlands, S. Ghane, A. M. Kolk, and P. M. Emmelkamp (2010) found that types of EMs elicited from ethnic minority respondents depended on the ethnicity of the interviewer. If the interviewer was ethnically similar, interpersonal, victimization, and religious/mystical causes were more reported.

Furthermore, B. Williams and D. Healy (2001) interviewed new referrals to a community mental health team. They found that individuals expressed a variety of causes throughout the interview and that beliefs were changeable. Another study by S. Jadhav, M. Weiss, and R. Littlewood (2001) investigated the "cultural experience of depression among white

Britons in London." A British version of the EMIC interview (Weiss 1997) was used to look at lay concepts and explanations of mental illness. A wide range of contradictory, overlapping, and linked explanations were found. While there was a "causal web" identified, there was no "explanatory model" of depression among white Britons.

There is then little evidence that EMs are discrete and independent variables that can be measured in specific ways with accurate tools.

Dr. Ahmed's study took place at the academic department of psychiatry at University College London and Camden and Islington National Health Service (NHS) Foundation Trust—the local provider of mental health care where Dr. Ahmed was based for specialist training in general adult psychiatry.

Eighteen men and women of Bangladeshi origin with a past or present diagnosis of psychotic illness were recruited through secondary mental health services in the London boroughs of Camden and Islington. Recruitment was by purposive sampling by directly approaching community mental health teams, early intervention teams, and hospital inpatient services. The inclusion criteria were (1) Bangladeshi ethnic origin and (2) psychotic illness falling into the *ICD-10* categories of schizophrenia, acute psychotic disorder, manic episode, bipolar affective disorder, or depressive disorder with psychosis.

All participants were currently engaged with mental health services. Sixty-six individuals that satisfied the inclusion criteria were approached. The researcher Dr. Ahmed liaised with the key workers, who asked individuals if they would be interested in taking part. Twenty people initially agreed to an interview. A participation fee of twenty British pounds was paid. Two interviewees who initially agreed to take part withdrew their consent. Informed and signed consent was obtained at the time of the interview.

Ethics approval was obtained from the Outer North East London Ethics Committee. Local approval and audit for the study came from the Camden and Islington NHS Foundation Trust research department (North Central London Research Consortium).

Demographic information was obtained from the participants at the time of the interview. This was age, gender, marital status, number of years spent in Bangladesh, and number of years spent in the United Kingdom. Electronic patient records were accessed later to obtain the psychiatric diagnosis, duration of illness, and time spent in the hospital.

2.3. Interviews

Sixteen participants were interviewed at home and four in hospital wards. As much as possible, interviews were conducted in nonclinical environments to counter potential bias of both participants and the interviewer in framing the interaction as a clinical session.

The interviews lasted around forty minutes and were recorded on a handheld digital sound recording device.

Dr. Ahmed then transcribed the material using the quantitative research software NVivo 8. The transcription phase was an important step in interpreting the interviews, allowing the researcher in-depth familiarity with the material.

The material was organized into themes of causation, naming, symptoms, and interaction with services.

Specific frequencies of words and descriptions were then obtained from the coding as part of the interview interpretation. These were (1) the name given by interviewees to their problems, (2) the symptoms experienced, and (3) the cause given to the illness.

3. Results

The information from the interviews is presented in three categories: (1) participant profile, (2) descriptive terminology obtained from the SEMI (naming, symptoms, and causes), and (3) case studies with contextualized narratives of the illness episode.

3.1. Participant Profile

Out of the eighteen participants, sixteen were men and two were women. The average age was 28.67 (SD 5.29). Eight were married, and ten described themselves as single. The majority (78 percent) had a diagnosis of schizophrenia. Eleven percent of the participants were diagnosed with bipolar affective disorder and 11 percent with depressive disorder with psychosis. The participants had spent a significant portion of their lives in Bangladesh—on average, a third of their lives. They had spent around nine months in total in a hospital for illness episodes.

3.2. Naming, Symptoms, and Causes

The SEMI provided narrative accounts from which the terms used to name the illness, its symptoms, and its causes were extracted.

Several names were given to their problems. Biomedical names were common, like *psychosis*, *paranoid schizophrenia*, *chronic psychosis*, and *depression*. More general terms such as *sickness*, *illness*, *going mad*, *mind disorder*, or *mental illness* were commonly used. The words *split personality* and *breakdown* were used once.

There was a huge variety of symptoms reported and how often each symptom was cited by the participants. The wide range seen could not be generalized or reduced easily into categories. However, paranoid symptoms were common, as were hearing voices, not sleeping, or becoming angry. The symptoms of stress, tension, worry, anxiousness, and nervousness could identifiably be clustered together. Somatic symptoms like having "pain in [their] heart," being "dizzy," and "somebody coming inside [them]" were also reported. Specific terms used were "microchip in the head," "memory loss," "low mood," "claustrophobia," and "feeling that seawater surrounds me." Only one person reported "a jinn inside me."

The cause of the illness and how often this cause was cited is shown in figure 17.1. Social and family causes were common, like bereavement, isolation, and financial difficulty. Jinn and black magic were not common causes reported. The causes with the highest frequencies were cannabis use and loneliness.

3.3. Case Studies

The following three case studies are descriptions of key aspects of illness experience to show the relationship between symptoms, perceived causation, and culture (KA = Khaldoon Ahmed).

Case 1: JG: "One Night I Came Home, I Was Shouting and Screaming"

JG, a thirty-year-old man diagnosed with psychosis and bipolar disorder, was interviewed at his home by the canal in Camden Town. After introductions, his wife made the interviewer, KA, a cup of tea. The interview came to an end when a maulana (mullah) arrived to help his daughter recite the Qur'an. JG described himself as a "liberal Muslim" and joked that he smoked cannabis but went for Friday prayers. He was wearing a *taveez* (amulet) around his neck and a turquoise-colored ring commonly worn by South Asian Sufis and Shiites. He said he was a "regular Sunni Muslim." JG was born in Sylhet and moved to London at age eleven, living in Hackney and then Camden. He was first hospitalized following a violent incident.

He was initially reluctant to talk about his illness but recounted the following:

KA: What happened?

JG: So much happened. . . . I have to go back. One night I came home, I was shouting and screaming. . . . I was taken to hospital by my family, and I ended up in mental hospital.

KA: How long were you in hospital for?

JG: I was there a good four to five months. They sent me home. When I first had my breakdown, I was there only for two weeks, then I came home. I had a relapse straightaway, then I was in hospital for four to five months. I came out, and after that, I was OK. In 2008, I had a second relapse. I was in hospital again.

KA: What was the cause of the breakdown?

JG: At that time, I was going through a really difficult time in my personal life . . . a lot of stress I was under. Before 2007, I was under a lot of stress, and debt, and then when it came to my personal life I was struggling to cope with the stress.

KA: What was the personal stress?

JG: Relationships. . . . At that time, I was not married.

Of his diagnosis, JG said, "I disagree with the doctors to a certain extent. They seem to believe I am hyperactive. I was always hyperactive. Sometimes I feel lazy; when I want to do things, I feel active. They think illness is being high, and I question them and ask what is normal?"

KA: Did other people think you had problems?

JG: Only medically trained people are able to tell.

He disputes his diagnosis of psychosis with bipolar disorder but accepts that he has a problem that only "medically trained" people can know. His descriptions use words like "stress," "relapse," and "breakdown." The account of his illness is structured around his hospitalizations. He connects his "breakdown" to social problems of debt and relationships. He also relates his problems to the stress of racism and anti-Muslim feeling: "It's bad, especially for Muslims since 9/11. On top of the normal life, they have to watch what they do and say. It's all that stuff affecting Muslims. The normal day-to-day life . . . on top of that, you have the new extra stress after 9/11. When you go out there, 20 percent of the world's cameras belong to the United Kingdom. Don't forget the big brother himself, the big satellite, to hear us. People cannot take it anymore, especially in the city."

He also related his illness to getting involved in violence:

> We lived in Hackney four years, then moved to Kentish [town], then to Wood Green because I had some problem with the local boys. The house we had in Kentish was from the council, I had some problems with boys, and we went to temporary accommodation. They were racist. I got into fights. They were Black boys. Since then he got shot dead. We moved before he got shot; I found out from news.
>
> My first breakdown was 2007. I was twenty-eight or twenty-nine. I always was a very normal person. I react normally to certain people. In the past, I stood up for things I believe in. With the racist guy, I just ignored it, but it was not much of a problem until I had a breakdown.
>
> But the guy was out of order completely, the way he was talking and just snapped. He called me Paki. . . . I was carrying this multitask knife. . . . I just took it out and said if you behave the way you did, I'll do you. That's why I got arrested, because he called me Paki.

While JG did not himself seek help from traditional Islamic or Bangladeshi practitioners, his family obtained a taveez for him, and he wore it for a while.

KA: Did your family help you?

JG: Yes, my family has always been there for me.

KA: Did they suggest anything?

JG: My mum said pray [JG laughs]. Someone gave me taveez! Maulanas from Bangladesh. My mum asked to get a taveez, my sister as well, because they believe in it. They called the Maulana on the phone. . . . In Bangladesh, he gave us a taveez. They posted it. Do you believe in taveez? It works, I think.

KA: How does it work?

JG: It's down to your belief. It's to do with how much faith you have. I used to wear it, but it dropped, and I lost it. It has a surah inside. I don't know which one.

Case 2: SC: "The Doctors Always Want to Diagnose You with Something No Matter What You Say"

SC is a twenty-three-year-old who was interviewed on a ward in a North London hospital. He was born female but wanted to be identified as male.

In appearance, he looked and dressed like a teenage boy with a slight build. He had a long-standing diagnosis of schizophrenia and had spent many years in and out of hospitals. His brother and mother were also diagnosed with schizophrenia.

KA: Do you have an illness?

SC: The first time I was diagnosed with something, it was psychosis. The doctors explained very little to me about it. I don't think every time I have psychosis, I have to come into this hospital. I come here sometimes to have some rest from my family and stuff.

KA: When did you first have problems?

SC: My brother was playing violent films and smoking all day, and we shared the same space at my mum's house. His habit of smoking and watching videos back to back, not being healthy, made me feel sick. My sister was very rude. Every time I see her, she is on my case, and she makes me feel very stressed.

KA: Do you think there is a name for the problem?

SC: The doctors always want to diagnose you with something no matter what you say, as you're their patient. But that's up to them, and if that helps me in the future, then that's something better for me, so I have to encourage a little bit of being looked at as a patient.

KA: What causes problems like schizophrenia or depression?

SC: I don't take that schizophrenia stuff seriously. I think if someone's not sleeping for a whole month . . . that person can develop cracks in their mind, in their psyche, just get paranoid. I saw my brother getting like that, and I saw how he is talking to himself. He was diagnosed with schizophrenia.

    I got isolated in uni [university], and my self-esteem got really bad. My mood got bad. I didn't have much work to do or speak to anybody. I was transgender and was finding out what that was. Before there wasn't much on TV. I didn't have much help, and my family forced me to wear earrings and female clothes and dress like a woman and be like a woman. They bullied me when I was child; they forced me to dress as a woman.

He pressed psychiatrists involved in his care to organize chromosome testing to see if he was male or female. He wanted to be referred for gender reassignment, but this did not go ahead. A gender specialist psychiatrist assessed SC and was of the opinion that the gender confusion was a psychotic symptom.

SC described himself as a "semireligious Muslim" and said the following when asked about jinn:

KA: Do you believe in jinn?

SC: I believe they exist, but I couldn't really care much for that. I wouldn't know. I don't think I'm a person that God is helping at the moment in my life. I've helped myself. I've had a hard life, and I've come through it by myself. It's my hard work and my strength. I've had hard times when I have had breaks and come to the hospital, but it's my hard work; God isn't helping me.

Case 3: MSR: "Can You Make Me into a Mutant?"

MSR is a twenty-nine-year-old man who was interviewed in a hospital ward. He was admitted for schizophrenia and was unwell with severe symptoms of thought disorder and delusions. In the interview, he listed various surahs (verses) of the Qur'an he knew by heart and how *zikr* (repetition of the names of Allah) helped him: "I go to the mosque when I need to. When I am away, I do *zikr*, I say, 'Allah Hu, Allah Hu, Allah Hu.'"

He then said,

MSR: When Satan is attacking me, I read that surah, and after that, I become clean.

KA: How do the surahs clean you?

MSR: These surahs come specially from the Qur'an; they came from the sifarah [chapter], then printed in the Qur'an. They are the best fighters in the world. They reach your mind and help you as well, because they are doctors, police, army, so many things; they help you read your mind and step-by-step go to jihad.

He thought there was a chip in his brain that recorded everything: "I had a baby tag from UCL [University College London Hospital]; it was on the leg. It's the chip in my brain in the leg."

KA: Do you believe in jinn?

MSR: There is a lot of jinn; there are jinn inside me. I see X-Men; it's a power, I can read minds, do things. I like this place; it's quiet. My ears hurt, but you can't see the pain; the prophet said no pain. Make me a mutant. Will you make me a mutant?

KA: Do you see jinn?

MSR: My friends left me in the car in Redhill in the dark. I was scared. A man and woman came beside me. I saw them in King's Cross as well. They came from inside me when I said Allah o Akbar [God is great].

During the interview, MSR became increasingly unintelligible: "Can you tell me if I am Indian? I might be Bangladeshi, Pakistani, or Indian. That's what I want to know. . . . What is my religion? I need to know."

4. Conclusions

Dr. Ahmed's study strikingly demonstrates that younger Bangladeshis living in inner-city London encode their experience of psychosis in the language of biomedical psychiatry. This is in contrast to studies by Dein and Khalifa where religious explanations and healing are sought. It is likely that in the second and third generations of the community, cultural assimilation and contact with health services make belief in jinn possession and the use of traditional healers less common. Dr. Ahmed's findings, however, do need to be seen in light of the limitations of his study. First, interviews were conducted in English, which might not capture Bengali idioms of distress that would point to alternative explanations of illness. Second, participants were recruited from mental health services and, as a cohort, had been exposed to medical treatment. One would expect their reports of illness understanding to be more "biomedical" as compared to individuals who did not come into contact with services.

The eighteen interviews conducted, however, do represent a fascinating interchange between a South Asian Muslim minority group and mental health services. While an individual may describe "anxiety" and "paranoia," it cannot be taken for granted that this corresponds in a similar way to biomedical categories of mental illness (this would of course apply to any other ethnic group). The samples in Dr. Ahmed's study show considerable ambivalence about their diagnoses. SC, for example, sees becoming a patient and accepting the diagnosis of schizophrenia as a strategy with the greater goal of being listened to for the person he really is. JG was taken to spiritual healers by his family and wore a taveez at the same time as taking medication and seeing psychiatrists for bipolar disorder. These interviews can be seen as representative of "therapeutic itineraries," pathways where individual illness experiences are shaped through contact with health services (Peglidou 2010, who describes this process in Greece).

The results of this study inevitably also bring us to the question of why rates of psychosis in British Bangladeshis are double that of the majority population. The participants themselves in the causation of their illnesses drew attention to racism, Islamophobia, and difficulties in integration (see figure 17.1). Problems for Muslims after 9/11 were cited, or social isolation and not speaking English properly. Low self-esteem, family problems, cannabis use, and sexual abuse were causes with a strong social dimension self-reported by interviewees.

While psychiatry has successfully given a framework and understanding to the study participants, it has arguably not been able to address or respond to the social causes of exclusion and marginality that the individuals cite themselves. This needs to be addressed as an issue of health justice.

References

Bhui, K., and D. Bhugra. 2002. "Explanatory Models for Mental Distress: Implications for Clinical Practice and Research." *British Journal of Psychiatry* 181:6–7.

Callan, A. 2003. "Mental Illness, Medical Pluralism and Islamism in Sylhet, Bangladesh." PhD thesis, University College London.

Callan, A., and R. Littlewood. 1998. "Patient Satisfaction: Ethnic Origin or Explanatory Model?" *International Journal of Social Psychiatry* 44:1–11.

Dein, S., M. Alexander, and D. Napier. 2008. "Jinn, Psychiatry and Contested Notions of Misfortune among East London Bangladeshis." *Transcultural Psychiatry* 45 (1): 31–55.

Eade, J., and D. Garbin. 2006. "Competing Visions of Identity and Space: Bangladeshi Muslims in Britain." *Contemporary South Asia* 15 (2): 181–193.

Fearon, P., J. B. Kirkbride, C. Morgan, P. Dazzan, K. Morgan, T. Lloyd, G. Hutchinson, J. Tarrant, W. L. Fung, J. Holloway, R. Mallett, G. Harrison, J. Leff, P. B. Jones, and R. M. Murray. 2006. "Incidence of Schizophrenia and Other Psychoses in Ethnic Minority Groups: Results from the MRC AESOP Study." *Psychological Medicine* 36:1541–1550.

Ghane, S., A. M. Kolk, and P. M. Emmelkamp. 2010. "Assessment of Explanatory Models of Mental Illness: Effects of Patient and Interviewer Characteristics." *Social Psychiatry and Psychiatric Epidemiology* 45 (2): 175–182.

Groleau, D., A. Young, and L. Kirmayer. 2006. "The McGill Illness Narrative Interview (MINI): An Interview Schedule to Elicit Meanings and Modes of Reasoning Related to Illness Experience." *Transcultural Psychiatry* 43 (4): 671–691.

Jadhav, S., M. Weiss, and R. Littlewood. 2001. "Cultural Experience of Depression among White Britons in London." *Anthropology and Medicine* 8 (1): 47–69.

Khalifa, N., T. Hardie, S. Latif, I. Jamil, and D. M. Walker. 2011. "Beliefs about Jinn, Black Magic and the Evil Eye among Muslims: Age, Gender and First Language Influences." *Journal of Culture and Mental Health* 4:68–77.

Kirkbride, J. B., D. Barker, F. Cowden, R. Stamps, M. Yang, and P. B. Jones. 2008. "Psychoses, Ethnicity and Socio-economic Status." *British Journal of Psychiatry* 193:18–24.

Kleinman, A. 1980. *Patients and Healers in the Context of Culture: An Exploration of the Borderland between Anthropology, Medicine, and Psychiatry.* Berkeley: University of California Press.

Lloyd, K. R., K. S. Jacob, V. Patel, L. St. Louis, D. Bhugra, and A. H. Mann. 1998. "The Development of the Short Explanatory Model Interview (SEMI) and Its Use among Primary-Care Attenders with Common Mental Disorders." *Psychological Medicine* 28 (5): 1231–1237.

London Borough of Camden (LBC). 2007. *2001 Census Factsheet No. 9: Bangladeshis in Camden.*

McCabe, R., and S. Priebe. 2004a. "Assessing the Stability of Schizophrenia Patients' Explanatory Models of Illness over Time." *Journal of Mental Health* 13 (2): 163–169.

——. 2004b. "Explanatory Models of Illness in Schizophrenia: Comparison of Four Ethnic Groups." *British Journal of Psychiatry* 185:25–30.

Mia, Shamea Yasmin. 2015. "Navigating Histories: An Exploration of Second Generation High-Achieving British Bangladeshi Muslim Young Women Living in North-East London." Doctoral thesis, University of London, Goldsmiths.

O'Connor, W., and J. Nazroo, eds. 2002. *Ethnic Differences in the Context and Experience of Psychiatric Illness: A Qualitative Study.* Department of Health by the National Centre for Social Research and the Department of Epidemiology and Public Health at the Royal Free and University College Medical School.

Office for National Statistics (ONS). 2011. "Ethnicity and National Identity in England and Wales 2011." Part of 2011 Census, Key Statistics for Local Authorities in England and Wales Release. Accessed October 10, 2020. https://tinyurl.com/hz7saup.

Peach, C. 2006. "South Asian Migration and Settlement in Great Britain 1951–2001." *Contemporary South Asia* 15 (2): 133–146.

Peglidou, A. 2010. "Therapeutic Itineraries of 'Depressed' Women in Greece: Power Relationships and Agency in Therapeutic Pluralism." *Anthropology and Medicine* 17 (1): 41–57.

Rudell, K., K. Bhui, and S. Priebe. 2009. "Concept, Development and Application of a New Mixed Method Assessment of Cultural Variations in Illness Perceptions: Barts Explanatory Model Inventory." *Journal of Health Psychology* 14 (2): 336–347.

Weich, S., J. Nazroo, K. Sproston, S. McManus, M. Blanchard, B. Erens, S. Karlsen, M. King, K. Lloyd, S. Stansfeld, and P. Tyrer. 2004. "Common Mental Disorders and Ethnicity in England: The EMPIRIC Study." *Psychological Medicine* 34 (8): 1543–1551.

Weiss, M. 1997. "Explanatory Model Interview Catalogue (EMIC): Framework for Comparative Study of Illness." *Transcultural Psychiatry* 34:235–263.

Wilce, J. M. 2004. "To 'Speak Beautifully' in Bangladesh: Subjectivity as Pagalami." In *Schizophrenia, Culture, and Subjectivity*, edited by J. H. Jenkins and R. J. Barrett, 196–218. Cambridge: Cambridge University Press.

Williams, B., and D. Healy. 2001. "Perceptions of Illness Causation among New Referrals to a Community Mental Health Team: Explanatory Model or Exploratory Map?" *Social Science & Medicine* 53 (4): 465–476.

Appendix

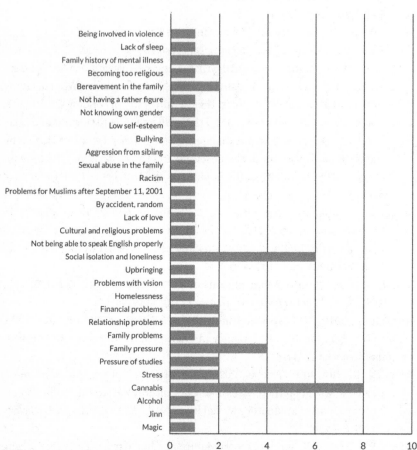

Figure 17.1: Cause of illness and frequency

18

The Freedom of Religion and the Right to Mental Health

CHALLENGES AND A QUEST FOR RECONCILIATION

Mari Stenlund

ABSTRACT

The relationship between freedom of religion and the right to mental health poses many challenges if people attend to such religious activity and hold such religious beliefs that might threaten their mental health. This chapter presents different ways to understand the freedom of religion and discusses how the right to mental health relates to these different views. The most useful approach would be to understand freedom of religion in terms of capability. If a capabilities approach is adopted, the individual's freedom of religion may be defined as the capability of choosing the religious beliefs to follow, belonging to the religious community, and living according to religious views. In this case, the conflict between freedom of religion and the right to mental health seems to disappear because the rights are interwoven with each other. It is suggested in this chapter that, on one hand, religious communities should have a right to teach about their views but, on the other hand, the state should have a duty to promote the capabilities of every human being—for example, by education, health care, and social services—in order to ensure that people are capable of making choices in their religious communities.

1. Introduction

The United Nations' international human rights covenants define that every human being has the right both to freedom of religion and to the enjoyment of the highest attainable standard of mental health—in brief, the "right to mental health" (see United Nations Human Rights 1966a, art. 18; 1966b, art. 12). It seems that when the right to mental health is discussed, the background supposition has been that enjoying civil liberties, freedom of religion included, protects also the right to mental health. Lawrence O. Gostin (2001) formulates this as follows: "Some measure of mental health is indispensable for human rights because only those who possess some reasonable level of functioning can engage in political and social life. Similarly, human rights are indispensable for mental health because they provide security from harm or restraint and the freedom to form, and express, beliefs that are essential to mental well-being" (266).

This holds true in most cases, since being religious or spiritual often promotes mental health (see, e.g., Koenig and Larson 2001). However, it is conceptually important to discuss also unfortunate conflicting cases. The relationship between freedom of religion and the right to mental health is challenging if people attend religious activities and hold such religious beliefs that might violate their mental health. For example, people adopt beliefs and make choices that cause them to be anxious or depressed. They may follow religious leaders who teach, or even pressure, them to choose a way of life that they would have not chosen "themselves" and that may restrict their possibilities to use their abilities and keep in contact with people they used to be close with. People may do so, for example, because they are afraid of ending up in hell, losing some kind of spiritual virtue, or losing all their close people in their community. If they have mental health challenges, they are not necessarily seeking any psychiatric help for those because their religious community may have a view that psychiatry should be avoided and spiritual help should be sought instead (see, e.g., Linjakumpu 2015; Ruoho 2013; Villa 2013).[1]

I see a problem in that people may attend to such religious communities freely and in this way use their freedom for something that hurts

---

[1] It is worth noting that the realization of an individual's rights in their community is mainly a Western discussion. Kristiina Kouros, who is the secretary general of the Finnish League for Human Rights, has noticed that bringing up the issue of pressured individuals in their religious communities resonates with her northern European and North American colleagues, while colleagues from many other countries find it difficult to see these issues as human rights problems. See Kouros (2011, 138).

their mental health. Or are they free when they end up doing so? Fruitfully understanding and protecting the right to mental health in these kinds of situations depend on how the concept of freedom is understood.

Understanding the relationship between freedom of religion and the right to mental health is challenging because, first, it is unclear what is meant by these rights and what these rights actually protect, and second, it is not self-evident how the conflicts between these rights, if there are such, can be resolved. In this chapter, I present different ways to understand the freedom of religion and discuss how the right to mental health relates to these different views. I consider these human rights in the juridical sense, which means that they impose juridical obligations on other people and the state. In the end, I present ideas about how both freedom of religion and the right to mental health could be protected as broadly as possible and what kinds of challenges these rights present to religious communities and public policy.

2. Freedom of Religion in Terms of Negative Liberty

In the discussion concerning human rights, the conception of negative liberty refers to the classical way to understand the meaning of civil and political rights (CP rights), of which freedom of religion is one. CP rights have traditionally been considered negative rights. This means that they are intended to protect the individual from government officials intruding into their life. The only positive obligation of the state is to ensure, by jurisprudence and, if needed, juridical punishment, that people do not violate each other's freedom (Stenlund and Slotte 2018, 431).[2]

When freedom of religion is interpreted as negative freedom, it means that other people may not interfere in concrete ways with another individual's belief and the manifestation of this belief. The individual may believe and practice their present beliefs, but on the other hand, the person need not believe or practice some beliefs if that is what they want at the time (Stenlund and Slotte 2018, 431; Stenlund 2014, 94–105).

When freedom of religion is understood in terms of negative liberty, it may be in clear conflict with the right to mental health if the person manifests their religion in a way that possibly harms their own or someone else's mental health. Most thinkers who defend understanding freedom in the negative sense also present acceptable reasons for

---

2 On negative liberty in the discussion of political philosophy, see, for example, Berlin (2005, 169–70) and Feinberg (1973, 7, 15).

restricting it. The most obvious reason for restricting negative liberty is the protection of other people's rights (Berlin 2005, 171–72; Feinberg 1973, 23). When it comes to freedom of religion, this approach is clearly seen in current human rights theory and human rights documents, since freedom of religion can be restricted when the purpose is to protect other people.[3]

It is clear that there is no right to endanger the life and safety of other people. However, in the context of people's mental well-being, it is challengingly unclear how we should understand and express the idea that other people's rights may restrict someone's freedom of religion. According to Lawrence O. Gostin (2001, 271), behavior and stressful conditions are factors outside of government's control. If I understand Gostin's point correctly, he seems to think that the state should not restrict by legislation the way people behave and create stressful conditions in religious communities, even if they might violate mental health. However, though there were no legal duties against the creation of such conditions, there might well be such a moral duty for religious communities and citizens in general. In addition, there might be a moral duty also to help people who have been suffering from stressful conditions, but the legal duty, if there is such, probably belongs to the state.

The problem seems to be that when people live together in communities, whether religious or not, it is part of normal human life that they may cause each other mental distress ranging from slightly hurt feelings and mild social coercion to all-out, total mental breakdowns (see Feinberg 1973, 27–29, 32). Restricting freedom of religion in order to protect people from all types of mental distress does not seem acceptable in liberal states, though conceptually, it would of course be possible for the state to take some kind of control over mental health–violating behavior and conditions—for example, by illegalization.

According to Joel Feinberg (1973, 27–29, 32), preventing a mental breakdown would be a justified reason for restricting other people's freedom. However, it is not clear what factors actually cause the breakdown and thus what the state should restrict. For example, to what extent should people, in exercising their freedom of religion, take into account the vulnerability of other people? Should people always consider whether there is somebody somewhere who might have a mental

---

3 Except it is not justified to interfere with the right to hold thoughts and opinions in one's mind in any circumstances. See Stenlund and Slotte (2018), Tahzib (1996, 25–26), Nowak (1993, 314–15), and Partsch (1981, 214, 217).

breakdown because of what they say or teach? How far can we assume that expressions of opinions in the course of teaching, for example, are the fundamental reasons for mental breakdowns? Even though we might think that everyone should avoid causing other people to have mental breakdowns, is it a moral or a legal failure if a mental breakdown occurs? Are there situations where it is not possible to avoid causing mental breakdowns, however hard one might try, without one's own area of freedom of religion becoming too narrow?

If the view of freedom of religion in terms of negative liberty is adopted, I suggest, first, that at least some kind of intentionality should be seen as one indicator for illegal behavior in a religious community, which means that there could be legal punishment for people who have caused a mental breakdown *intentionally*. Second, it might be that especially vulnerable groups (at least children and people with serious mental health disorders or mental disabilities) should be protected from such abuse. This could be done partly also by taking the vulnerable person's view carefully into account. For example, it should be determined if a person who is a patient in a mental health facility really welcomes visitors from their religious community or whether they actually would not like to see them.[4] Taking the vulnerability and possible incompetence of people into account is important because the background supposition of the view of negative liberty is often that people are competent.

3. Freedom of Religion in Terms of Authenticity

The approach of understanding freedom of religion in terms of negative liberty has been, however, criticized by the accusation that it is too narrow and does not take into account that people may be influenced also by different social and mental restrictions that make them unfree to believe and practice their own beliefs. It has been presented that freedom of religion should be understood primarily in terms of authenticity. In this case, freedom of religion seems to signify the right to hold one's own beliefs, which are themselves the results of an authentic believing and thinking process. Thus freedom of religion signifies the right to be the author of one's beliefs and opinions. Freedom of religion also

---

4 In Finland, a support group for the victims of religions reports the case where the judicial committee of Jehovah's Witnesses visited the patient twice in the "closed" psychiatric ward, and it is not clear whether the patient actually wanted them to visit her. See Uskontojen uhrien tuki ry ([UUT] 2014, 12–13).

signifies the right to self-fulfillment—namely, the right to a life where one's manifestations and expressions are in harmonious relationship with one's authentic beliefs (Stenlund and Slotte 2018, 435; Stenlund 2014, 172–91).[5]

Since the concept of authenticity refers to the internal or psychological dimension of a person, the restrictions of authenticity are also internal and psychological even though the source of these restrictions seems to be external to the person. When freedom of religion is understood in terms of authenticity, the potential threat to the individual would appear to be communities that could manipulate their members or potential members.

Unfortunately, when people refer to manipulation as a form of interference with someone's authenticity, they do not always explain what they mean by that term. However, when the various views concerning manipulation are collected together and reflected upon in relation to the view that freedom in terms of authenticity is a human right, it seems that conceptually, the central features of manipulation are, first, that the manipulator has the intention to manipulate and, second, that the person who is being manipulated changes their beliefs and thoughts and acts involuntarily, against their real will (see, e.g., Langone n.d.; Zimbardo 2007, 258–59).

It has also been claimed that the manipulator hides some significant information from the person they want to manipulate. According to Dennis Wrong, manipulation is a form of power that is connected to a tendency to hide some information. In manipulation, the person who is the object of manipulation does not know that they are the object of such an influence. The manipulator makes the person act in the way the manipulator wants them to act by hiding some decisive information (Wrong 2002, 28–29). The case is different in everyday influencing phenomena, in persuasion and pressure to conform, where no significant information has been intentionally hidden.

When freedom of religion is understood in terms of authenticity, there seems to be no conflict in relation to the right to mental health, since authentic beliefs are thought to be "healthy." On the other hand, if the person is manipulated, they necessarily cannot be said to be a mentally healthy person. Susana Beltran notes how heavy psychological

5 On political philosophical discussion concerning authenticity, see, for example, Oshana (2007), Dworkin (1985, 353–59), Scanlon (1972, 215–16), and Berlin (2005, 178).

manipulation violates the freedom of religion, because people are prevented from leaving a group and from freely changing their religion. In addition, severe manipulation may, according to Beltran (2005, 289–90), cause physical or psychological damage and may contravene the prohibition against subjecting a person to torture or cruel, inhuman, or degrading treatment. It is crucial that when Beltran discusses manipulation as a restriction of freedom of religion, she considers it as a form of coercion that is fundamentally psychological. If people were prevented from leaving a group or changing their views physically or by legal constraints, it would be a restriction in the negative sense as well.

According to Beltran, the realization of the freedom of religion requires that people are prevented from being manipulated and from any form of dependence generated by manipulative groups (Beltran 2005, 289–90). Preventing manipulation does not even restrict the manipulator's freedom of religion, since they were allowed to express their authentic views but not lies.

It is worth noting that when the freedom of religion is being discussed, manipulation should be clearly distinguished conceptually from persuasion and conforming, which are normal influencing methods. For example, if a religious leader claims that people who believe a certain thing and behave in a certain way may end up in hell, it is not a case of manipulation since the leader themself really believes that there is such a risk. It is persuasion since the religious leader does not hide any information but invokes the beliefs that the other people (at least if they get distressed) share. However, outsiders might easily consider this manipulation if they think that the threat of ending up in hell is not real.[6]

The problem of understanding freedom of religion in terms of authenticity is, however, that it is more philosophically than juridically inclined and too idealistic to be applied as such in the discussion concerning juridical rights. The result is that it may be even dangerous because it would be allowed to intrude on people's negative liberty in order to protect their authenticity, which might result in a totalitarian state. Second, people's agency is not supported if they are defined as pure victims without any interests or reasons for ending up or staying in a

---

6 Thanks to Kimmo Ketola, who explained the difference between manipulation and persuasion in this context.

community where their mental health was violated. These reasons lead me to suggest that even though authenticity is a philosophically interesting theme, freedom of religion as a juridical human right should not be discussed in terms of authenticity.

4. Freedom of Religion in Terms of Capability

The approach of understanding freedom of religion in terms of capability seems to be more promising. The capability approach toward freedom has been presented, for example, by Amartya Sen (2000, 9–10), who argues that a person is free when they are able to lead their life in such a way that life is valuable to them. According to Martha Nussbaum (2011, x, 18–19), the capability approach, also known as the capabilities approach and the human development approach, is interested in what people are actually able to do and to be and what real opportunities are available to them. When freedom is understood in terms of capability, different aspects of human life are brought together. Sen's (2000, 3–11) central claim is that the different kinds of freedoms strengthen each other, while Nussbaum (2011) emphasizes that "the most important elements of people's quality of life are plural and qualitatively distinct: health, bodily integrity, education, and other aspects of individual lives cannot be reduced to a single metric without distortion" (18). The intertwining nature of human rights has also been recognized in human rights theory. For example, CP rights and economic, social, and cultural rights (ESC rights) are often reconciled in the international research on human rights. The purpose of all human rights has been seen to be the same, and they are considered to be interdependent and interrelated (see, e.g., Whelan 2010).

When it comes to freedom of religion, it might signify in terms of capability that the individual is capable of choosing which religious beliefs to follow, belonging to the religious community, and living according to religious views. When freedom of religion is understood in terms of capability, it is meaningful to consider the alternatives that a person within a religious community has and their capability to make choices (see Stenlund and Slotte 2018, 438–39).

We may suppose that, in general, there are no conflicts between membership in some religious community and being sufficiently capable to make choices. Equally, one could discuss whether the state could cooperate more with religious communities in order to promote its citizens' capabilities.[7] Nussbaum (2006, 297) also emphasizes that people who adhere to authoritarian religions should also be respected without being made to feel denigrated.

However, there are also situations where the individual's capabilities to choose their beliefs and lifestyle are limited in a religious community for social and psychological reasons. Social reasons may limit a person's capability to make a choice, for example, if the individual was born and grew up in a religious community closed off from the outside world. Even though this individual could, in principle, leave the community and choose some other beliefs and lifestyle, they may, in practice, consider it almost impossible to leave the community and their relationships there. In extreme cases, the members of a religious community may also decide to cut their contacts with a person who does not follow the rules and beliefs of the community even though the person who has left might be a family member. Therefore, it is meaningful to ask whether the individual's freedom of religion can be realized in such a closed community. The individual who has grown up in a more open community and who has a social life also outside it has, in practice, more opportunities to change their beliefs and lifestyle and the abilities needed to do so.[8] The possibility of choice is central in the capabilities approach, as the following example given by Nussbaum (2006) shows: "A Muslim woman may prefer to remain veiled, and the approach says nothing against this, provided that there are sufficient political, educational, and other capabilities present to ensure that the choice is a choice" (298).

Psychological reasons may weaken a person's capabilities for choice if their religiosity is so undeveloped that it does not meet the challenges of adult life (see Teinonen 2007, 114, 122, 125). The person may also find it psychologically difficult to give up some doctrine or idea. For example, if the person is distressed about the possibility of ending up in hell if they do not adopt some particular beliefs, they might lack capability. The individual's freedom of religion in terms of capability can also be seen as restricted in the situation where a poor individual receives charity from a religious community and becomes in this way

---

7 For example, Päivänsalo (2014) has suggested the possibility of collaborating with religious actors in order to protect and promote the right to health.
8 See Nussbaum (2008, 140–45), who considers the capability of the choice of children who have grown up in an Amish community.

dependent and adopts some of their views, even though they were not, in principle, forced to adopt them.

When it comes to potential conflicts between different human rights, such as freedom of religion and the right to mental health, the capabilities approach seems to be challenging conceptually. There seem to be two levels in the capabilities approach. Because the view of negative liberty is a part of the view of freedom in terms of capability, this part of freedom of religion may conflict on the first level with the right to mental health. However, fundamentally on the second level, there should be no conflicts because being capable of choosing requires sufficient mental health, and the person who is deeply distressed because of their beliefs and religious lifestyle cannot be defined as being free in terms of capability. It seems actually impossible to say where the right to freedom of religion ends and where the right to mental health begins, which seems similar to the way Lawrence Gostin (2001, 266) describes the relationship between the right to mental health and other human rights.

The question about the opportunities available to an individual to make choices and act upon them in a religious community is conceptually challenging. One could pose the question of whether it should be the legal duty of a religious community not to weaken its members' capability. It seems that this sort of suggestion is included, for example, in a memorandum of the Finnish League of Human Rights (2009) about the teachings of the Laestadian revival movement. This movement, which acts in the Lutheran Church of Finland, considers birth control a sin. The Finnish League of Human Rights argues against the Laestadian movement here, claiming that the birth-control-as-a-sin view violates the human rights of the members of the movement. If the view of freedom of religion in terms of capability is adopted, I would prefer an approach that gives negative liberty to religious communities to teach about their views but at the same time sees enhancing the capabilities of every human being as the duty of the state. This would mean that the state would have to ensure the right of every citizen to education, where capabilities would be improved, and would also ensure that there was sufficient health care and social services for everyone. If people grow up to be capable, they are also sufficiently capable of dealing with a religious teaching that, for example, might promote the view that birth control is a sin. If this was the case, there would be no need to interfere with negative liberty and restrict the right of religious communities and individuals to teach their religious views.

A more difficult question is how to teach and raise children and other vulnerable citizens whose capabilities for choice are not sufficiently developed. Even though it might be allowed to teach about hell, sin, and other similar themes, should the state somehow restrict the way such themes are taught? For example, if the reality of hell is described in a vivid way, the question arises whether some kind of emotional damage is being inflicted on a child. Jonathan Wolff (2012, 130–31) highlights a similar theme by noting that some people with mental health problems may be vulnerable, for example, to forced exorcism, which he calls also "therapeutic violence."

The way humanity is dealt with in the capabilities approach recognizes, however, that people are social by their nature and need each other (see Nussbaum 2006, 159–60). Thus even though the focus in this chapter has been on the conflicts where individuals' rights might be violated by their religious communities, the capabilities approach also seems to note the important role of communities in living a worthwhile life. Despite the risks discussed in this chapter, belonging to communities—and in many cases, religious ones—may improve the individual's chances of finding a worthwhile life. Moreover, the right to mental health probably would not flourish if people lived noncommunal and individualistic lives in order to avoid pressure or other questionable forms of power. So it seems that the risks for mental health in the context of religious communities are interwoven with the vast potential for improving mental health and attaining a life worth living.

5. A Quest for Reconciliation

If freedom of religion and the right to mental health are understood in terms of capability, the conflict between them seems to disappear. However, this means that, even though the idea is that the area of negative liberty could be relatively large, some areas of it must be restricted. For example, children might have a right to such education that promotes their capabilities for choosing, which means that their parents could not decide completely if their children go to school or not.

When freedom of religion and the right to mental health are understood from the viewpoint of the capabilities approach, the obligation arises to the state to arrange such conditions (capabilities increasing education included) that ensure the capabilities for everyone. Since obligations of the state increase, it might be relevant to work with religious communities that share the goal of promoting capabilities.

References

Beltran, Susana. 2005. "The International Protection of Human Rights versus Groups Employing Psychological Manipulation." *International Journal of Human Rights* 9 (3): 285–305.

Berlin, Isaiah. 2005. *Liberty*. Edited by Henry Hardy. Oxford: Oxford University Press.

Dworkin, Ronald. 1985. *A Matter of Principle*. Cambridge, MA: Harvard University Press.

Feinberg, Joel. 1973. *Social Philosophy*. Foundations of Philosophy Series. Upper Saddle River, NJ: Prentice Hall.

Finnish League of Human Rights. 2009. "Ehkäisykielto loukkaa ihmisoikeuksia." *Taustamuistio* (memorandum), March 4, 2009. Accessed September 12, 2019. https://tinyurl.com/yyhhmm5k.

Gostin, Lawrence O. 2001. "Beyond Moral Claims: A Human Rights Approach to Mental Health." *Cambridge Quarterly of Healthcare Ethics* 10 (3): 264–274.

Koenig, Harold G., and David B. Larson. 2001. "Religion and Mental Health: Evidence for an Association." *Internal Review of Psychiatry* 13 (2): 67–78.

Kouros, Kristiina. 2011. "Kuka on vastuussa?" In *Iloisen talon kellareissa*, edited by Kristiina Kouros, 137–146. Helsinki, Finland: Like.

Langone, Michael D. n.d. "Cults: Questions and Answers." International Cultic Studies Association. Accessed September 12, 2019. https://tinyurl.com/y4jw77ob.

Linjakumpu, Aini. 2015. *Uskonnon varjot: Hengellinen väkivalta kristillisissä yhteisöissä*. Tampere: Vastapaino.

Nowak, Manfred. 1993. *U.N. Covenant of Civil and Political Rights*. CCPR Commentary. Kehl, Germany: N. P. Engel.

Nussbaum, Martha C. 2006. *Frontiers of Justice: Disability, Nationality, Species Membership*. Cambridge, MA: Belknap Press of Harvard University Press.

———. 2008. *Liberty of Conscience: In Defense of America's Tradition of Religious Equality*. New York: Basic Books.

———. 2011. *Creating Capabilities: The Human Development Approach*. Cambridge, MA: Belknap Press of Harvard University Press.

Oshana, Marina. 2007. "Autonomy and the Question of Authenticity." *Social Theory & Practice* 33 (3): 411–429.

Päivänsalo, Ville. 2014. "Fragile Health Justice: Cooperation with Faith Organizations." In *Religion and Development: Nordic Perspectives on Involvement in Africa*, edited by Tomas Sundnes Drønen, 109–125. New York: Peter Lang.

Partch, K. J. 1981. "Freedom of Conscience and Expression, and Political Freedoms." In *The International Bill of Rights: The Covenant on Civil and Political*

Rights, edited by Louis Henkin, 209–245. New York: Columbia University Press.

Ruoho, Aila. 2013. *Päästä meidät pelosta: Hengellinen väkivalta uskonnollisissa yhteisöissä*. Helsinki, Finland: Nemo.

Scanlon, Thomas. 1972. "A Theory of Freedom of Expression." *Philosophy and Public Affairs* 1 (2): 204–226.

Sen, Amartya. 2000. *Development as Freedom*. New York: Anchor Books.

Stenlund, Mari. 2014. "Freedom of Delusion—Interdisciplinary Views Concerning Freedom of Belief and Opinion Meet the Individual with Psychosis." PhD diss., University of Helsinki. Accessed September 12, 2019. http://urn.fi/URN:ISBN:978-952-10-9747-8.

Stenlund, Mari, and Pamela Slotte. 2018. "Forum Internum Revisited: Considering the Absolute Core of Freedom of Belief and Opinion in Terms of Negative Liberty, Authenticity, and Capability." *Human Rights Review* 19 (4): 425–446.

Tahzib, Bahiyyih G. 1996. *Freedom of Religion or Belief: Ensuring Effective International Legal Protection*. International Studies in Human Rights. Vol. 44. Hague: Martinus Nijhoff.

Teinonen, Timo. 2007. *Terveys ja usko*. Helsinki, Finland: Kirjapaja.

United Nations Human Rights. 1966a. *International Covenant on Civil and Political Rights*. Accessed September 12, 2019. https://tinyurl.com/lh96aub.

———. 1966b. *International Covenant on Economic, Social and Cultural Rights*. Accessed September 12, 2019. https://tinyurl.com/qxqfpj5.

Uskontojen uhrien tuki ry (UUT). 2014. *Jehovan todistajien oikeuskomiteoiden toiminta ja karttamisrangaistukset: "Rakkaudellinen järjestely" vai rikos ihmisyyttä vastaan*. Accessed September 12, 2019. https://tinyurl.com/y2gkk5w9.

Villa, Janne. 2013. *Hengellinen väkivalta*. Helsinki, Finland: Kirjapaja.

Whelan, Daniel J. 2010. *Indivisible Human Rights: A History*. Philadelphia: University of Pennsylvania Press.

Wolff, Jonathan. 2012. *The Human Right to Health*. New York: W. W. Norton.

Wrong, Dennis H. 2002. *Power: Its Forms, Bases, and Uses*. 3rd ed. New Brunswick: Transaction.

Zimbardo, Philip. 2007. *The Lucifer Effect: How Good People Turn Evil*. London: Rider.

19

Global Burden of Disease, Addiction, and the Role of Religion

Janne Nikkinen

ABSTRACT

In the twentieth century, public health research began to produce evidence of lifestyle-related risks for noncommunicable diseases (NCDs). These include arteriosclerotic vascular disease, heart diseases and stroke, osteoporosis, and type 2 diabetes. The evidence base on the ways in which disease is associated with certain behavioral choices and lifestyles is constantly growing. According to Eurostat and the World Health Organization (WHO), life expectancy in Europe is decreasing for the first time in a century due to smoking, drinking, and obesity: approximately 30 percent of Europeans smoke, and 60 percent are obese or overweight. Addiction is also a global challenge to public health systems. Lifestyle-related diseases are also among the leading causes of death in occidental countries. This contribution explores the role of religion in this context. So-called faith-based nongovernmental organizations (NGOs) play an important part in the treatment of addiction. In this framework, addiction is viewed not merely dichotomously as a disease or choice but as a habit that exhausts one's mental and moral resources. This may bring added value to a treatment that focuses mostly on cravings and physical symptoms. However, it remains somewhat unclear what exactly is the added value of religiously affiliated addiction treatment. This chapter addresses this issue using lifestyle-related diseases and addictive behavior as examples. Good practices might be applied to other contexts, in case it is possible to point out the benefits. If this task is not accomplished, research and treatment resources may be misallocated. Further, addictive behaviors could continue to consume numerous quality-adjusted health years (QALYs) on a global level.

1. Introduction: Addiction and Lifestyle-Related Diseases

In discussions about mental health and health justice, the issue of addiction cannot be avoided. The phenomena that are now medicalized under the labels *addiction* and *disease* were for thousands of years labeled as *sin* or *vice*. In the past, the lack of self-control or the inability to resist harmful substances were attributed to moral failings that could be overcome with divine assistance (Madueme 2008). In modern times, alcohol misuse, tobacco, and even the use of marijuana (in some jurisdictions where the use is legal) often are viewed only as "bad habits," unless (substantial) social costs are involved or other kinds of "harm to others" are present. For example, gambling is now accepted almost everywhere. There is an interesting chapter about the legalization of gambling in the US with the title "The Culture War Issue That Never Was: Why Right and Left Have Overlooked Gambling" by Alan Wolfe in *Gambling-Mapping the American Moral Landscape* (2009). Laws authorizing casino and racetrack operations were often passed through "stealth" campaigns without much publicity or scrutiny. In the US state of Pennsylvania in 2004, a major gambling bill was passed through both chambers in a speedy fashion over the Fourth of July weekend without any hearings or input from citizenry (Teague 2007). Furthermore, in those US states where the issue was on the ballot, there was not much public debate about the limits for gambling offers and marketing after legalization. Governments are keen to stress that the public good should be understood as fiscal good and overlook the harm gambling causes since social costs are often misunderstood (Grinols 2004; Nikkinen and Marionneau 2014).

It is increasingly the case that lifestyle-related diseases, resulting from the use of sugar, alcohol, tobacco, and illegal drugs, are a public health priority. Diabetes and lung cancer (the result of smoking) are acknowledged as serious health issues. Worldwide, approximately 5.9 percent of all deaths are related to the use of alcohol (WHO 2015). The use of alcohol is also the third leading cause of poor health and premature death globally, after low birth weight and unsafe sex (Anderson et al. 2012). Nevertheless, in many countries, effective alcohol policies are not implemented, even though alcohol kills more people in the world annually than

AIDS, tuberculosis, and violence combined (Organization for Economic Co-operation and Development [OECD] 2015). In the twentieth century, tobacco use has caused one hundred million premature deaths worldwide, and in this century, it is estimated that the number will be as high as one billion (Freudenberg 2016). In China alone, two out of three Chinese men become smokers; half of them will eventually die due to tobacco smoking (Chen et al. 2015). Still, it is more common to see advertising and campaigns raising funds for the fight against breast cancer, even though in the developed countries, lung cancer resulting from smoking kills more women than breast cancer (Torre et al. 2015). New forms of addictive behavior have also emerged within the last few decades, such as excessive gambling (due to the recent global gambling expansion), creating dependency and contributing to the global burden of disease in an unforeseen manner (Adams 2008; Orford 2011; Sulkunen et al. 2019).

However, it is possible to reduce the consumption of addictive substances through public policies and legislative actions focused on effective prevention. These policies should not rely on information and "awareness" campaigns that can be exploited by conflicting interests. For example, support of the alcohol and brewery industry has been shown to influence "responsible drinking campaigns" (Barry and Goodson 2009). Similarly, "responsible gambling" is promoted by the international gambling industry, even though the concept is even more unclear than is the case with the use of alcohol (Hancock and Smith 2017). Since both alcohol and gambling create important economic revenues for governments, the industry lobbyists are capable of influencing government officials (Adams 2008; Orford 2013; Freudenberg 2016). Advertising alcohol is often permitted at sports events where they can influence an underage audience, and the effective curbing of drinking is often difficult due to the prevailing notions about individualism. This is the case even though it has been possible to show that one of the most effective ways to reduce the consumption of alcohol is to lower the consumption of alcohol in the entire population (for the so-called total consumption or single-distribution theory, see Babor et al. 2010). However, since effective restrictions are placed in more mature markets such as Europe and North America, the global alcohol industry moves its focus increasingly to developing nations, including Africa (Babor, Robaina, and Jernigan 2015).

The harm resulting from the use of tobacco products has been recognized for decades, yet still one-fifth of adults in the world continue to use them. In developed countries, the use of tobacco is decreasing, but at the same time, the burden of disease is shifting to developing nations. It is estimated that by 2030, tobacco-related deaths will decrease by 9 percent from the level in 2002 in high-income countries, and the number of deaths will more than double in low-income countries within a similar time frame. In China, the use of tobacco is already the leading cause of death, as mentioned earlier. In Africa, it has been pointed out that Ebola has been the focus of media attention, but little attention is paid by the governments of the continent to the fact that both the number of smokers and also the number of consumed cigarettes are increasing (Blecher and Ross 2013).

The question of why producers of "coercive commodities" (Young and Markham 2017) can avoid public health regulations and effective prevention is a complex one and not easily answered. One would expect that considering all the evidence that the use of tobacco has killed more people in the twentieth century than all wars combined (including such man-made disasters as the two world wars), the public health authorities would protect the people efficiently from the harms of tobacco. The partial answer to this, provided by Nicholas Freudenberg and other similar commentators, is that tobacco corporations use lobbying effectively, and this undermines international health treaties aimed at reducing smoking (Freudenberg 2016). To provide a complete answer to the challenge of coercive commodities would be out of the scope of this chapter. Instead, the purpose of this contribution is to discuss addiction and substance use in relation to the global burden of disease and explore what role religious-based approaches may offer in order to alleviate the situation. This is because, first, as also already pointed out, much of the global burden of disease is attributable to mental and substance use disorders (Whiteford et al. 2013). Second, mental disorders create enormous costs, either directly through public health-care systems or indirectly as lost productivity and lower quality of life (Trautmann, Rehm, and Wittchen 2016). Third, the issue might be that since much of substance abuse and addiction treatment is provided by NGOs operating through voluntary work, including faith-based organizations, they have not obtained the academic research attention that would be the case if the treatment had been provided by government workers only. In the US there exists a substantial research base about faith-based addiction treatment, with over six hundred academic articles starting from the 1940s (Ruotsila 2016). Christopher Cook (2004) has suggested that academic viewpoints, which often emerge in a clinical setting, tend to regard the so-called moral model of addiction, often preferred by religious-based actors, as somewhat outdated. In this moral model of addiction, when the desire is at the same time to continue and to discontinue the use of addictive substances, addiction is explained primarily in moral terms and notions (i.e., personal failing and a lack of character), often using a religious framework and the explanations it provides as assistance. This leads to an unnecessary stigma for those who are treated due to addictive behavior (Leshner 1997; qtd. in Heather 2017). It is increasingly the case that researchers and those advancing public health see products as dangerous and blame the people for their problems as an industry tactic to avoid responsibility (Orford 2011; Freudenberg 2016; Orford 2019).

However, in order to address the issue of whether religious-based actors are successful in the treatment of addiction, it is not necessary to first take a stand on what theoretical approach to the issue of addiction works best. Initially, accomplishing such a task may provide more material for the debate regarding theoretical approaches on the issue of addiction. Globally, most of the people lack access to quality mental health services (Wainberg et al. 2017). If it is recognized that faith-based actors and religion in general may have a major, positive role in reducing the global burden of disease that results from addictive behavior and substance use, it would also enable a more nuanced discussion about the impact of religion on society.

2. The Role of Religion in Addiction Treatment

In the following, I discuss addiction mostly in relation to Christianity, given space limitations. Research in other religious traditions can be found: Paramapandhu Groves (2014) writes with regard to Buddhist perspectives, Kate Loewenthal (2014) considers addiction in the context of Judaism, and Mansur Ali (2014) frames the issue in relation to Islam. From the vantage point of the research, the difficulty is that the impact of religion and spirituality on any human condition is difficult to measure in a meaningful manner because even for religion, there are numerous definitions, and combining spirituality with religious activity further complicates the matter. In the case of addiction and dependency, there are no commonly accepted definitions for either of these concepts. Christopher Cook (2004) has provided one often-cited definition of spirituality as related to a "universal dimension of human experience" that has been used in the context of health research. This definition involves three aspects: inner subjective awareness, communal relationships, and a general understanding that there is something that is transcendent and exceeds the realm of the human self (Borras et al.

2010). From the vantage point of religious ideologies, the study by Barbara Lorch and Robert Hughes (1985) that explored the issue with young people noted that the function of religion as a deterrent to the use of harmful substances is mostly due to its influence on personal values and norms (Lorch and Hughes 1985). Attending church or being a member of a religious community had less effect on actual youth behavior in the United States in the 1980s.

According to Laurence Borras and his colleagues (2010), who cite studies involving alcohol and drug abuse (Larson and Wilson 1980; Hilton 1991), and a national US study conducted in the 1990s (Midanik and Clark 1995), the protective role of spirituality and religiosity regarding addictive behavior has been well established. Furthermore, Laurence Borras et al. refer to studies conducted by Richard Gorsuch (1995) pointing out that religious groups have less alcohol misuse than secular ones. However, some alcoholics also do hold negative beliefs about religion, such as the image of God as a ruthless judge, which may influence their drinking patterns. Thus Borras and his colleagues state that "religious-based social control" may not only alleviate the problems related to alcohol use but also complicate them. On the individual level, Borras et al. also note that those who profess religious beliefs use less alcohol and fewer drugs compared to nonreligious persons (here Borras et al. refer to Khavari and Harmon 1982). The Christian faith may have also influenced how those people in recovery deal with their feelings of guilt and shame (Lund 2017).

On the population level, the major US study that established the relationship between conservative religious affiliation and lower risk for alcohol and nicotine dependencies was research involving more than two thousand all-female twins (Kendler et al. 2003). In addition, Borras et al. (2010) state that over a dozen studies have associated excessive alcohol and drug abuse with "a lack of sense of meaning," when the Life Purpose Scale has been used (for the LPS, see Crumbaugh and Maholick 1969). Furthermore, private religious practices (such as prayer and Scripture reading) have been associated with less alcohol misuse (Koenig et al. 1994, although the authors stress the need for longitudinal research). In the field of problem gambling, dual problem users in the case of substance abuse and gambling have been noted to be more secular, at least in one study available from the United States (Feigelman, Wallisch, and Lesieur 1998).

Although most of these studies are based on the Anglo-American context only, it may be possible to suggest that religion and spirituality have important implications for understanding addiction. It is equally important to consider the religious dimension in treatment, as this also defines possible responses to the issue. In case we understand the issue of addiction as a medical problem and/or malfunction of the brain (the so-called brain disease model of addiction, or BDMA), the response will be a medical one. However, in the case in which the issue emerges in a more spiritual framework, the medical response alone will be inadequate. Much of the problem gambling treatment research focuses on understanding psychological well-being and correcting false beliefs about gambling, including the odds of winning (Ghezzi et al. 2006). However, in an anthropological study that drew on fifteen years of field research in Las Vegas, it was observed that many of those who had issues with gambling did not necessarily gamble primarily to win money but in order to get in the "zone," as they often disregarded winnings or losses (Schüll 2012). Trance-like states and dissociation have been reported in several gambling surveys and publications (see Binde 2007, which includes references to a dozen different studies from Sweden, the United States, and Canada). If this kind of religious and spiritual experience is present in addictive behavior, the secular care providers and social workers might benefit from co-operation with faith-based organizations. It is also convenient to suggest that faith-based organizations may be in a better position to provide an adequate treatment response if a religious dimension is present in the formation of addiction. At the very least, they can note all the relevant factors that influence treatment.

3. Faith-Based Organizations and Addiction Treatment Today

Since the 1990s, faith-based prevention of addiction has drawn increasing amounts of political support and research attention. For example, the US federal government has invested heavily in the Faith-Based Initiative launched in 2001, providing federal funding for religious-based social services and substance abuse treatment. In the period between 2003 and 2007 alone, this funding accounted for $10.4 billion in the United States (Adrian 2010). At the beginning, the initiative was claimed to be politically motivated, and it also created much controversy among academics (Carlson-Thies 2009). Nowadays, the program is an integral part of service funding in the United States, although it has been renamed as the White House Faith and Opportunity Initiative in May 2018 through an executive order issued by President Donald J. Trump. One should note that there is no separate funding for religious providers of addiction treatment; they are only allowed to apply on the same grounds as other applicants. Similarly, in Southern European countries such as in Italy, much of the social welfare is provided through organizations affiliated with the Catholic Church. It is perhaps noteworthy that in some areas of cocaine production in Latin America, the faith-based organizations may be almost the only ones who operate in the field of addiction treatment (Delaporte 2018).

Assessing the effectiveness of faith-based treatments, Johnson, Tomkins, and Webb (2008) have reviewed 669 studies (conducted in English) in order to establish the relationship, first, between religion and health outcomes and, second, religion and well-being. In relation to health outcomes, the explored research (overwhelmingly) supports the conclusion that "higher levels of religious involvement and practices make for an important protective factor that buffers or insulates individuals from deleterious outcomes." With regard to well-being, they state, "Religious commitment or practices make for an important factor promoting an array of prosocial behaviors and thus enhancing various beneficial outcomes" (Johnson, Tomkins, and Webb 2008, 7). For example, in the case of drugs and alcohol, people participating in religious activities show fewer tendencies to use drugs (87 percent of the studies show this) or alcohol (94 percent). Adults who do not attend religious services regularly are twice as likely to use or consume alcohol, thrice as likely to consume tobacco products, over five times more likely to be users of hard drugs, and eight times more likely to smoke marijuana/cannabis (Ruotsila 2016).

It is worthwhile to note that not all commentators see the role of religion as only a positive one. Concerns related to evaluation of outcomes, treatment effectiveness, and best practices have been raised in relation to faith-based treatment providers (Adrian 2010). It is difficult to establish a positive correlation with spiritual orientation and decreased drug use and abstinence (Murray, Goggin, and Malcarne 2006). The attitude of staff in secular addiction treatment centers and among medical and nursing staff toward religion is somewhat negative (Borras et al. 2010). Borras et al. list several reasons for this: little religious affiliation within certain professional groups involved in addiction treatment such as psychiatrists in North America and the United Kingdom, lack of knowledge about religious affairs, and "a tendency to perceive as being pathologic all thoughts and behavior of patients referring to spiritual dimension" (Borras et al. 2010, 2366). Perhaps the gravest issue for research that evaluates the matter is a recognized lack of common concepts and definitions that hinders almost all measurement, evaluation, and definitive conclusions (Montagne 2010). For example, religion and spirituality are highly elusive concepts that can be used in literature in a variety of ways: Montagne (2010) counts over sixty differing terms, words, and phrases that have been used in Borras et al. (2010) to describe "religion."

Without specific definitions and concepts, it is still possible to assess the role of faith-based organizations, since they continue to operate in numbers in addiction treatment, and there are also those that have their roots in religion, such as Alcoholics Anonymous (AA), even though they nowadays present themselves publicly as a more secular organization. Although the role of religion is increasingly recognized in research, the service providers seem to find it difficult to acknowledge their religious roots. In the United Kingdom, the Young Women's Christian Association (YMCA) removed the word "Christian" from its name in 2011 after more than 150 years of existence and preferred to be called Platform 51 instead. The change sparked criticism from other representatives of religion, although the YWCA of England and Wales explained that the word "Christian" does not represent the organization properly anymore, since it is an organization to assist and represent all women. However, in the United Kingdom, this was also seen as an expression of interest in continuing to receive state support in the future (Doughty 2011). In Sweden, many Christian-based NGOs operating have discontinued personnel recruitment based on Christian faith (Larsson, Letell, and Thörn 2012).

4. Conclusions

In the last few decades, the role of faith-based NGOs has been recognized, especially in the United States and the United Kingdom. Change in US politics due to then-President George W. Bush in 2001 was seen by many faith-based organizations as the recognition of the important work that they perform. From the mid-1990s to 2010 in the United Kingdom, New Labour (party) added faith-based social services to its "Third Way" approach. The governmental Faith Communities Capacity Building Fund delivered over £12 million between 2006 and 2008 to faith-based organizations (Fentener, Daly, and Forster 2008). Later, over £10 million were delivered via other channels to over five hundred faith-based actors. According to Markku Ruotsila, faith-based organizations produce approximately 40 percent of all social work accomplished in the United Kingdom (Ruotsila 2016).

However, there are some concerns that must be addressed. First, in the case that faith-based organizations choose to rely on public funding in the United States and elsewhere, the question arises whether this also influences their freedom to act according to their own principles. In the United Kingdom, the example of the YWCA indicates that not all faith-based NGOs are confident that secular governments are willing to support them without an explicit breakaway from their religious roots.

This leads to a second concern: if public funds are accepted to finance activities, the NGOs may not be capable of advancing the cause of the addicts in a public realm against the government. For example, in some countries, the public profit that emanates from hypothecated taxation of gambling activities is used as earmarked payments for alcohol and drug treatment NGOs (including faith-based ones, such as the Christian-based Blue Ribbon in Finland). Accepting such funds de facto creates a conflict of interest (Adams 2016).

Third, and perhaps the most complicated of the related concerns, are the questions: What kind of funds are used to support research in the field of addiction, and who accomplishes the research? Faith-based organizations often operate with small grants and relatively minor subsidies that are primarily used to enhance treatment and not for accomplishing high-level research that is conducted mostly in academic or research institutions. The available funding sources may not be interested in financing research on the role of faith-based providers, who may already have a fiscal conflict of interest of their own because they provide treatment through the support of the very same government that supports the addiction industries. The profits from the sale of addictive products are often used not only to block effective prevention but also to influence the available research and the public debate (Adams 2013).

The public discourse about addiction tends to favor the notion that "addicts" are the ones who are "responsible" for their illness and somehow "vulnerable" or "prone" to addiction. This diverts attention from the responsibilities borne by those who benefit from addictive products, including alcohol, tobacco, and games of chance (Orford 2013). The research that is supported by funds that are derived from the sales of addictive products (through hypothecated taxation or levies) often does not evaluate the government-industry relationship, which is crucial in enabling the availability of addictive products (Cassidy, Loussouarn, and Pisac 2013). Without ever-increasing availability of gambling products, there would be fewer people who are labeled as gambling addicts (Sulkunen et al. 2019).

Since the burden of taxation is increasingly on individuals as the portion of corporate tax is decreasing, governments in Europe (and elsewhere) are tempted to use sales and excise taxes to collect revenue (Egerer, Marionneau, and Nikkinen 2018). Thus various taxes on alcohol, tobacco, and especially gambling are increasing. The arguments that were used to justify taxes on gambling activities are increasingly present in the context of the legalization of recreational cannabis use in the United States (Nikkinen 2017). The legalization of recreational cannabis in Canada, multiple US states, and Uruguay leads to a new cycle of revenue from addicts to governments through taxation, which is not easily broken even though the harms may increase in the future. Since most faith-based organizations are focused on enhancing the situation of an individual, they may not be able to address the root cause of addictive behavior: the availability of coercive commodities and governmental support of the use of addictive products, when viewed primarily as an industry capable of producing employment and tax revenue.

In order to move forward, I would make three recommendations: The first is to raise the quality of the research, which is in need of clarity on research topics when the role of religion is explored. There are studies that deal with the conceptual base of Christian, faith-based substance abuse rehabilitation programs (e.g., McCoy et al. 2004), but more attention should focus on the efficacy in treatment since it seems that there is such to be found (e.g., Johnson, Tomkins, and Webb 2008). In case the strength of the faith-based treatment is that it fills a certain spiritual "void" that has been earlier filled with substance abuse and then replaces it with religious recovery through salvation and a "long-term relationship with God," it limits the role of religion only as a crutch for those who try to be sober or otherwise lack the willpower to resist harmful substances or excessive behaviors.

Geoffrey Lyons, Frank Deane, and Peter Kelly (2013) have noted that currently most of the research in this field revolves around AA-based twelve-step programs. This is not desirable, since most Christian-based substance abuse treatment programs are not based on this approach. If there are true psychological and other benefits from faith-based addiction treatment, determining these factors could also enhance secular treatments (e.g., Lund 2016, 2017).

My second recommendation is related to research funding: conflicts of interest should be declared when engaging in addiction research. Thomas Babor and Peter Miller (2014) noted in the journal *Addiction* that out of thirty studies selected randomly from those supported by the American

Gambling Association (AGA), only one (Kessler et al. 2008) cited proper references to the funding source when published. In tobacco research, the fact was that "the doubt was the product" for the industry; that is, it was assumed that it was the industry's task to question research that points out the harmful nature of addictive products. In the field of alcohol studies, the situation in research may be improving due to a longer debate about conflict of interest, but in gambling research, it is just emerging (Livingstone et al. 2018). A new issue in this context is the study of the use of medical cannabis. Although medical cannabis has been legalized in thirty-three US states (as of 2019) and in many European countries, its medical impacts may not be as beneficial as many proponents seem to suggest and are mostly unknown due to insufficient research. The legalization of recreational cannabis will most likely create adverse situations to already vulnerable population groups (Volkow et al. 2014). A recent report by National Science Academies in the United States stressed the need for diverse research funding (NASEM 2017) in order to avoid a situation in which the researchers have fiscal or other interests that influence their research.

Third, one should critically evaluate the possible difference in treatment outcomes and results between the ordinary care providers and faith-based addiction treatment providers. The difficulty is that many of the faith-based treatment statistics are currently provided by the organizations themselves. The organizations have an interest in presenting their own treatment results in a favorable light (Ruotsila 2016). The faith-based treatment facilities may also sometimes cater to a different clientele, a factor that could influence the results. The measurement of success in addiction treatment is difficult, especially if the goal of the treatment is often unclear. Some programs may seek abstinence, while others have a goal of "moderate" use, whatever that means for an individual. Lack of adequate definitions is prevalent in all research in this field, so faith-based organizations should not be the only ones to face unrealistic demands about their results. After all, especially in developing countries, faith-based organizations may be among the few free or low-cost providers of assistance to certain underprivileged population subgroups who may receive little assistance or support from governments.

Acknowledgments

The author obtained the following financial support for the research, authorship, and/or publication of this chapter: Academy of Finland gambling research project funding. The academy obtains a share of its annual funding from the Finnish gambling monopoly (Veikkaus), although indirectly through the Ministry of Education and Culture. The Centre for Research on Addiction, Control, and Governance (CEACG) at the Faculty of Social Sciences, University of Helsinki, obtains a substantial part of its annual operating budget from the National Institute for Health and Welfare (THL) in Finland. These funds emanate from hypothecated gambling taxes (legal agreement; the Ministry of Social Affairs and Health charges the costs of research from Veikkaus).

References

Adams, Peter. 2008. *Gambling, Freedom, and Democracy*. Abingdon, UK: Routledge.

———. 2013. "Addiction Industry Studies: Understanding How Pro-consumption Influences Block Effective Interventions." *American Journal of Public Health* 103 (4): e35–e28. https://doi.org/10.2105/AJPH.2012.301151.

———. 2016. *Moral Jeopardy: Risks of Accepting Money from the Alcohol, Tobacco, and Gambling Industries*. Cambridge: Cambridge University Press.

Adrian, Manuella. 2010. "If We Spend $10 Billion on Faith-Based Interventions, Will They Work? A Comment on the Relationship between Addiction and Religion and Its Possible Implication for Care." Dialogue. *Substance Use & Misuse* 45:2390–2393. https://www.tandfonline.com/toc/isum20/current.

Ali, Mansur. 2014. "Perspectives on Drug Addiction in Islamic History and Theology." *Religions* 5:912–928. https://doi.org/10.3390/rel5030912.

Anderson, Peter, Lars Moeller, and Gauden Galea, eds. 2012. *Alcohol in the European Union: Consumption, Harm, and Policy Approaches*. Geneva, Switzerland: World Health Organization Regional Office in Europe.

Babor, Thomas, Raul Caetano, Sally Casswell, Griffith Edwards, Norman Giesbrecht, Kathryn Graham, Joel Grube, Linda Hill, Harold Holder, Ross Homel, Michael Livingston, Esa Österberg, Jürgen Rehm, Robin Room, and Ingeborg Rossow. 2010. *Alcohol: No Ordinary Commodity*. 2nd ed. Oxford: Oxford University Press.

Babor, Thomas, and Peter Miller. 2014. "McCarthyism, Conflict of Interest and Addiction's New Transparency Declaration Procedures." *Addiction* 109 (3): 341–344. https://doi.org/10.1111/add.12384.

Babor, Thomas, Katherine Robaina, and David Jernigan. 2015. "The Influence of Industry Actions on the Availability of Alcoholic Beverages in the African Region." *Addiction* 110:561–571. https://doi.org/10.1111/add.12832.

Barry, Adam, and Patricia Goodson. 2009. "Use (and the Misuse) of the Responsible Drinking Message in Public Health and Alcohol Advertising: A Review."

Health Education and Behavior 37 (2): 288–303. https://doi.org/10.1177/1090198109342393.

Binde, Per. 2007. "Gambling and Religion: Histories of Concord and Conflict." *Journal of Gambling Issues* 20:145–166. https://doi.org/10.4309/jgi.2007.20.4.

Blecher, Evan, and Hana Ross. 2013. *Tobacco Use in Africa: Tobacco Control through Prevention.* Atlanta, GA: American Cancer Society. https://doi.org/10.13140/RG.2.1.1038.2247.

Borras, Laurence, Yasser Khazaal, Riaz Khan, Sylvia Mohr, Yves-Alexandre Kaufman, Daniele Zullino, and Philippe Huguelet. 2010. "The Relationship between Addiction and Religion and Its Possible Implications for Care." *Substance Use & Misuse* 45:2357–2375. https://www.tandfonline.com/loi/isum20.

Carlson-Thies, Stanley. 2009. "Faith-Based Initiative 2.0: The Bush Faith-Based and Community Initiative." *Harvard Journal of Law and Public Policy* 32:931–947. https://tinyurl.com/y2ee3zrq.

Cassidy, Rebecca, Claire Loussouarn, and Andrea Pisac. 2013. *Fair Game? Producing Gambling Research.* Goldsmiths Report. London: University of London, European Research Council. https://tinyurl.com/yyvgjorr.

Chen, Zhengming, Richard Peto, Maigeng Zhou, Andi Iona, Margaret Smith, Ling Yang, Yu Guo, Zheng Biang, Garry Lancaster, Paul Sherliker, Shutao Pang, Hao Wang, Hua Su, Ming Wu, Xiaping Wu, Junshi Chen, Rory Collins, and Liming Li. 2015. "Contrasting Male and Female Trends in Tobacco-Attributed Mortality in China: Evidence from Successive Nationwide Progressive Cohort Studies." *Lancet* 386:1447–1456. https://doi.org/10.1016/S0140-6736(15)00340-2.

Cook, Christopher. 2004. "Addiction and Spirituality." *Addiction* 99:539–551. https://doi.org/10.1111/j.1360-0443.2004.00715.x.

Crumbaugh, James, and Leonard Maholick. 1969. *Manual of Instructions for the Purpose-in-Life Test.* Munster, IN: Psychometric Affiliates.

Delaporte, Pablo. 2018. "We Will Revive: Addiction, Spirituality and Recovery in Latin America's Cocaine Production Zone." *Third World Quarterly* 39 (2): 298–313. https://doi.org/10.1080/01436597.2017.1328275.

Doughty, Steve. 2011. "YMCA Drops the Word Christian from Its Historic Name to Call It Platform 51." *Daily Mail,* January 7, 2011. https://tinyurl.com/yx8t7t7o.

Egerer, Michael, Virve Marionneau, and Janne Nikkinen, eds. 2018. *Gambling and European Welfare States: Current Challenges and Future Prospects.* London: Palgrave Macmillan.

Feigelman, William, Lynn Wallisch, and Henry Lesieur. 1998. "Problem Gambler, Problem Substance Users, and Dual-Problem Users: An Epidemiological

Study." *American Journal of Public Health* 88 (3): 467–470. https://doi.org/10.2105/ajph.88.3.467.

Fentener, Rita, Penelope Daly, and Robert Forster. 2008. *Faith Groups and Government: Faith-Based Organizations and Government at Local and Regional Levels.* Faiths and Communities Series. London: Community Development Foundation.

Freudenberg, Nicholas. 2016. *Lethal but Legal: Corporations, Consumption, and Protecting Public Health.* Oxford: Oxford University Press.

Ghezzi, Patrick, Charles Lyons, Mark Dixon, and Ginger Wilson, eds. 2006. *Gambling: Behavior Theory, Research, and Application.* Reno, NV: Context.

Gorsuch, Richard. 1995. "Religious Aspects of Substance Abuse and Recovery." *Journal of Social Issues* 51:65–83. https://tinyurl.com/y3ype38z.

Grinols, Earl. 2004. *Gambling in America: Costs and Benefits.* Cambridge: Cambridge University Press.

Groves, Paramapandhu. 2014. "Buddhist Approaches to Addiction Recovery." *Religions* 5 (4): 985–1000. https://doi.org/10.3390/rel5040985.

Hancock, Linda, and Garry Smith. 2017. "Critiquing the Reno Model I–IV International Influence on Regulators and Governments (2004–2015): The Distorted Reality of Responsible Gambling." *International Journal of Mental Health and Addiction* 15 (6): 1151–1176. https://doi.org/10.1007/s11469-017-9746-y.

Heather, Nick. 2017. "Q: Is Addiction a Brain Disease or Moral Failing? A: Neither." *Neuroethics* 10 (1): 115–124. https://doi.org/10.1007/s12152-016-9289-0.

Hilton, Michael. 1991. "The Demographic Distribution of Drinking Problems in 1984." In *Alcohol in America: Drinking Practices and Problems,* edited by Walter Clark and Michael Hilton, 87–101. New York: State University of Albany Press.

Johnson, Byron, Ralph Tomkins, and Derek Webb. 2008. "Objective Hope: Assessing the Effectiveness of Faith-Based Organizations: A Review of the Literature." In *Baylor Institute for Studies in Religion.* Waco, TX: Baylor University. http://www.baylorisr.org/wp-content/uploads/ISR_Objective_Hope.pdf. Accessed October 5, 2020.

Kendler, Kenneth, Kristen Jacobson, Carol Prescott, and Michael Neale. 2003. "Specificity of Genetic and Environmental Risk Factors for Use and Abuse/Dependence of Cannabis, Cocaine, Hallucinogens, Sedatives, Stimulants, and Opiates in Male Twins." *American Journal of Psychiatry* 160:687–695. https://doi.org/10.1176/appi.ajp.160.4.687.

Kessler, Richard, Irving Havang, Richard LaBrie, Maria Petukhova, Nancy Sampson, Ken Winters, and Howard Shaffer. 2008. "DSM-IV Pathological

Gambling in the National Comorbidity Survey Replication." *Psychological Medicine* 38:1351–1360. https://doi.org/10.1017/S0033291708002900.

Khavari, Khali, and Theresa Harmon. 1982. "The Relationship between the Degree of Professed Religious Belief and Use of Drugs." *International Journal of Addiction* 17:847–857. https://doi.org/10.3109/10826088209056331.

Koenig, Harold, Linda George, Keith Meador, Dan Blazer, and Stephen Ford. 1994. "Religious Practices and Alcoholism in Southern Adult Population." *Hospital & Community Psychiatry* 45 (3): 225–231. https://doi.org/10.1176/ps.45.3.225.

Larson, David, and William Wilson. 1980. "Religious Life of Alcoholics." *Southern Medical Journal* 73:723–727. https://doi.org/10.1097/00007611-198006000-00011.

Larsson, Bengt, Martin Letell, and Håkan Thörn, eds. 2012. *Transformations of the Swedish Welfare State: From Social Engineering to Governance?* Basingstoke, UK: Palgrave Macmillan.

Leshner, Alan. 1997. "Addiction Is a Brain Disease, and It Matters." *Science* 278 (5335): 45–47. https://doi.org/10.1126/science.278.5335.45.

Livingstone, Charles, Peter Adams, Rebecca Cassidy, Francis Markham, Gerda Reith, Angela Rintoul, Natasha Dow Schüll, Richard Woolley, and Martin Young. 2018. "On Gambling Research, Social Science and the Consequences of Commercial Gambling." *International Gambling Studies* 18 (1): 56–68. https://doi.org/10.1080/14459795.2017.1377748.

Loewenthal, Kate. 2014. "Addiction: Alcohol and Substance Abuse in Judaism." *Religions* 5:972–984. https://doi.org/10.3390/rel5040972.

Lorch, Barbara, and Robert Hughes. 1985. "Religion and Youth Substance Abuse." *Journal of Religion and Health* 24:197–208. http://www.jstor.org/stable/27505831.

Lund, Pekka. 2016. "Christianity in Narratives of Recovery from Substance Abuse." *Pastoral Psychology* 65 (3): 351–368. https://doi.org/10.1007/s11089-016-0687-3.

———. 2017. "Christian Faith and Recovery from Substance Abuse, Guilt, and Shame." *Journal of Religion & Spirituality in Social Work* 36 (3): 346–366. https://doi.org/10.1080/15426432.2017.1302865.

Lyons, Geoffrey, Frank Deane, and Peter Kelly. 2013. "Faith-Based Substance Abuse Programs." In *Interventions for Addiction: Comprehensive Addictive Behaviors and Disorders*, edited by Peter Miller, vol. 3, 147–153. San Diego, CA: Academic.

Madueme, Hans. 2008. "Addiction and Sin: Recovery and Redemption." *AMA Journal of Ethics* 10 (1): 55–58. https://tinyurl.com/y2g4u8sg.

McCoy, Lisa, John Hermos, Barbara Bokhour, and Susan Frayne. 2004. "Conceptual Basis of Christian, Faith-Based Substance Abuse Rehabilitation Programs: Qualitative Analysis of Staff Interviews." *Substance Abuse* 25 (3): 1–11. https://www.tandfonline.com/toc/wsub20/current.

Midanik, Lorraine, and Walter Clark. 1985. "Drinking-Related Problems in the United States: Description and Trends, 1984–1990." *Journal of Studies on Alcohol* 56:395–402. https://doi.org/10.15288/jsa.1995.56.395.

Montagne, Michael. 2010. "The Science of Spirituality and Addiction: What Is Being Measured? What Does It Mean?" *Substance Use & Misuse* 45:2357–2410. https://www.tandfonline.com/loi/isum20.

Murray, Thomas, Kathy Goggin, and Vanessa Malcarne. 2006. "Development and Validation of the Alcohol-Related God Locus of Control Scale." *Addictive Behaviors* 31:553–558. https://doi.org/10.1016/j.addbeh.2005.12.023.

National Academies of Sciences, Engineering, and Medicine (NASEM). 2017. *The Health Effects of Cannabis and Cannabinoids: The Current State of Evidence and Recommendations for Research.* Washington, DC: National Academies Press. https://doi.org/10.17226/24625.

Nikkinen, Janne. 2017. "The Legalization of Dangerous Consumption: A Comparison of Cannabis and Gambling Policies in Three US States." *Addiction Research & Theory* 25 (6): 476–484. https://doi.org/10.1080/16066359.2017.1366455.

Nikkinen, Janne, and Virve Marionneau. 2014. "Gambling and the Common Good." *Gambling Research* (National Association for Gambling Studies in Australia) 1:3–19. https://tinyurl.com/y3lxwo7h.

Orford, Jim. 2011. *An Unsafe Bet? The Dangerous Rise of Gambling and the Debate We Should Be Having.* Chichester, UK: Wiley-Blackwell.

———. 2013. *Power, Powerlessness and Addiction.* Cambridge: Cambridge University Press.

———. 2019. *Gambling Establishment: Challenging the Power of the Modern Gambling Industry and Its Allies.* London: Routledge.

Organization for Economic Co-operation and Development (OECD). 2015. *Tackling Harmful Alcohol Use: Economics and Public Policy.* Paris: OECD. https://doi.org/10.1787/9789264181069-en.

Ruotsila, M. 2016. "Uskoon pohjautuva sosiaalityö: Toimikenttä, tutkimus ja tulokset Yhdysvalloissa" [Faith-based social work: Field, research, and results in the United States]. In *Anna meidän nähdä* [Let us see], 79–135. Helsinki, Finland: Sininauhaliitto [Finnish Blue Ribbon].

Schüll, Natasha Dow. 2012. *Addiction by Design: Machine Gambling in Las Vegas.* Cambridge, MA: MIT Press.

Sulkunen, Pekka, Thomas Babor, Jenny Cisneros-Örnberg, Michael Egerer, Matilda Hellman, Charles Livingstone, Virve Marionneau, Janne Nikkinen, Jim Orford, Robin Room, and Ingeborg Rossow. 2019. *Setting Limits: Gambling, Science and Public Policy*. Oxford: Oxford University Press.

Teague, Matthew. 2007. "Gaming the System." *Philadelphia Magazine*, May 23, 2007. https://tinyurl.com/y6sutl8e.

Torre, Lindsey, Freddie Bray, Rebecca Siegel, Jacques Ferlay, Joannie Lortet-Tieulent, and Ahmedin Jemal. 2015. "Global Cancer Statistics 2012." *CA Cancer Journal for Clinicians* 65 (2), 87–108.

Trautmann, Sebastien, Jürgen Rehm, and Hans-Ulrich Wittchen. 2016. "The Economic Costs of Mental Disorders." *EMBO (European Molecular Biology Organization) Reports* 17 (9): 1245–1249. https://doi.org/10.15252/embr.201642951.

Volkow, Nora, Ruber Baler, Wilson Compton, and Susan Weiss. 2014. "Adverse Health Effects of Marijuana Use." *New England Journal of Medicine* 370 (23): 2219–2227. https://doi.org/10.1056/NEJMra140230.

Wainberg, Milton, Pamela Scorza, James Schulz, Liat Helpman, Jennifer Mootz, Karen Johnson, Yuval Neria, Jean-Marie Bradford, Maria Oquendo, and Melissa Arbuckle. 2017. "Challenges and Opportunities in Global Mental Health: A Research-to-Practice Perspective." *Current Psychiatry Reports* 19 (5). https://doi.org/10.1007/s11920-017-0780-z.

Whiteford, Harvey, Louisa Degenhart, Jürgen Rehm, Amanda Baxter, Aliza Ferrari, Holly Erskine, Fiona Charlson, Rosana Norman, Abraham Flaxman, Nicole Johns, Roy Burstein, Christopher Murray, and Theo Vos. 2013. "Global Burden of Disease Attributable to Mental and Substance Disorders: Findings from the Global Burden of Disease Study 2010." *Lancet* 382:1575–1586. https://doi.org/10.1016/S0140-6736(13)61611-6.

Wolfe, A. 2009. "The Culture War Issue that Never Was: Why Right and Left Have Overlooked Gambling." In *Gambling: Mapping the American Moral Landscape*, edited by Alan Wolfe and Erik Owens, 373–394. Waco, TX: Baylor University Press.

World Health Organization (WHO). 2015. "Alcohol." Last modified January 2015. https://tinyurl.com/um38wjs.

Young, Martin, and Francis Markham. 2017. "Coercive Commodities and the Political Economy of Involuntary Consumption: The Case of Gambling Industries." *Journal of Environment and Planning* 49 (2): 2762–2779. https://doi.org/10.1177/0308518X17734546.

Contributors

The following list is in the order of the book chapters:

Ville Päivänsalo, ThD, adjunct professor (docent) in theological and social ethics, University of Helsinki, has previously served in the same university as acting university lecturer in systematic theology and as assistant professor in global theology, worldviews, and ideologies. Päivänsalo, the author of *Balancing Reasonable Justice* (2007), *Maallinen oikeudenmukaisuus* (Earthly Justice; 2011), and *Justice with Health* (2020) as well as the first editor of *Tolerance* (2017), has also served, since 2018, as part-time Evangelical-Lutheran pastor and part-time lecturer.

Josephine Sundqvist (PhD) works for the Swedish International Development Cooperation Agency (Sida) as a program manager for global capacity development. She has a background as a peace and development researcher, and she holds a PhD in the sociology of religion from Uppsala University and a MA in global studies from Gothenburg University. She has previously worked with development cooperation in Southeast Asia and sub-Saharan Africa for the United Nations and Civil Society Organisations (CSOs). In recent years, she has conducted research on the religion/development nexus and the role of religious actors in public-private partnerships (PPPs) in Eastern Africa.

Dr. **Thomas Ndaluka** is a senior lecturer at the Mwalimu Nyerere Memorial Academy. He is the founder and first director of the Society and

Religion Research Centre. Ndaluka is the author of *Religious Discourse, Social Cohesion and Conflict in Tanzania: Muslim-Christian Relations in Tanzania* and has coedited a book entitled *Religion and State Revisited in Tanzania: Reflection from 50 Years of Independence.* He has published several articles in local and international journals.

Elina Hankela (ThD, University of Helsinki, 2013) is a senior lecturer at the University of Johannesburg, South Africa. In her academic work, Hankela draws on liberation theologies both methodologically and theoretically. She has conducted ethnographic research in urban South Africa for different projects, engaging in particular with questions related to religion, religious communities, and/or social justice.

Alok Chantia, PhD (anthropology), PhD (sociology), was a faculty member in sociology at Lucknow University, Lucknow, in 2006 and at Bhimrao Ambedkar Central University, Lucknow, in 2008–9; in human rights in the Social Work Department at Lucknow University, Lucknow (2005–6); and in anthropology at Jai Narain Post Graduate College, Lucknow University, Lucknow (2015). Presently, he is a counselor in sociology of religion at Indira Gandhi National Open University in Lucknow and is president of and an anthropologist at the All Indian Rights Organization-Chapter of Naina Dayal Foundation, India. He has been working for a human rights awareness program, which includes researching health justice, terminal diseases, blood donation, and HIV/AIDS. He has had more than one hundred research papers published in reputed national and international journals. *Viklap Ka Samaj* is his sole published book.

Preeti Misra, LLD, is professor in the Department of Human Rights, School of Legal Studies, Babasaheb Bhimrao Ambedkar Central University, Lucknow, and also served as assistant professor in Jai Narayan Post Graduate College, Lucknow, and in Shia Post Graduate College, Lucknow. Professor Misra is the author of *Domestic Violence against Women* (2006) and coauthor of *Textbook on Indian Penal Code* (2016) and *Law Relating to Protection of Women* (2018). He is also coeditor of *Ratanlal and Dhirajlal's Law of Crimes* (2018).

S. N. Among Jamir, doctor of theology in systematic theology (awaiting confirmation) from United Theological College, Bangalore, served as a coordinator of Ecumenical Solidarity for HIV and AIDS (ESHA), a program of the National Council of Churches in India (NCCI), from 2010 to

2012. Jamir is currently serving as a pastor for Kohima Ao Baptist Church, Nagaland, India (affiliated with Nagaland Baptist Church Council).

Ronald Lalthanmawia, MBBS, FHM, IPCHIV, is a medical doctor currently working as coordinator of HIV and AIDS Program, Christian Conference of Asia (CCA), Chiang Mai, Thailand. He was previously the head of Community Health Department of Christian Medical Association of India (CMAI), New Delhi, India. He has authored several articles in various publications, including *A Theological Reader on Human Sexuality and Gender Diversity: Envisioning Inclusivity* and *Christian Response to Issues of Human Sexuality*, in the area of community health, HIV and AIDS, and human sexuality.

Dr. Md. **Abu Sayem** (PhD, the Chinese University of Hong Kong, 2020) is a faculty member of the World Religions and Culture Department at the University of Dhaka (Bangladesh). He is the author of two dissertations, "Religious Perspectives on Environment Issues: A Comparative Study of John B. Cobb, Jr. and Seyyed Hossein Nasr" (PhD diss., Chinese University of Hong Kong, 2020) and "The Monotheistic Concept in Judaism and Islam: A Comparative Study" (MPhil diss., University of Dhaka, 2010), as well as two book chapters and twenty-two journal articles.

Dr. **Thomas Renkert** is a postdoctoral researcher at Diakoniewissenschaftliches Institut, Heidelberg. His current work is preliminarily titled "Transformative Testimony—Diakonia as an Ecclesiological Category." He studied Protestant theology in Heidelberg, where he received his PhD with a study on Wolfhart Pannenberg's concept of time and eternity in 2014. He is also one of the founders and editors of the open-access journal *Cursor_Journal for Explorative Theology* (cursor.pubpub.org).

Rev. Dr. **Arul Dhas T.** is an ordained minister of the Church of South India. His PhD is from the Department of New Testament Language, Literature and Theology, University of Edinburgh. He has been serving in the Christian Medical College, Vellore, as the chaplain since 1989 and is presently the Reader of Pastoral Counseling. He is on the teaching faculty for bioethics in Christian Medical College, Vellore, and a CPE supervisor. He is an active member of the Christian Medical Association of India.

Dr. **Henrietta Grönlund** is professor of urban theology at the University of Helsinki, Finland. Her research interests include civic engagement, prosocial behavior, and welfare. She has researched these themes in several national and international research projects, especially in relation to religion and values and in urban contexts. Grönlund's work has been awarded national and international awards and published in Finnish and international journals, edited volumes, and monographs.

Dr. **Jibon Nesa** is an independent scholar and a social activist on humanitarian, social welfare, and human development. In 2018, she was awarded a PhD degree in Islamic studies at the University of Dhaka. As an Erasmus Mundus Exchange researcher, she worked in intercultural theology at the University of Göttingen. She is the author of *Holy Mary in Christianity and Islam: A Comparative Study* (2011) and four research papers in referred journals on religion, culture, and society.

Dr. **Hana Al-Bannay** is a consultant of health promotion, cross-cultural communication, and training at Sorouh Management Consultations in Saudi Arabia. She obtained a PhD in rehabilitation sciences from the University of British Columbia in Canada, where she studied Saudi women lifestyle–related health beliefs and behaviors and conducted a pilot diabetes education program adapted to the cultural and religious contexts of women in Saudi Arabia.

Rev. Dr. **Sahaya G. Selvam** holds a PhD in psychology of religion from the University of London. The study of religion has been his academic focus since his postgraduate studies. He has a master of arts in philosophy of religion and another master of arts in psychology of religion. His current research focuses on character development of youth in Africa using cultural and religious frameworks.

Dr. **Auli Vähäkangas** is a professor in practical theology at the University of Helsinki, Finland. Vähäkangas's research has focused on those in vulnerable situations: HIV-positive and childless people in their communities. She led an international research project, Youth at the Margins (2013–16), which was funded by the Academy of Finland. Between 1998 and 2005, she taught at Makumira University College of Tumaini University in Tanzania.

Dr. **George Zachariah** serves the Trinity Methodist Theological College, Auckland, Aotearoa New Zealand, on the faculty for theological studies. He has also served as professor of theology and ethics at the United

Theological College, Bangalore, India, and the Gurukul Lutheran Theological College and Research Institute, Chennai, India. He is the author of *Alternatives Unincorporated: Earth Ethics from the Grassroots* (London: Equinox Press, 2011) and *Gospel in a Groaning World: Climate Injustice and Public Witness* (Tiruvalla: CSS, 2012). He has edited several volumes and published articles in international journals.

Dr. **Ayesha Ahmad** is a lecturer in global health, St. George's, University of London, and honorary lecturer in global health, University College London. She specializes in religion and culture in mental health and gender-based violence during conflict, disasters, and humanitarian crises. Her forthcoming book, *Humanitarian Action and Ethics* (Zed), is coedited with Dr. James Smith. She has published widely in edited book volumes and peer-reviewed academic journals as well as media articles. She is frequently requested as an invited speaker on topics relating to Islam and ethics, war and storytelling, and gender-based violence in Afghanistan.

Dr. **Khaldoon Ahmed** is a consultant psychiatrist working in the NHS in East London. He has an interest in the health of ethnic minorities and has completed an MSc in medical anthropology at University College London. Khaldoon is a filmmaker and has made numerous creative nonfiction films that have screened internationally, including at the Berlinale. He believes strongly in the power of creativity in mental illness and is a trustee of the charity Mental Fight Club. Khaldoon was born and brought up in London, is of Muslim Pakistani heritage, and lived for a while in Mexico City.

Dr. **Simon Dein** is a consultant psychiatrist and honorary professor at Durham University and honorary professor in medical anthropology and education at Queen Mary's University, London.

Dr. **Mari Stenlund** is a Finnish social ethicist and doctor of theology. As a researcher, Stenlund specialized in religion, mental health, and human rights. She has published several international articles concerning the ethical and philosophical challenges of psychotic delusions, psychiatric involuntary treatment, and human rights theory. She also has clarified human rights issues in spiritual abuse and worked on alternative and complementary therapies with experts on mental health. Currently, Stenlund works as a religion teacher at a secondary school.

Janne Nikkinen, ThD, is a university researcher at the University Helsinki Centre for Research on Addiction, Control and Governance (CEACG). He is coauthor of *Setting Limits: Gambling, Science and Public Policy* (Oxford University Press, 2018) and coeditor of *Gambling Policies and European Welfare States* (Palgrave, 2018). He has addressed numerous audiences in addiction and gambling-related conferences across the globe (e.g., IGT Auckland 2010, APPGAC Hong Kong 2011, ICJ Cancun 2013, IAGR Johannesburg 2017, and DC16 Melbourne 2018).

Index of Names

Index of Subjects